CURRENT CONCEPTS IN DRUG METABOLISM AND TOXICOLOGY

CURRENT CONCEPTS IN DRUG METABOLISM AND TOXICOLOGY

Edited by

Gabrielle M. Hawksworth

Professor of Molecular Toxicology
Division of Applied Medicine, and School of Medical Sciences
University of Aberdeen
Foresterhill, Aberdeen, United Kingdom

Serial Editor

S. J. Enna

Department of Molecular and Integrative Physiology
Department of Pharmacology, Toxicology and Therapeutics
University of Kansas Medical Center
Kansas City, Kansas, USA

Managing Editor

Lynn LeCount

University of Kansas Medical Center, School of Medicine
Kansas City, Kansas, USA

ADVANCES IN

PHARMACOLOGY

VOLUME 63

ELSEVIER

AMSTERDAM • BOSTON • HEIDELBERG • LONDON
NEW YORK • OXFORD • PARIS • SAN DIEGO
SAN FRANCISCO • SYDNEY • TOKYO
Academic Press is an imprint of Elsevier

Academic Press is an imprint of Elsevier
525 B Street, Suite 1900, San Diego, CA 92101-4495, USA
225 Wyman Street, Waltham, MA 02451, USA
32, Jamestown Road, London NW1 7BY, UK
Radarweg 29, PO Box 211, 1000 AE Amsterdam, The Netherlands

First edition 2012

British Library Cataloguing-in-Publication Data
A catalogue record for this book is available from the British Library

Library of Congress Cataloging-in-Publication Data
A catalog record for this book is available from the Library of Congress

ISBN: 978-0-12-398339-8
ISSN: 1054-3589

For information on all Academic Press publications
visit our website at store.elsevier.com

Printed and bound in United States in America
Transferred to Digital Printing, 2012

Contents

Contributors

Numbers in parentheses indicate the pages on which the authors' contributions begin.

Sotiria Boukouvala (169) Department of Molecular Biology and Genetics, Democritus University of Thrace, Alexandroupolis, Greece

Kevin Brady (257) Bicycle Therapeutics Ltd., Cambridge, United Kingdom

Ping Cai (81) Department of Pharmaceutical Sciences, Leslie Dan Faculty of Pharmacy, University of Toronto, Toronto, Ontario, Canada

Xin Chen (81) Department of Pharmaceutical Sciences, Leslie Dan Faculty of Pharmacy, University of Toronto, Toronto, Ontario, Canada

Ian M. Copple (43) The University of Liverpool, MRC Centre for Drug Safety Science, Department of Molecular & Clinical Pharmacology, Liverpool, United Kingdom

M. J. Cross (207) MRC Centre for Drug Safety Science, Department of Molecular and Clinical Pharmacology, University of Liverpool, Liverpool, United Kingdom

Ann K. Daly (137) Institute of Cellular Medicine, Newcastle University Medical School, Framlington Place, Newcastle upon Tyne, United Kingdom

Giannoulis Fakis (169) Department of Molecular Biology and Genetics, Democritus University of Thrace, Alexandroupolis, Greece

C. E. P. Goldring (207) MRC Centre for Drug Safety Science; and Stem Cells for Safer Medicine, Department of Molecular and Clinical Pharmacology, University of Liverpool, Liverpool, United Kingdom

N. Hanley (207) Stem Cells for Safer Medicine, Department of Molecular and Clinical Pharmacology, University of Liverpool, Liverpool; and Manchester Academic Health Science Centre, University of Manchester, Manchester, United Kingdom

J. Heslop (207) MRC Centre for Drug Safety Science, Department of Molecular and Clinical Pharmacology, University of Liverpool, Liverpool, United Kingdom

Julia Ip (81) Department of Pharmaceutical Sciences, Leslie Dan Faculty of Pharmacy, University of Toronto, Toronto, Ontario, Canada

L. Kelly (207) MRC Centre for Drug Safety Science; and Stem Cells for Safer Medicine, Department of Molecular and Clinical Pharmacology, University of Liverpool, Liverpool, United Kingdom

J. P. Keogh (1) Independent DMPK Consultant, Hitchin, Hertfordshire, United Kingdom (formerly Mechanisms and Extrapolations Technologies, Drug Metabolism and Pharmacokinetics, GlaxoSmithKline, R&D Ltd.)

R. Kia (207) MRC Centre for Drug Safety Science, Department of Molecular and Clinical Pharmacology, University of Liverpool, Liverpool, United Kingdom

N. R. Kitteringham (207) MRC Centre for Drug Safety Science; and Stem Cells for Safer Medicine, Department of Molecular and Clinical Pharmacology, University of Liverpool, Liverpool, United Kingdom

Nicola Laurieri (169) Department of Pharmacology, University of Oxford, Mansfield Road, Oxford, United Kingdom

Jinze Li (81) Department of Pharmaceutical Sciences, Leslie Dan Faculty of Pharmacy, University of Toronto, Toronto, Ontario, Canada Current address: Department of Immunotoxicology, Drug Safety Evaluation, R&D, Bristol-Myers Squibb Company, New Brunswick, New Jersey, USA

Yan Li (81) Therapure Biopharma Inc, Mississauga, Ontario, Canada

Feng Liu (81) Department of Pharmaceutical Sciences, Leslie Dan Faculty of Pharmacy, University of Toronto, Toronto, Ontario, Canada

Alexandra R. M. Lobach (81) Department of Pharmaceutical Sciences, Leslie Dan Faculty of Pharmacy, University of Toronto, Toronto, Ontario, Canada

Imir G. Metushi (81) Department of Pharmacology and Toxicology, Faculty of Medicine, University of Toronto, Toronto, Ontario, Canada

Tetsuya Nakagawa (81) Department of Pharmaceutical Sciences, Leslie Dan Faculty of Pharmacy, University of Toronto, Toronto, Ontario, Canada Current address: Dainippon Sumitomo Pharma Co., Osaka, Japan

Winnie Ng (81) Department of Pharmaceutical Sciences, Leslie Dan Faculty of Pharmacy, University of Toronto, Toronto, Ontario, Canada

Maria Novalen (81) Department of Pharmaceutical Sciences, Leslie Dan Faculty of Pharmacy, University of Toronto, Toronto, Ontario, Canada

B. K. Park (207) MRC Centre for Drug Safety Science; and Stem Cells for Safer Medicine, Department of Molecular and Clinical Pharmacology, University of Liverpool, Liverpool, United Kingdom

Marija Popovic (81) Department of Pharmaceutical Sciences, Leslie Dan Faculty of Pharmacy, University of Toronto, Toronto, Ontario, Canada Current address: Non-Clinical Safety Assessment, Eli Lilly & Co., Indianapolis, IN, USA

C. Rowe (207) MRC Centre for Drug Safety Science; and Stem Cells for Safer Medicine, Department of Molecular and Clinical Pharmacology, University of Liverpool, Liverpool, United Kingdom

Amy Sharma (81) Department of Pharmaceutical Sciences, Leslie Dan Faculty of Pharmacy, University of Toronto, Toronto, Ontario, Canada

Edith Sim (169) Department of Pharmacology, University of Oxford, Mansfield Road, Oxford; and Faculty of Science, Engineering and Computing, Kingston University, Kingston, United Kingdom

R. L. C. Sison-Young (207) MRC Centre for Drug Safety Science; and Stem Cells for Safer Medicine, Department of Molecular and Clinical Pharmacology, University of Liverpool, Liverpool, United Kingdom

Tadatoshi Tanino (81) Department of Pharmaceutical Sciences, Leslie Dan Faculty of Pharmacy, University of Toronto, Toronto, Ontario, Canada Current address: Faculty of Pharmacy, Kinki University, Osaka, Japan

Jack Uetrecht (81) Department of Pharmaceutical Sciences, Leslie Dan Faculty of Pharmacy; and Department of Pharmacology and Toxicology, Faculty of Medicine, University of Toronto, Toronto, Ontario, Canada

Rob Webster (257) Pfizer Global Research and Development, Sandwich, Kent, United Kingdom

Xiaochu Zhang (81) Department of Pharmaceutical Sciences, Leslie Dan Faculty of Pharmacy, University of Toronto, Toronto, Ontario, Canada

Xu Zhu (81) Department of Pharmaceutical Sciences, Leslie Dan Faculty of Pharmacy, University of Toronto, Toronto, Ontario, Canada

J. P. Keogh

Independent DMPK Consultant, Hitchin, Hertfordshire, United Kingdom (formerly Mechanisms and Extrapolations Technologies, Drug Metabolism and Pharmacokinetics, GlaxoSmithKline, R&D Ltd.)

Membrane Transporters in Drug Development

Abstract

Membrane transporters have wide, but specific tissue distributions. They can impact on multiple endogenous and xenobiotic processes. Knowledge and awareness within the pharmaceutical industry of their impact on drug absorption, distribution, metabolism and elimination (ADME) and drug safety is growing rapidly. Clinically important transporter-mediated drug–drug interactions (DDIs) have been observed. Up to nine diverse transporters are implicated in the DDIs of a number of widely prescribed drugs, posing a significant challenge to the pharmaceutical industry. There is a complex interplay between multiple transporters and/or enzymes in the ADME and pharmacogenomics of drugs. Integrating these different mechanisms to understand their relative contributions to ADME is a key challenge.

Many different factors complicate the study of membrane transporters in drug development. These include a lack of specific substrates and inhibitors, non-standard *in vitro* tools, and competing/complementary mechanisms (e.g. passive permeability and metabolism).

Discovering and contextualizing the contribution of membrane transporters to drug toxicity is a significant new challenge.

Drug interactions with key membrane transporters are routinely assessed for central nervous system (CNS) drug discovery therapies, but are not generally considered across the wider drug discovery. But, there is interest in utilizing membrane transporters as drug delivery agents.

Computational modeling approaches, notably physiology-based/pharmacokinetic (PB/PK) modeling are increasingly applied to transporter interactions, and permit integration of multiple ADME mechanisms. Because of the range of tissues and transporters of interest, robust transporter, *in vitro*

Advances in Pharmacology, Volume 63 1054-3589/12 $35.00

http://dx.doi.org/10.1016/B978-0-12-398339-8.00001-X

to *in vivo*, scaling factors are required. Empirical factors have been applied, but absolute protein quantitation will probably be required.

I. Introduction

A. What are Drug Transporters?

Compartmentalization at intracellular, cellular and tissue levels is fundamental to the function and well being of living organisms. Higher organisms contain a complex system of physical barriers, which help to control systemic, tissue and cellular exposure to both xenobiotics and endogenous molecules. Specific mechanisms have evolved which selectively absorb nutrients and excrete waste products across these barriers, and to ensure that endogenous substances are maintained at normal levels in the body. These same systems can also modulate the absorption, distribution, metabolism and elimination (ADME) of xenobiotic substances. Molecules with a net charge (positive or negative) will have restricted access to cells and tissues, unless facilitated by uptake transporters, because of their inability to cross the plasma membrane. Conversely highly permeable molecules should generally have good penetration, unless restricted by the activity of efflux transporters. Most endogenous molecules exist as charged species. Small changes in pH, differences in protein binding and/or relative solubility between extra- and intracellular milieu may also influence the net concentrative effect of a transporter. Both uptake and efflux transporters are present in most, if not all, cell types. Whilst the overall transporter complement will influence intracellular drug concentrations, their effects may also be quite subtle. The fundamental action of a membrane transporter protein is either to maintain a substrate in equilibrium, or to establish a concentration gradient across a membrane, or tissue barrier, which could not otherwise be achieved.

There are approximately 400 transporter-like genes expressed in humans. These are categorized into two major superfamilies: the solute carrier (SLC) (Heddiger, 2010) and ATP-binding cassette (ABC) transporters (Muller, 2006). The ABC superfamily is significantly smaller (48 members) than the SLC (over 300 members). Both superfamilies are further categorized, based on similarity of function and/or gene sequence. Both transporter superfamilies appear to have broad substrate specificities, ranging from metal ion transport, bile salts, sugars, hormones, amino and nucleic acids, small peptides and nucleosides, and of course, xenobiotics. All the ABC and many of the SLC transporters behave as active transporters. It is convenient to think of ABC transporters as maintainers of low intracellular concentration of their substrates (i.e. efflux transporters), and SLC transporters as establishers of high intracellular concentrations (i.e. uptake transporters), but there are exceptions. ABC transporters (e.g. P-glycoprotein, also referred to as Pgp or MDR1) directly hydrolyze ATP, SLC transporters create concentration gradients by co-transport and/or exchange of ions, or act as facilitative transporters. Although it is generally accepted that Pgp (and perhaps other ABC transporters) takes its substrates from the plasma membrane, and solute transporters from the free fraction in the blood or cytosol, crystal structures are not available and so the precise mechanisms involved are still a matter of investigation.

II. Key Features of Transporters

A. Location, Orientation, and Function

Membrane transporters are membrane bound proteins with multiple trans-membrane spanning domains and specific cellular locations and membrane orientations, which define their tissue/cellular function. Knowledge of transporter tissue distribution and cellular localization is essential if one is to understand the role of a particular transporter in a given organ or cell. For example, Pgp is a luminally expressed efflux transporter. It is widely expressed in tissues, most notably in the gastrointestinal tract (GIT), liver, brain and kidney. As an efflux transporter, it maintains low intracellular concentrations of its substrates. In the GIT and central nervous system (CNS), Pgp effluxes molecules into the gut lumen or into the blood, limiting cellular exposure, oral absorption or CNS exposure to drugs, and protecting the body and CNS from significant exposure. By contrast, in the kidney and liver, Pgp expels its substrates (in this instance already present in the cell) into the urine and bile.

Transporters are also differentially distributed across tissues and organs. For instance OATP1B1 and OATP1B3 are essentially specific to the liver, whereas OATP4C1 is specific to the kidney. However, other transporters have a far more widespread distribution, e.g. Pgp, OCT3, and MRP4 (Fig. 1).

B. Differential Distribution and Interplay/Redundancy

There is interplay between efflux and uptake transporters, which depend on their differential distribution in the cell, tissue or physiological location. Many drugs are substrates and/or inhibitors of multiple transporters. Some scenarios are outlined below:

1. *Same cell surface location, different function*: both uptake and efflux transporters with similar substrate specificities can be located on the same cell surface. For example, the organic anion efflux transporters MRP3 and MRP4 and organic anion uptake transporters OATP1B1 and OATP1B3 are all expressed on the sinusoidal surface of hepatocytes. The relative affinities, local substrate concentrations, and relative expression

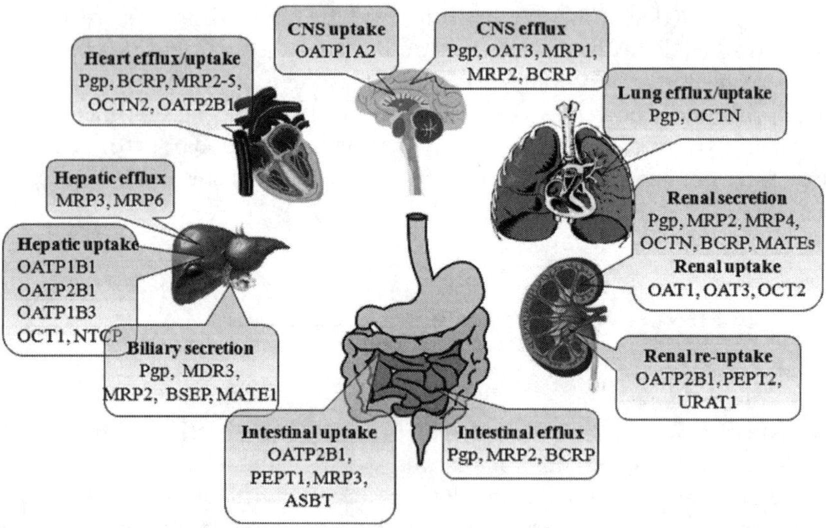

FIGURE 1 Schematic (not comprehensive) illustrating the extensive distribution of membrane transporters *in vivo*, and their basic function in each tissue. The precise cellular localization will also impact on net effect in the organ.

levels of these complementary transporters will influence the net impact on the intracellular and extracellular concentration of a given co-substrate, such as bile salts (Keppler, 2011; Svoboda, 2011).

2. *Opposite cell surface location, complementary function*: the apical facilitative glucose/galactose transporter on the apical (luminal) surface of the enterocyte SGLT1 (SLC5A1) is complemented by SLC2A2 (GLUT2) on the basolateral surface to facilitate the oral absorption of glucose and other monosaccharides.
3. *Complex distributions across multiple tissues and cell locations*: enterohepatic cycling of bile acids is highly regulated by multiple GIT and hepatic uptake and efflux transporters (as well as metabolizing enzymes) (Dawson et al., 2010). Also, transporter-mediated disposition, pharmacology and elimination of the glycemic drug metformin are driven by different transporter isoforms, differentially distributed across multiple tissues (Nies et al., 2011; Yonezawa & Inui, 2011) (Fig. 2).

Definitive evidence of cellular locations for some transporters in some tissues is available, but there is no definitive source that describes the location of all transporters in all tissues for any species. Some useful public resources are available, e.g. Human Protein atlas (Knut & Alice Wallenberg Foundation, 2011), Human ABC transporters (Muller, 2006), and the Bioparadigms websites (Heddiger, 2010). Much of this information is drawn from various other public resources (e.g. PubMed). The content is not

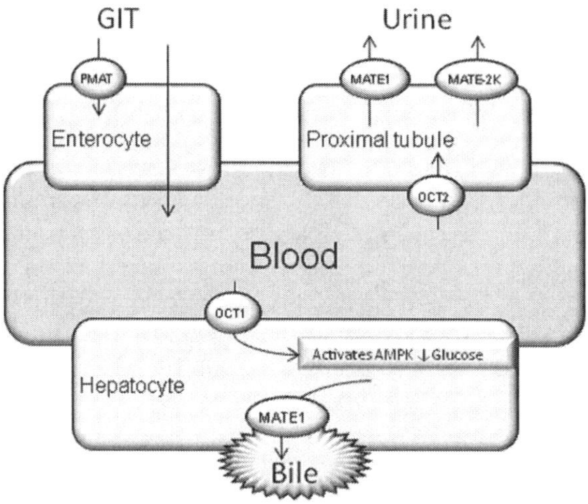

FIGURE 2 Proposed transporter-mediated disposition, pharmacology and elimination of metformin showing interplay between multiple transporters, differentially distributed across multiple tissues: In humans, OCT1 is exclusive to hepatocytes and OCT2 to the kidney, whereas MATEs are present in both organs. OCT1 and OCT2 are virtually absent in other tissues.

always well curated, however, and if not, should be used with some caution, making reference to relevant expert groups, as necessary.

It appears that there is some redundancy and/or compensatory regulation of endogenous transporter activity. Most genetically modified animals are viable and fertile, e.g. mdr1a/mdr1b knockout animals are generally healthy (although highly sensitive to ivermectin exposure compared to wild-type littermates; Lankas et al., 1997). TR-rats which are natural mutants lacking functional mrp2 on the apical surface of hepatocytes, compensate for reduced biliary elimination of bile acids by expressing higher levels of mrp3 on the basolateral surface resulting in increased bile acids in the blood (Johnson et al., 2006). Human populations possessing functional mutations of transporters have also been identified. For example, those with functional SNPs which result in reduced activity of OATP1B1 have reduced capacity for the statin class of drugs (Wen & Xiong, 2010), and those with genetic variants in bile salt export pump (BSEP) have increased susceptibility to cholestasis (Keppler, 2011).

It should also be noted that functional SNPs may result in enhanced and/or reduced activity of the transporter for its substrates. A recent review of OATP1B1 clinically relevant SNPs by Niemi et al. (2011) covers the area well. Although the science is advancing rapidly in many areas, the majority of transporters have yet to be thoroughly characterized, and their endogenous functions have to be determined. The complexity of the interplay among multiple transporters, metabolizing enzymes, and other processes is only beginning to be appreciated, and is a major challenge to industry and academia in understanding the overall impact on ADME of drugs.

C. Transporter Expression Levels

Expression levels of transporters in tissues are usually low as a proportion of the total genomic or proteomic material. Furthermore, in a whole tissue (e.g. tissue homogenates), it is possible that a transporter may be below the limits of detection, however, this does not necessarily indicate lack of functional activity. A recent analysis of protein levels of a number of important drug metabolizing enzymes (DMEs) and transporters in human liver samples from 17 donors gave a range for transporters of 0.06–7.35pmole/mg protein versus a DME range of 2.4–114pmole/mg protein (Ohtsuki et al., 2012; Schaefer et al., 2012). As transporter expression is limited to specific locations on the plasma membrane, it is not unreasonable to expect that relatively small amounts of transporter protein will be highly effective.

Whilst there are a number of published values for genomic expression levels of some transporters in some tissues, there is a much smaller body of work describing their protein expression levels in human tissues and cells. Furthermore, it appears that there is poor correlation between genomic and protein expression levels of transporters (Ohtsuki et al., 2012). Recent advances in absolute immunoquantification methodologies provide an alternative to isolated membrane preparation (Tucker et al., 2012). An understanding of the functional levels of transporters *in vitro* versus *in vivo* is generally lacking, and needs to be addressed if routine extrapolation of *in vitro* data to predict *in vivo* outcomes has to be successful.

D. Species Differences

There is good information on the transporter gene profiles in rodents and in humans, however there are many gaps in our knowledge of cross-species expression and functionality; in particular comparisons of non-rodent and non-human transporter gene profiles, expression and function are patchy. From the information available, there seem to be similar transporter complements across species; however there are many instances where there is no direct homology in expression or function. For instance, in rodents there are five hepatic oatp transporters (1a1, 1b2, 1a4, 1a5, and 1a6) compared to three human hepatic OATPs (1B1, 1B3 and 2B1). There is a single Pgp protein (MDR1) expressed in humans, whereas rodents express two proteins (mdr1a and mdr1b), which are differentially distributed across tissues (Shirasaka et al., 2011). In dogs, oatp1b4 appears functionally homologous to OATP1B1 and OATP1B3 (Wilby et al., 2011). To further complicate cross-species comparison, it appears that even where transporters are well conserved across species (e.g. OCT1 and OCT2), their relative tissue distribution may not be. In humans, OCT1 appears to be highly expressed in liver and OCT2 in kidney, whereas in rodents both homologues are substantially expressed in both the tissues. OAT transporters show similar differences. Translation of preclinical findings to predict human outcomes is therefore very challenging. Digoxin, rosuvastatin and metformin – drugs which are well recognized *in vivo* substrates of transporters – have markedly different PK and ADME in rodents versus humans.

Species differences in drug toxicity may also be related to differences in membrane transporter sub-cellular expression. For instance human SLC29A1 (ENT1), an equilibrative nucleoside transporter widely expressed in tissues, has been shown to localize to mitochondrial and plasma membrane *in vitro*, whereas the murine form localizes only to the plasma membrane (Lee et al., 2006). Thus the enhanced mitochondrial toxicity of nucleoside drugs such as fialuridine (a known in vitro substrate of ENTs) observed in humans may be due to species differences in sub-cellular expression of this transporter.

III. Transporters and the Pharmaceutical Industry

A. Historical Perspective

Active drug transport *in vivo* was first observed many decades ago. It was of particular interest for renally cleared molecules where altered renal function was associated with disease states (e.g. uric acid clearance and gout; Gutman & Yu, 1957, 1958). Although the precise mechanisms remained unknown, in the 1950s scientists and clinicians successfully extended the elimination half-life of, the then rare drug, penicillin to extend its therapeutic window by co-administration of probenecid (Burnell & Kirby, 1951). Probenecid was subsequently shown to be a potent inhibitor of members of the renal organic anion transporters (OATs). During the 1980s drug transporters were identified as mediators of cancer chemo-resistance (refs), in particular P-glycoprotein (Pgp, MDR1). These discoveries sparked great interest in the oncology field, and were considered a breakthrough in the understanding of cancer multiple drug resistance. Although the impact of efflux transporters such as MDR1 on tumor exposure to drugs was readily demonstrated *in vitro*, no successful clinical applications have been licensed thus far, despite three generations of increasingly potent and selective inhibitors (Kelly et al., 2011; Tamaki et al., 2011).

Over the last 10–15 years, the potential and reality of transporter involvement in the ADME of xenobiotics has become widely accepted (Ayrton & Morgan, 2008; Giacomini et al., 2010). After oncology, probably the earliest appreciation of transporters in drug disposition and efficacy, and where major effort is still applied in the drug industry, is the delivery of CNS drugs across the blood–brain barrier (BBB) (Potschka, 2011). Pgp was identified as a major barrier protein for many CNS drug substances, and to this day, Pgp substrate activity (or lack of it) remains a key selection target for CNS drug discovery groups.

Since the initial discovery of the Pgp efflux transporter, several other efflux and uptake transporters involved in chemotherapy drug resistance have been identified, using experimental and empirical approaches.

The potential for transporters to be mediators of pharmacokinetic (PK) drug–drug interactions (DDIs) was appreciated relatively soon after the discovery of Pgp, and was adopted as a regulatory requirement for DDI investigation during the 1990s (Food and Drugs Administration, 2006). However, the discovery that some HMG-CoA inhibitors (e.g. rosuvastatin, pravastatin) were substrates of the organic anion transporter protein (OATP) family, and that inhibition of these transporters could lead to clinically significant PK DDI has arguably been the biggest driver for incorporating transporter science into mainstream drug development (Shitara & Sugiyama, 2006). Table I lists transporters which are of current relevance or interest in the drug development field.

In more recent times, toxicity as a result of modulation of transporter activity by drugs has been postulated. For example, modulation of multidrug resistance protein 2 (MRP2, ABCC2) and the BSEP (ABCB11) by xenobiotics is now believed to be significant in drug induced liver injury (DILI) (Dawson et al., 2012). This is not at all surprising, as these transporters (amongst a number of others, as well as certain DMEs) regulate intracellular exposure to toxic bile salts and acids (Dawson et al., 2010).

With the notable exception of CNS drug discovery and delivery, there has yet to be widespread industry application of transporter science to improve drug efficacy or delivery in the pharmaceutical industry, although some companies have successfully exploited transporters for drug delivery (Xenoport's Gabapentin pro-drug Enacarbil is the most recent example). Given the rapid development and acceptance of transportology by the wider scientific community, appreciation of their potential to impact on drug efficacy in tissues other than the CNS and tumors will continue to increase.

B. Challenges and Opportunities for Drug Development

Clinical safety concerns, notably PK DDI and DILI have proven to be the greatest drivers for expansion of knowledge and activity for drug transporters in drug development. DDI is more advanced of the two areas, and will be focused on for the remainder of this chapter.

Drug transporters also offer opportunities to preferentially deliver drugs to their site of action, or to improve oral bioavailability. But there are significant challenges to making these strategies a reality. Nonetheless there have been successes resulting in improved delivery of some otherwise poorly bioavailable compounds (e.g. Gabapentin and some antiviral medications). However, discovery of new CNS drugs has (and still is) severely hampered

TABLE I Listing of Transporters of Current Interest in the Pharmaceutical Industry

Transporter	*Gene*	*Tissue location*	*Direction of transport or orientation*	*Endogeneous substrate(s)*	*Clinically relevant substrates (victim)*	*Clinically relevant inhibitors (perpetrator)*	*Clinical relevance*		
							DDI	*Toxicity*	*Disease associations*
OCT2	SLC22A2	Kidney	Blood→cell	Creatinine, small organic cations	Metformin, Varenicline, Antiretrovirals, Gabapentin, Lamotrigine, Pyrimethamine	Cimetidine	Y	Renal tox, antivirals	N
OATP1B1	SLCO1B1	Liver	Blood→cell	Bile salts	Statins (e.g. Rosuvastatin, Pravastatin) Repaglanide, Olmesartan	Cyclosporine, Gemfibrozil, Eltrom-bopag, Rifampicin, Lopinavir/ Ritonavir	Y	Hyperbiliru-binemia	Rotor syndrome
OATP1B3	SLCO1B3	Liver	Blood→cell	Bile salts					
BCRP	ABCG2	GIT, CNS. liver, kidney, others	Cell→lumen	Lipids/cholesterol?	Rosuvastatin, Topotecan	GF120918	Y		N
OAT1	SLC22A6	Kidney	Blood→cell	Organic anions, polyspecific, e.g. α-ketoglutarate	Methotrexate. Antiretrovirals (e.g. Zidovu-dine, Acyclovir), NSAIDs	Probenecid	Y	Renal	N
OAT3	SLC22A8	Kidney	Blood→cell	Organic anions, polyspecific	Methotrexate	Probenecid	Y	Renal	N

(continued)

TABLE I Listing of Transporters of Current Interest in the Pharmaceutical Industry *(continued)*

Transporter	*Gene*	*Tissue location*	*Direction of transport or orientation*	*Endogeneous substrate(s)*	*Clinically relevant substrates (victim)*	*Clinically relevant inhibitors (perpetrator)*	*Clinical relevance*		
							DDI	*Toxicity*	*Disease associations*
Ppg/MDR1	ABCB1	GIT, CNS. liver, kidney, others	Cell→lumen	Lipids/cholesterol?	Digoxin	Quinidine, Ritonavir	Y		N
OCT1	SLC22A1	Liver	Blood→cell	Organic cations, polyspecific	Metformin, Antiretroviral drugs	Not demonstrated	Y		N
BSEP	ABCB11	Liver	Cell→bile	Bile salts	unproven	Lapatinib	N	DILI	Unk
NTCP	SLC10A1	Liver	Blood→cell	Na-taurocholate, bile salts	Not demonstrated	Bosentan	N	DILI	Unk
MATE1	SLC47A1	Kidney, liver	Cell→lumen	Organic cations	Metformin	Cimetidine?	Suspected		N
MATE2	SLC47A2	Kidney, testis, colon	Cell→lumen	Organic cations	Metformin	Cimetidine?	Suspected		N
OAT4	SLC22A11	Kidney	Cell→urine	Organic anions, polyspecific, e.g. urate	Methotrexate	Probenecid	Y		N
OAT2	SLC22A7	Liver	Blood→cell	Organic anions, polyspecific, e.g. cGMP	Not demonstrated	Not demonstrated	N		N
OCT3	SLC22A3	Ubiquitous	Blood→cell	Organic cations, polyspecific	Not demonstrated	Not demonstrated	N		N
OCTN1	SLC22A4	Ubiquitous	Blood→cell	Ergothionine	Not demonstrated	Not demonstrated	N		Unk

(continued)

TABLE I Listing of Transporters of Current Interest in the Pharmaceutical Industry *(continued)*

							Clinical relevance		
Transporter	*Gene*	*Tissue location*	*Direction of transport or orientation*	*Endogeneous substrate(s)*	*Clinically relevant substrates (victim)*	*Clinically relevant inhibitors (perpetrator)*	*DDI*	*Toxicity*	*Disease associations*
OCTN2	SLC22A5	Heart, lung, wide-spread	Blood→cell	Carnitine	Not demonstrated	Not demon-strated	N	Carnitine deficiency	Y
PEPT1	SLC15A1	GIT	Gut→cell	Di/tri-peptides	B-Lactam antibiotics. Valacyclovir	Not demon-strated	N		N
MCT1	SLC16A1	Ubiquitous	Lumen→cell	Lacate, pyruvate, ketone bodies	Gabapentin-Enar-cabil	Not demon-strated	N		Unk
MRP2	ABCC2	GIT, liver, kidney, others	Cell→lumen	Bilirubin glucs,	Not demonstrated	Not demon-strated	Suspected	DILI	Dubin-Johnson Syndrome
MRP3	ABCC3	GIT, liver, kidney	Cell→blood (liver)	Glutathione conjugates, bile salts	Ethynyl estradiol metabolites	Not demon-strated	Suspected	Cholestasis, DILI	Unk
MRP4	ABCC4	Many tissues	Cell→blood (liver)	Cyclic nucleotides, bile salts	Not demonstrated	Not demon-strated	N	Cholestasis, DILI	Unk
GLUTs	SLC2 family	Wide-spread	Cell→blood	Glucose and other sugars	Not demonstrated	Not demon-strated	N		Type 2 diabetes
SGLTs	SLC5 family	Wide-spread	Lumen→cell	Glucose and other sugars	Not demonstrated	Not demon-strated	N		Type 2 diabetes
ASBT	SLC10A2	GIT	Gut→cell	Bile salts	Not demonstrated	Not demon-strated	N		Unk

(continued)

TABLE I Listing of Transporters of Current Interest in the Pharmaceutical Industry *(continued)*

Transporter	*Gene*	*Tissue location*	*Direction of transport or orientation*	*Endogeneous substrate(s)*	*Clinically relevant substrates (victim)*	*Clinically relevant inhibitors (perpetrator)*	*Clinical relevance*		
							DDI	*Toxicity*	*Disease associations*
OSTα/β	SLC51A1 and A1BP	GIT	Cell→blood	Bile acids	Not demonstrated	Not demonstrated	N		Unk
OATP1A2	SLCO1A2	Brain, kidney, liver	Blood→cell	Bile salts	Not demonstrated	Not demonstrated	Suspected		Unk
OATB2B1	SLCO2B1	Liver, intestine	Blood→cell		Not demonstrated	Not demonstrated	Suspected		Unk

Bolded entries are implicated in DDI for important drug classes, and regulatory authorities recommend the NCE be assessed for DDI liability against these. Others are of lesser DDI importance and/or are implicated in drug delivery or drug toxicity. Some transporters may have wider tissue distribution than indicated. Where multiple tissue expression is listed, "Lumen" has generally been used to indicate that substrates may be transported from/to different compartments (e.g. blood, bile or urine).

by the action of efflux transporters at the BBB notably Pgp, which protect the brain from xenobiotic exposure. Although there is significant investigation in this area by specialized drug delivery groups based both on the industry and academia, targeted drug delivery to patients remains an aspiration rather than a reality.

C. The Clinical Relevance of Membrane Transporters and Their Impact on the Pharmaceutical Industry

PK DDI occur for many marketed drugs. Some are sufficiently marked so as to require dose adjustments or exclusions in the clinic. DDIs occur when two (or more) co-administered drugs interact with a common pathway which results in greater or lesser systemic exposure of one or more drug (the victim). They are considered clinically relevant when the change in drug exposure is sufficient to exceed safe levels, or to reduce concentrations to sub-therapeutic levels. Most DDIs have traditionally been ascribed to DMEs, but increasingly transporters are implicated. We now appreciate that transporters impact on oral absorption of important therapeutic drugs (e.g. digoxin, sulfasalazine and fexofenadine), first pass extraction (statins), tissue distribution (e.g. methotrexate), and biliary and urinary excretion (e.g. digoxin, metformin, penicillins and antivirals), and that many co-administered drugs modulate these transporters, leading to clinically relevant DDIs (Ayrton & Morgan, 2008).

D. Drivers Which Make Transporter DDI Investigation Necessary

There are two distinct aspects of DDI risks which must be considered for new chemical entities (NCEs) drugs – firstly whether the pharmacokinetics of the NCE will be impacted by co-administration of other drugs, the so-called "victim" scenario. Secondly, whether the NCE itself will impact the PK of a co-administered drug, termed the "perpetrator" scenario. Consideration of each aspect is necessary for a reasoned and comprehensive assessment of the risks of adverse events (AEs) in the clinic. To do this not only the knowledge of the mechanisms which the NCE interacts with is required, but also the knowledge of the mechanisms which potential co-meds modulate or use. Interaction of a victim and perpetrator with a common clearance mechanism is the key driver for investigation of DDI, regardless of whether this is a transporter or metabolic mechanism. This is a well-established approach in the pharmaceutical industry for metabolism-based DDI, and the same general principles are applied for drug transporters.

Statins (rosuvastatin, pitavastatin, simvastatin, atorvastatin) are one of the most widely prescribed medications in the western world, and some are now available as over the counter preparations. Because of this widespread use, statin DDIs are not only of interest to regulators, clinicians and patients, but also represent a significant developmental risk to pharmaceutical companies, as contra-indication against such a major drug class will inevitably reduce market penetration, or render the NCE unmarketable.

1. *Passive Membrane Permeability*

Passive membrane permeability is the diffusion of drug across tissue barriers and cell membranes. Barrier tissues (e.g. GIT, BBB, kidney, etc.) typically feature tight intercellular junctions at the epithelial and/or vascular endothelial layers, which severely restrict paracellular transfer of molecules. This serves to protect the body or tissue from exposure to potentially toxic substances. Therefore, molecules generally need to pass through the cell in order to cross the barrier, and must cross the plasma membrane to access the interior of the cell. Small lipophilic molecules with no net charge are more likely to permeate across cell barriers than those which are charged and hydrophilic. Systemically acting, orally dosed drug molecules must be able to cross at least the GIT to reach their site of action.

Depending on their function, drug transporters will either enhance or limit drug permeability across barriers and cells. But the balance between active and passive permeability events will influence a drug's ADME properties. For highly passively permeable drugs, the predominant process for cell permeation may be passive, more so if the available drug concentration is greater than its affinity (Km) for a given transporter (i.e. when the transporter is saturated). This is often the scenario in the GIT for orally administered drugs. However, when drug concentrations are at or below the Km (e.g. at the BBB), the contribution of the transporter element may predominate over the permeability fraction. At the other extreme, poorly passively permeable molecules may be heavily reliant on uptake transporter mechanisms for oral absorption and for tissue penetration.

Although there are some controversies in the contributions of unidentified transporters to *in vitro* measurements of permeability (Kell et al., 2011; Sugano et al., 2010), within an industry setting, ranked passive permeability measurements are often used to select drug candidates with greater permeability, so as to reduce the impact of transporter mechanisms (uptake or efflux) on drug ADME and PD. This is a useful strategy as it gives generally greater confidence that the selected candidate is less likely to be limited in its PK or PD profile by the action of transporters.

2. *Transporter-Metabolism Interplay*

Transporter-metabolism interplay has long been acknowledged as likely to occur, particularly in the GIT, where it is postulated that Pgp and CYP3A4 in particular will act together to limit the absorption of xenobiotics from the gut (Benet et al., 2008; Van Waterschoot et al., 2010). Pgp and CYP3A4 have very broad substrate specificities, and many shared substrates and inhibitors. When Pgp and CYP3A4 are expressed separately and together in the same systems, there is clearly a relationship between transporter and metabolic activities. Usually the effect is that less drug reaches the receiver chamber when both Pgp and CYP3A4 are expressed than when just one or the other is expressed. Additionally, preclinical *in vivo* experiments using knockout mice also demonstrate a relationship. However, the nature of the interplay (whether synergistic or additive) is the subject of debate and discussion in the transporter community (Van Waterschoot et al., 2010). The clinical implications of Pgp/CYP3A4 interplay may be significant, however conclusive clinical studies demonstrating their dual impact have yet to be published. This is partly because it has not been possible, thus far, to identify suitable and selective clinical inhibitors of Pgp which are not also inhibitors of CYP3A4, and vice versa. Although some recommendations have been made, based on comparison of relative *in vitro* inhibition profiles of drugs for CYP3A4 and Pgp, these have yet to be tested in controlled clinical trials (Zhang et al., 2008). An excellent review of the nature of Pgp/CYP3A4 interplay has recently been published (Van Waterschoot et al., 2010).

Transporter-metabolism interplay is likely to occur in other tissues, particularly in the liver. Recent publications have cited hepatic interplay between CYP2D6 and OCT1 for Ondansetron (Tzvetkov et al., 2012), and Tramadol (Tzvetkov et al., 2011).

3. Range and Selectivity of Transporters – Specific Substrates and Inhibitors

Using the outputs from the most comprehensively characterized transporters (OATPs, OATs, OCTs, Pgp, BCRP, BSEP and MRP2), it is clear that although general substrate and inhibitor features can be cited, few useful substrates or inhibitors are truly exclusive to just one transporter. This is true within a particular transporter sub-family, where substrate/inhibitor redundancy is often observed, and across families (e.g. BCRP and Pgp), particularly where the transporter has a very broad substrate specificity.

When selecting a probe substrate or inhibitor, one should thoroughly review the profile of the molecule across a range of transporters, particularly those which are also likely to be expressed in the chosen systems. A further complication in a DMPK setting is that DME affinities also need to be considered. It may be possible to select substrates or inhibitors which are essentially selective due to different affinities for a given transporter. In this instance, however, the experimenter should characterize the substrate/inhibitor in the chosen system.

Whilst many hundreds of drugs have been tested as Pgp substrates and/or inhibitors, this is not true for the majority of other drug transporters. Where drugs have been tested against multiple transporters or DMEs, there are few if any instances where they are shown to interact (as substrate and/

or inhibitor) with just a single one. Cyclosporine is a potent inhibitor of Pgp, BCRP, OATPs, MRPs and CYP3A4 amongst others (Foti et al., 2010; Jemnitz et al., 2010; Kajosaari et al., 2005; Morjani & Madoulet, 2010; Niemi et al., 2011; Wolf et al., 2010), methotrexate is a substrate of multiple OATs, OATPs, Pgp and MRPs (Takane, 2011; Vlaming et al., 2011). Digoxin is a notable clinical substrate of Pgp, but is believed to be a substrate of other, as yet unidentified uptake transporters (Acharya et al., 2008; Taub et al., 2011). Sulfasalazine is a substrate of BCRP and MRP2 (Adkison et al., 2010; Jemnitz et al., 2010). Although it can be reasonably postulated that other transporters may be less promiscuous than Pgp, which likely has a very broad substrate specificity, to test the interplay between specific transporter and metabolism mechanisms, it is preferable (though not always possible) to have a good understanding of all the mechanisms involved in the molecules ADME.

4. *Genetic Polymorphisms*

Functional genetic polymorphisms have been described for a number of clinically relevant transporters. Polymorphisms of OATP1B1 are associated with altered PK (Ieiri et al., 2009; Wen & Xiong, 2010) and altered toxicology (Vladutiu & Isackson, 2008) of statin drugs. OATP1B1 and OATP1B3, and MRP2 and BCRP are variously associated with altered pharmacokinetics or efficacy of a number of statin drugs in Asian populations (Ieiri et al., 2009; Wen & Xiong, 2010). Polymorphisms in OCT1 and OCT2, and possibly MATEs are associated with altered efficacy and renal elimination of Metformin (although there are some conflicting results) (Tzvetkov et al., 2009; Wang et al., 2008; Zolk et al., 2009). The Tramadol metabolite, O-desmethyltramadol is a substrate of OCT1 (Tzvetkov et al., 2011). Subjects with non-functional OCT1 polymorphisms have been observed to have higher blood concentrations of the metabolite and significantly longer duration of opioidergic effects. These studies illustrate the need to understand which transporters are involved in delivering drugs to their site of action, metabolism and elimination.

5. *Membrane Transporter Regulation*

Molecular mechanisms of drug transporter regulation have recently been reviewed (Tirona, 2011). Although it is possible to explore up or down regulation of transporter (and DMEs) on the bench, the clinical impact is more challenging to predict and demonstrate, although there are some published clinical studies (Akamine et al., 2011; Kharasch et al., 2008; Yamada et al., 2011). This is because inducers are often also inhibitors, and the impact of induction may be offset by inhibition effects. It is difficult to predict the balance of these effects, as dynamic modeling tools are required to simultaneously model both mechanisms, thus often the only way forward is to progress to a clinical study to explore the interaction.

IV. Studying and Contextualizing Transporter Interactions: Application and Interpretation of Data

Currently, nine membrane transporters (Pgp, BCRP, OATP1B1, OATP1B3, OCT1, OCT2, OAT1, OAT3, and BSEP) are considered by transporter DDI specialists and/or regulators as important DDI investigation targets for new drugs. The International Transporter Consortium (ITC) have endeavored to contextualize the risks posed through DDI (Giacomini et al., 2010), and to provide both commercial organizations and regulatory bodies with guidelines on when and how to investigate transporter DDI liabilities. Regulatory agencies have also updated their guidances to address these recent advances in understanding (European Medicines Agency, 2010; Food and Drugs Administration, 2012). However, the science and our understanding of it is still evolving, and it will be several years, perhaps decades, before the field matures, at least as it impacts on drug development.

Investigating transporter interactions is somewhat more complicated than metabolism DDI investigation. This is due to many factors, e.g. the types and number of different transporters which are now implicated in DDI, their sequential arrangement and actions in the cell and organs.

A. When to Assess Drug Transporter Interactions

There are no hard and fast rules for timings to investigate DDI during development, apart from those stipulated by regulatory agencies in their guidances. In the drug industry, two major considerations apply – firstly, what are the known DDI risks associated with key co-meds for the target patient population, and secondly at what time of the development process will the drug be administered to patients taking these co-meds? For instance in a rheumatoid arthritis patient population, methotrexate is a widely prescribed co-med. This is a narrow therapeutic index (NTI), chronically dosed medication with rare, but sometimes fatal DDI with non-steroidal anti-inflammatory drugs (NSAIDs), penicillins and probenecid. Methotrexate is renally eliminated by OATs, and the DDIs observed have been ascribed to interference with these mechanisms. Thus if the NCE is intended for this population, OAT inhibition is undesirable, as it may not be possible to eliminate the risk of a DDI, or monitor for it in clinical use. Digoxin is another NTI, Pgp substrate, widely prescribed in heart disease populations, and eliminated virtually unchanged in urine. Co-dosed potent Pgp inhibitors such as quinidine and verapamil are contra-indicated, as fatally high exposures to digoxin can occur, so introducing a NCE which is a potent Pgp inhibitor to this population is risky. Statin medications are increasingly prescribed in middle aged and elderly populations to reduce cholesterol. They are substrates of OATPs, and DDIs which can lead to myopathy and rhabdomyolysis over a prolonged period on co-administration with OATP inhibitors, thus additional monitoring and/or dose adjustment may be necessary if the statin is co-dosed with a potent OATP inhibitor.

Next, consider the characteristics of the NCE. Is it a high or low dose drug, chronic or short-term medication, how potently does it inhibit (or induce) transporters *in vitro*? The risk of DDI or AEs tends to be greater for high dose, chronically administered medicines, because the body burden and systemic exposures are also generally higher, thus even moderate *in vitro* transporter inhibition may translate into significant clinical inhibition. Further studies may be warranted to obtain more comprehensive information on the mechanisms involved (e.g. transporter-metabolism interplay). Ultimately, however a clinical DDI study may be the only way to conclusively mitigate the risk.

The ITC guidelines (Giacomini et al., 2010), and the latest FDA guidance (Food and Drugs Administration, 2012), provide some useful decision trees to guide drug development scientists in this area. There are also a number of published quantitative predictive tools for some transporters (primarily OATPs) (Kusuhara & Sugiyama, 2009; Watanabe et al., 2011). The guideline and guidances are valuable, and predictive modeling approaches are the way forward, although significant refinements are required, and users would be well advised to take a pragmatic view in applying to a given NCE.

V. The Transporter Toolkit, its Opportunities and Challenges

Although the transporter toolkit is extensive, the availability, utility, and throughput of the tools is mixed, and translation of output for human outcomes is variable (Table II). The experimental study of transporters is probably the most challenging of the DMPK sciences for a host of reasons:

- The transporter must be expressed in a membrane, in the correct orientation, and if in a polarized system, at the correct location on the plasma membrane.
- Drug substance must be measured either disappearing from one compartment or appearing in another, or often both, and sometimes simultaneously.
- Very few, if any truly specific substrates or inhibitors have been identified for transporters.
- The absolute amount of transported drug is generally very small in relation to that applied, particularly in any given *in vitro* system – typically two or more orders of magnitude lower than that applied initially for *in vitro* assays, thus even very small amounts of cross-contamination are unacceptable.
- *In vitro* assay samples may contain high concentrations of drug in very small sample volumes, or conversely much lower levels of drugs in larger volumes, therefore accurate and sensitive assays for drug levels in samples, minimizing potential cross-contamination with drug from other sources, is essential for successful transporter experimentation and interpretation. For example, the intracellular volume of one million hepatocytes (a typical

TABLE II Tools Available for Investigation of Transporter Interactions, Their Availability, Utility and Translatability to Human Outcomes

		Availablility		*Throughput and utility*			*Translation*[a]			
System type	*Technique/tool*	*Human*	*Preclinical*	*Ease of use*	*Routine work*	*Bespoke work*	*Mechanistic*	*IVIVE*	*Predictive*	*Representative*
In vitro	Overexpressed cell lines	H	L	Good	Yes	Yes	Yes	Maybe	Maybe	No
	Isolated 1° hepatocytes	H	H	Good	Yes	Yes	Yes	Maybe	Yes	Somewhat
	Other isolated 1° cells	L	L	Medium	No	Yes	Yes	Maybe	Yes	Somewhat
	Vesicles	H	L	Good	Yes	Yes	Yes	Maybe	Maybe	No
	Oocytes	L	L	Low	No	Yes	Yes	Maybe	Maybe	No
	SiRNA (use with 1° cells)	M	L	Low	No	Yes	Yes	Maybe	Yes	No
	2D/3D cell systems	M	L	Medium	No	Yes	Yes	Maybe	Yes	Somewhat
	Derived/ immortalized cell lines	M	L	Medium	Yes	Yes	Yes	Maybe	No	Somewhat
Ex vivo	Tissue slices	L	M	Low	No	Yes	Yes	Maybe	Yes	More so
	Ussing techniques	L	M	Low	No	Yes	Yes	Maybe	Yes	More so
	Perfused organs	L	M	Low	No	Yes	Yes	Maybe	Yes	More so
	Tissue drug concentration/ mapping	L	M	Low	No	Yes	Yes	Maybe	Yes	Yes
	Dissected tissue components	L	L	Low	No	Yes	Yes	Maybe	Yes	Yes

(continued)

TABLE II Tools Available for Investigation of Transporter Interactions, their Availability, Utility and Translatability to Human Outcomes *(continued)*

		Availablility		*Throughput and utility*			*Translation*[a]			
System type	*Technique/tool*	*Human*	*Preclinical*	*Ease of use*	*Routine work*	*Bespoke work*	*Mechanistic*	*IVIVE*	*Predictive*	*Representative*
In vivo	Chemical/KO/transgenics/humanized	–	M	Low	No	Yes	Yes	–	Maybe	Yes
	Preclinical imaging	–	L	Low	No	Yes	Yes	–	Maybe	Yes
	Clinical imaging	M	–	Low	No	Yes	Yes	–	Maybe	Yes
	Clinical DDI/PK	H	–	Low	No	Yes	Yes	–	–	Yes
In silico	PBPKPD modeling/prediction	M	L	Medium	–	–	No	Yes	Maybe	Yes
	Structure-based interaction prediction	M	–	Good	–	–	No	Maybe	No	No
Other	Genomic expression levels	H	L	–	–	–	Yes	–	–	Yes
	Protein expression levels	L	L	–	–	–	Yes	–	–	Yes
	Cellular localization/tissue distribution	M	M	–	–	–	Yes	–	–	Yes
	Metabolomics	L	L	–	–	–	Maybe	–	–	Yes

Key:
Availability - considers whether tool exists, and industry access to it as a service or as a reagent (note that many larger pharmaceutical companies have developed in-house tools to meet their needs):
H—high availability, good access for most transporters of interest for DDI investigation; L—low availability with limited access from commercial or academic sources; M—moderate availability, meaning some access, but limited in range, quality or quantity.
Throughput - considers commercial availability, assay costs, and adaptability to medium and high throughput applications:
Ease of use - level of specialized laboratory set-up required, level of operative expertise or maintenance; Routine work - applicability to routine or high-throughput applications, providing a defined level of data; Bespoke work - appropriate for in-depth investigation of transporter interactions (e.g. kinetics, multiple mechanisms).
Translation, considers the utility of data to evaluate and predict human or clinical outcomes:
Mechanistic - provides qualitative evidence/description of transporter interactions; IVIVE - can be configured to provide data for quantitative extrapolation from *in vitro* to *in vivo*; Predictive - allows comparison of transporter interactions across species, including man (e.g. comparative safety assessment); Representative - relevance of tool to the corresponding native tissue/organ (e.g. hepatocytes = liver, proximal cells = kidney, etc.).
[a]Clarification of comments:
Maybe - additional information (e.g. scaling factors, validation or ranking) is likely required to refine extrapolations or predictions; Somewhat - tool derived from native tissue, but post-isolation processing may impact on transporter expression, function or location; More So - tool presumed to preserve the integrity of transporter expression, location and function.

number of cells used for *in vitro* hepatic uptake assays) is approximately 1μL. A transporter-mediated 2-fold concentrative effect from a 1μM donor solution (i.e., 1nmole/mL) will yield a sample with a total of 2pmole of drug substance for analysis.

- High specific activity, high purity radiolabels are required for *in vitro* measurements, as low levels in samples make confirmation of the identity of transported radioactivity challenging. Additionally, total counts are typically assumed to be equivalent to total drug (i.e. radiolabel drug is assumed to be 100% pure). In cell-based systems, metabolism of radiolabeled substrates (particularly at extended incubation times) needs to be considered. As metabolites are generally more hydrophilic (and therefore generally less permeable than the parent molecule), they may be trapped within cells, thus creating a radioactivity, but not a drug, concentration gradient.
- Other processes which are compound-specific, and therefore difficult to predict or control (e.g. non-specific binding to apparatus, lipophilicity and passive permeability) can result in assays with poor dynamic range, even though transporter interactions may still be important.
- *In vivo* experimentation in preclinical species generally requires measurement of drug in multiple tissue compartments, often at low levels and with the risk of blood contamination.
- Clinical studies measure circulating blood and sometimes urine concentrations, which will not give information on changes in tissue exposure.

It is also difficult to apply transporter assays in a drug discovery setting, as high throughput is generally required. The most amenable high-throughput assays measure inhibition/antagonism of the mechanism tested. This is acceptable where the intent is to screen out potent inhibitors of a transporter (e.g. DDI risk for OATP1B1). However, inhibition of transport is not an appropriate surrogate for substrate activity (of particular interest for CNS therapies), and in practice, "poor" competitive inhibitors may in fact be "good" substrates, as these may not saturate the transporter readily. To confirm substrate activity, sensitive, direct measurement of transported drug is required. The resource needed for this quality of analysis for even a relatively small number of potential drug candidates is large, and only a few molecules in a drug screen will be characterized to this extent.

In a drug development setting however, the imperative is to understand the mechanisms which the NCE engages, and to apply this to assess DDI risk and impact on PK. In this situation, testing against a selection of transporters as an inhibitor and a substrate may be appropriate.

A. *In Vitro* Techniques

In vitro DME assays have gained wide acceptance in industry, academia, and most importantly with the regulatory agencies which license new drugs (e.g. the FDA and EMEA). *In vitro* approaches provide the opportunity to explore the interaction of drugs with human and preclinical transporter proteins, and represent the most useful experimental tools to the pharmaceutical industry. Unlike enzymology, where drug substrate is metabolized to an entirely new species, transportology explores the movement of drug substrate from one compartment to another with no change in the substrate itself. Therefore the well-established *in vitro* enzymology tools used across industry (e.g. microsomes) are largely irrelevant for transporter work. Multi-compartmental systems are required for virtually all transporter investigations, and many different configurations and systems have been established (Table II). There is no consensus in the industry at this time on the most appropriate system to explore any given type of interaction, although some general principles are becoming routine.

Although any cell can theoretically be used to measure drug transport of some sort (all living cells will have their own complement of transporters after all), well-characterized systems tend to give the most reliable outputs, and those which overexpress the transporter of interest are probably the most robust and reproducible.

Oocytes expressing the transporter of interest are considered the purest tool for study of transporters (particularly uptake transporters), however they are very low throughput and can be difficult to establish and maintain, and thus are rarely applied in an industrial setting. The workhorse tools used in industry and academia are either cell (gene transfected over-expressing cells, isolated primary cells, or immortalized cell lines, see Table I), or isolated plasma membrane vesicle (vesicles) based, as these maintain transporter directionality and function. There are many different ways to apply these *in vitro* tools, although cell-based assay use and utility are somewhat dependent on the cell type and cell polarity. Whereas uptake transporters are often investigated in (non-polarized) cells grown on standard tissue culture plates, cell-based efflux transporter experiments typically use polarized cell lines, grown on semi-permeable supports, allowing measurement of drug transport in both apical to basolateral (A>B) and basolateral (B>A) directions, This allows directional efflux measurements across both sides of the cell layer, which is essential to understand the impact of efflux transporters on passive permeability. The Caco2 and MDCK immortalized polarized cell lines are particularly popular in industry, variously used to measure both passive membrane permeability and the impact of efflux transporters (typically Pgp, but also MRP2 and BCRP) on drug permeability. Whereas the Caco2 cells are a human-derived cell line, MDCK are canine in origin, but are often used following transfection with human Pgp (MDCK-MDR1) or other human transporter genes.

Primary cell systems are more often applied in a qualitative, or semi-quantitative manner to gain understanding of mechanisms (particularly for human transporters), although there are examples of quantitative approaches (Paine et al., 2008; Poirier et al., 2009b). For example, hepatocytes can be grown in collagen sandwich cultures (allowing them to establish the bile canaliculi necessary for directional flux) to explore the impact of inhibitors on bile acid transporters (Kotani et al., 2011; Maeda & Sugiyama, 2010; Marion et al., 2011; Nakanishi et al., 2011). In addition to primary hepatocytes (used as suspensions, plated or sandwich cultured formats), renal proximal tubule cells, brain microvessel endothelial cells and some more complex co-cultures of primary cells are also used in industry to mimic particular tissue barriers (Brown et al., 2008; Lippmann et al., 2011).

Ex vivo tissues have been traditionally used to measure drug permeability and transporter mechanisms, primarily using rabbit gut mucosa mounted in Ussing chambers. Since the emergence of human over-expressing cell lines, and for reasons of ethical animal use, these models have generally fallen out of favor in industry. Fresh tissue slices have not been used extensively thus far for transporter work, however as imaging technologies advance, these may become an appropriate tool for use in understanding transporter mechanisms in relatively intact human tissues.

All of the above methods can be, and in many instances are, used to generate quantitative (IC_{50},Ki, Km, Vmax, etc.) or semi-quantitative (efflux ratio, intrinsic permeability) measurements. Cost and complexity may render this impractical in some instances however. Michaelas–Menten kinetics are generally used to describe transporter interactions, although in time, these may prove not to be the most appropriate descriptors as the science develops and evolves (Agnani et al., 2011; Kolhatkar & Polli, 2010).

Most assay formats, particularly uptake transporter and vesicle experiments require sensitive and specific drug assays, as the volume of the receiving compartment (i.e. the volume of the cell or vesicle) is very small (nL to μL volumes), and the absolute amount of drug available for measurement is also very small (although the actual drug concentration in the compartment may be very high). Radiolabeled (^{14}C or ^{3}H) versions of substrates are widely used, as are sensitive LC-MS/MS assays. In all systems, contamination of samples with unwanted drug substance must be minimized as even very low levels of contamination from stock solutions, dirty pipettes or analytical equipment may render data interpretation impossible.

B. Limitations of *In Vitro* Transporter Assays

Across the pharmaceutical industry and academia, there are no agreed standards for assay components, design, outputs or interpretation. This renders cross-assay comparisons rather difficult, and this is important when the data are intended to be used to predict DDI risks. Although lab-

TABLE III Comparison of OCT2 IC_{50} Literature Data from Various Investigators

Test inhibitor	*Probe substrate*	*Concentration (μM)*	*Cell line*[a]	*IC_{50} (μM)*	*Ref*
Cimetidine	Ethidium bromide	1	CHO	1380	Lee et al. (2009)
Cimetidine	MPP+	10	HEK	126	Zolk et al. (2009b)
Cimetidine	MPP+	Not stated	HEK293	1650	Umehara et al. (2007)
Cimetidine	Amiloride	Not stated	HEK293	14	Biermann et al. (2006)
Cimetidine	ASP	Not stated	HEK293	26	Biermann et al. (2006)
Cimetidine	Creatinine	Not stated	HEK293	27	Urakami et al. (2004)

[a] Background cell line transfected with the human gene SLC22A2.

to-lab variability is a well-established phenomenon for many techniques, this may well be more pronounced for transporter assays using live cells, as many variables will impact on assay outputs (e.g. expression levels of the transporter of interest, potentially interfering endogenous transporters, passage number, assay formats, etc.). Indeed, a recent cross-pharma comparison of quantitative *in vitro* Pgp inhibition assays using a common test substrate digoxin, with Caco2, MDCK-MDR1 or Pgp vesicles, numerous assay end points, and data calculation methods showed limited cross-correlation between assay outputs (Lee, 2011). The results indicate that the sources of the variability are multi-factorial (cell type, assay format and data manipulation). It is rare to see such a comprehensive comparison, but one might expect similar results from other transporter assays. For instance, a simple comparison of cimetidine inhibition of various substrates of OCT2 indicates three orders of magnitude difference in reported IC_{50} values (Table III).

The value of *in vitro* assay outputs in drug development is to enable prediction of clinical DDI risk. To extrapolate clinical DDI outcomes, in addition to good quality, robust and reproducible *in vitro* data, the cellular/tissue locations and amounts of each potential transporter, and how that transporter operates are important factors, as are the range of different transporters which may be relevant to the molecule's disposition. Harmonization of *in vitro* approaches is an important challenge to the industry which will be very difficult to achieve. In the interim, by using well-designed, robust and reproducible tools with demonstrated validation against known (preferably clinically relevant) substrates and inhibitors, the risk of misinterpretation can be reduced. Tables IVa and b list some basic aspects of *in vitro* transporter assay design, which the author believes are important for robust and interpretable *in vitro* assays.

Lack of lab-to-lab reproducibility is manageable where the assay output is ranked within the assay against a calibration dataset, and conclusions are drawn solely from this output (e.g. if ranking potential new drug

TABLE IVA Suggested Basic Requirements and Study Designs for Robust and Reproducible *In Vitro* Investigations of Drug Interactions with Membrane Transporters – Transporter Transfected or (Over-Expressing) Immortalized Cell Lines, and Membrane Vesicles Prepared from Transporter Transfected Cells

Experiment	*Minimum requirements*	*Binary assay (yes or no) application*	*Parameter generating (e.g. IC_{50} or Km) application*
Transporter Inhibition	Characterized control probe substrate(s) and inhibitors (initial rates, Km, Vmax, IC_{50} robustly reproduced), should be sufficient to allow ranking of output against relevant (clinical) substrates or inhibitors. Additional for cell-based assays: cell and/or membrane/monolayer integrity test/marker in presence of test compound, integrated into assay, with established acceptance criteria. Directional flux assay preferred for efflux transporter assays. Additional for vesicles "No vesicle" or control vesicle assays to assess non-specific binding of test and controls. AMP can replace ATP as an additional control.	Single probe substrate conc. (at or below Km) ± control inhibitor (sufficient to cause complete inhibition – 10 or more times IC_{50}), 3 concs. (high, medium and low)of test inhibitor – check solubility. A–B and B–A measurements if flux assay. Output: percent or net inhibition	Minimum of 7 test inhibitor concentrations (including "no-drug" control). Single probe substrate concentration at or below Km. If flux assay, can be basolateral to apical (B to A), or A–B only, or both (efflux ratio, ER). Provide evidence that design is viable and robust. Same for control inhibitor, unless validation data available, when a single concentration ± control inhibitor is acceptable. Output: IC_{50} value
Uptake substrate	Characterized control probe substrate and inhibitor (initial uptake rates, Km, Vmax, IC_{50} robustly reproduced). Radiolabeled (high purity, high specific activity) or non-radiolabeled test compound with specific, sensitive assay. Additional for cell-based assays: Assess mass balance/ non-specific binding in system, and cell/ monolayer integrity in presence of test compounds. Additional for vesicle "No vesicle" or control vesicles to assess non-specific binding of test and controls. AMP can replace ATP as an additional control.	Single, low as practicable concentration of test substrate (e.g. equivalent to unbound circulating concentration) ± control inhibitor (sufficient to cause complete inhibition – 10 or more times IC_{50}) over a timecourse (min of 3 timepoints to allow calculation of initial rate). Same for control substrate, at non-saturating concentration. Output: Initial uptake rate in the presence and absence of inhibitor	Multiple concentrations (at least 7) of test substrate (covering therapeutic range and as high as practically possible) ± control inhibitor (sufficient to cause complete inhibition – 10 or more times IC_{50}). Single or multiple timepoints (multiple timepoints provide initial rates and more robust data). Similar data for control substrate, if not previously validated, otherwise single concentration of characterized control substrate ± inhibitor. Output: Km/Vmax/Pdiff.

(continued)

TABLE IVA Suggested Basic Requirements and Study Designs for Robust and Reproducible *In Vitro* Investigations of Drug Interactions with Membrane Transporters – Transporter Transfected or (Over-Expressing) Immortalized Cell Lines, and Membrane Vesicles Prepared from Transporter Transfected Cells

Experiment	*Minimum requirements*	*Binary assay (yes or no) application*	*Parameter generating (e.g.* IC_{50} *or Km) application*
Efflux substrate	As above, additionally: cell-based assays: polarized system preferred.	As above, but single timepoint assay may be acceptable for polarized systems. Cell-based assays: assess passive permeability in the presence of inhibitor, if required. Use Pexact to compensate for mass balance. Outputs: cell-based assays - A–B and B–A transport rates, ER with and without inhibitor, ER collapses to ~1 in the presence of inhibitor. Apparent passive permeability (Pexact or Papp). Vesicle assays - net transport rate (total transport minus control transport)	Preliminary assessment in binary assay recommended. Set up as above except, single timepoint may be acceptable for polarized systems. Outputs: A–B and/or B–A transport rates, ER, passive permeability (cell-based assays), Km/Vmax/Passive permeability (cell and vesicle assays).

TABLE IVB Suggested Basic Requirements and Study Designs for Robust and Reproducible *In Vitro* Investigations of Drug Interactions with Membrane Transporters – Transporter Assessments Using Primary Cells, e.g. Hepatocytes (Fresh, Frozen, Plated or Sandwich Cultured)

Experiment	*Minimum requirements*	*Binary assay (yes or no) application*	*Parameter generating (e.g. IC_{50} or Km) application*
Bespoke assay systems. If intended for routine use, proceed as guided above for other system.	Use multiple (human) donors, and design work to investigate specific theses. Positive controls and inhibitors for known transporter processes (e.g. Estradiol glucuronide for OATPs) should be used to demonstrate viability, and if possible, activity for the target transporter(s). If cryopreserved hepatocytes, batches characterized by suppliers are preferred. Cells can be used in multiple formats (plates, suspension, matrigels. Radiolabel test compound (high specific activity) usually preferred, but non-radiolabeled may be appropriate for some designs. Integrity assessment of cells in presence of test compound, and assessment of stability in system should be considered	Include appropriate controls to demonstrate and rank functionality from batch to batch and experiment to experiment – uptake of probe/test substrate ± test/control inhibitor(s) at concentrations at or below Km (substrate) and 10 or more times higher than IC_{50} (inhibitors). Demonstrate vectorial transport from medium into bile for sandwich cultured hepatocytes.	Km, Vmax, Pdiff. Area is developing and a number of different approaches possible – explore literature for appropriate study designs. Simultaneous mechanistic modeling of data may be appropriate. Include appropriate controls.

candidate potency against a target). However, in the DDI field, we need to apply *in vitro* data to quantitative extrapolations of clinical DDI risk. Thus *in vitro* assay outputs must be calibrated against known clinical outcomes. For DMEs, the extrapolation tools are advanced and generally reliable, there are relatively few tools (primarily microsomes and hepatocytes) used in reasonably standard formats, and their kinetics are well understood and characterized. Additionally, the major enzymes are readily available in recombinant and native forms, extrapolation factors are well established and tested, and the enzyme mechanisms of actions themselves are sufficiently similar to each other that, for the purposes of DDI extrapolation, much of the same parameters can be used for multiple or integrated predictions. This means that the Pharma industry and the drug licensing agencies have an expectation that the same level of certainty can be applied to transporter DDI risk evaluation. However the reality is that the necessary information is not readily available for most of the growing number of drug transporters of interest to the industry. The ITC Whitepaper (Giacomini et al., 2010), swiftly followed by the European Regulatory Agency (EMA) (European Medicines Agency, 2010) and more recently the US Food and Drugs Administration (FDA) (Food and Drugs Administration, 2012) have made certain recommendations for the evaluation of transporter DDI risk, making good use of the available knowledge to give the best possible advice to drug developers. However, given that many of the *in vitro* tools are not of themselves thoroughly characterized, specific *in vitro* and/or clinical probe substrates or inhibitors are yet to be identified, and the lack of consensus in the industry on how to apply and interpret the *in vitro* tools, one can expect that the landscape and advice will continue to shift for some time.

C. *In Vivo* Techniques

1. *Preclinical Techniques*

Preclinical species are widely used for DMPK work, providing important information on drug absorption, circulating concentrations, pharmacokinetics, metabolic routes and overall excretion, and facilitate interpretation of other preclinical data and design of clinical programmes. Although preclinical PK data are routinely used to predict clinical PK profiles, in general, preclinical data are considered only qualitatively predictive of clinical outcomes. The utility for DMEs and transporters is limited because of the extensive species differences in expression, function, and location (for transporters).

Quantitative whole body autoradiography (QWBA) of drug-related radiolabel in rodent species is a commonly applied drug development tool to visualize the distribution of drugs *in vivo*. QWBA illustrates the distribution characteristics of the drugs and drug-related materials, and thus is an indication of potential transporter-mediated distribution (Fig. 3). A general principle is that if a drug has good passive permeability characteristics then it should distribute relatively freely into tissues (notwithstanding the effects of protein binding, etc.), the converse is also true. Where tissues show very high (uptake transporter) or very low (efflux transporter) drug-related material concentrations, this is taken as an indicator of a potential transporter-mediated effect, which may require further investigation.

Genetically modified mice (so-called knockout or knock-in mice) have been enormously valuable in illustrating the *in vivo* impact of transporters

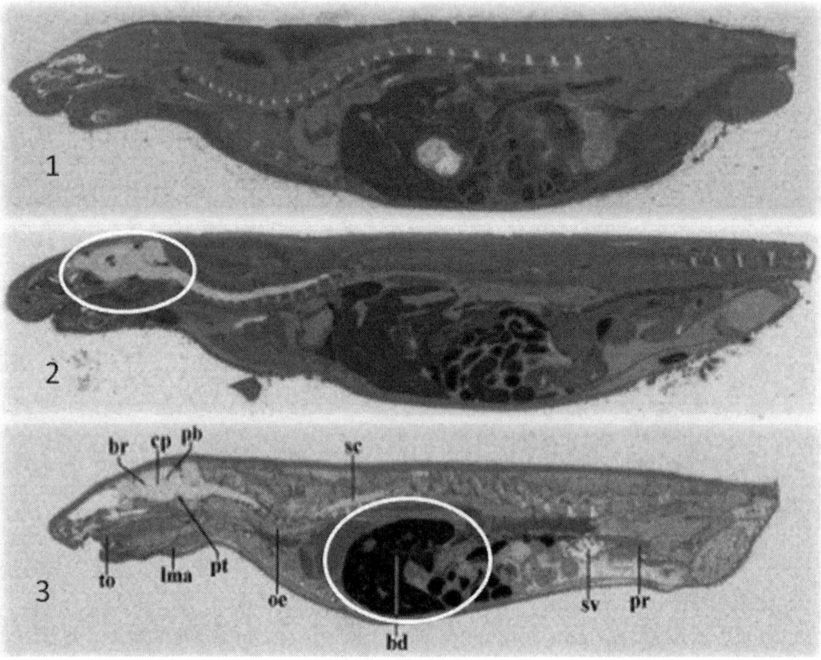

FIGURE 3 Rat Quantitative Whole Body Autoradiography (QWBA) following oral dosing of three different radiolabeled small drug-like molecules, showing the typical distribution that might be observed for: (1) a highly permeable molecule with no obvious influence of transporters on distribution; (2) an efflux transporter substrate (e.g. Pgp) on CNS distribution (circled area); (3) an uptake transporter substrate (e.g. OATP) on hepatic distribution (circled area).

on drug pharmacokinetics and drug disposition. The general approach is to compare and contrast parameters between the modified animal and a back-crossed "normal" strain. Although tissues and isolated cells can be taken from these animals for experimentation, most investigations are carried out using intact mice, or occasionally isolated in-situ tissues (however this is technically challenging). The animals are relatively expensive, and conclusive experiments may require a significant numbers of animals.

The most widely used knockout mice in industry have been the mdr1a/1b dual knockout, and the mdr1a/1b/bcrp triple knockout mice, as they are particularly useful to illustrate the role of Pgp and bcrp in distribution of drugs to the CNS (Agarwal et al., 2011; Polli et al., 2009; Yang et al., 2010). Mdr1a and mdr1b are the murine orthologues of human MDR1. It appears that there is reasonable homology in substrate specificity for these transporters between these species. Other knockout animals are available both commercially (e.g. http://www.taconic.com), and from some academic groups, and have also demonstrated utility. For instance, methotrexate (a substrate of multiple uptake and efflux transporters) has been extensively investigated in a range of single and multiple transporter knockout mice, and in some transgenic models (van de Steeg et al., 2010; Vlaming et al., 2009; Wang et al., 2011).

Other experimental approaches using preclinical approaches are well documented, notably measurement of steady state drug levels in rat brain tissue (Jeffrey & Summerfield, 2010; Summerfield et al., 2008), and use of in-situ liver and kidney to explore the handling of drugs and its modulation by other drugs (Hobbs et al., 2011; Tamhane et al., 2010). Some natural mutants, notably rats lacking mrp2 (TR- and EISAI rats) have also provided valuable insights (Hobbs et al., 2011).

2. *Limitations of Preclinical* In Vivo *Tools*

Although animals provide important *in vivo* mechanistic insights for transporters, which are unlikely to be obtained by any other means, their utility to the pharmaceutical industry and drug development is limited. Apart from the expense of generation and husbandry of genetically modified animals, transporter tissue distribution and expression levels (as well as differences in metabolism) are sufficiently different across species to confound direct translation from preclinical species to humans, which is of fundamental importance to the industry. Additionally, although gene-altered mice are generally fit and healthy, there is little information on changes in regulation of compensatory mechanisms (e.g. upregulation of MRP3 in response to knockout of MRP2 to protect liver from exposure to damaging levels of bile acids). Transgenic mice, where the equivalent murine genes have been replaced with the human orthologues, may ultimately prove to be superior to knockouts, however unless the mouse is fully humanized (i.e. all the murine orthologues are replaced with the human gene), these are unlikely to be tools which can be routinely applied in the industry.

3. *Clinical Tools*

The objective of drug discovery and development is to create safe and efficacious medicines to treat human diseases, thus the success of the industry hangs on demonstrating these properties in man to the satisfaction of patients, clinicians, regulatory authorities and bill payers. Clinical study outcomes trump earlier preclinical findings. Transporters impact on both safety and efficacy in humans, however demonstrating their impact clinically can be challenging. Typically, blood concentration over time data is used to estimate many PK parameters such as bioavailability and apparent volume of distribution, and these are then related to the pharmacodynamic effect observed, but it is generally not possible to measure tissue levels of drugs in humans, and therefore the differential impact drug transporters may have on distribution and elimination processes, and on efficacy or toxicology which may not be readily monitored in a clinical setting.

The most commonly applied protocol in industry to investigate transporter interactions use the classical DDI study design, where healthy volunteers are dosed (usually to steady state) with the drug of interest (victim drug), and then challenged with a co-administration of a competing drug (perpetrator drug). Comparative blood concentration–time profiles are then used to demonstrate the impact on the PK of the victim drug.

Probably the clearest demonstration of transporter-mediated DDI relates to the statin class of medicines. Cyclosporine, eltrombopag, gemfibrozil, lopinavir and ritonavir, tacrolimus, and tripanavir and ritonavir have all been observed to increase circulating concentrations of rosuvastatin in the clinic. The consequences of increased systemic exposure to statins are increased risk of myopathy and potentially fatal rhabdomyolysis. Because of the widespread and rapidly increasing use of statins in the developed world, understanding the mechanism(s) underlying the observed DDIs is important, as other new drugs entering clinical use may interact with the same mechanisms, which may impact on their safe clinical use. Rosuvastatin is a lipophilic acid which has poor passive membrane permeability; it is eliminated in humans as primarily unchanged drug in faeces. Although metabolized *in vitro*, rosuvastatin is a substrate of numerous drug transporters *in vitro*. Rosuvastatin was firstly found to be a substrate of hepatic OATP transporters (OATP1B1, 1B3), and then of other uptake and efflux transporters such as OATP1A2 and 2B1, NTCP, MRP2, MDR1 and BCRP (Ho et al., 2006; Kitamura et al., 2008). Although it was believed that the interactions observed related primarily to inhibition of hepatic uptake via OATP1B1, it is now more likely that the DDIs observed are a result of inhibition of a combination of multiple transporters distributed in the GIT (predominantly BCRP) and liver (OATP1B1, OATP1B3 and NTCP) (Generaux et al., 2011). Cyclosporine is a notable inhibitor of a broad range of enzymes and transporters and has the most profound clinical effect on rosuvastatin PK (about 6-fold change in AUC). Statins act on the hydroxylmethylglutaryl CoA (HMG-CoA) enzyme in the liver, and the impact on the PD of the statins has long been of concern to investigators and clinicians (Generaux et al., 2011; Link et al., 2008). A recent review of the overall impact of OAP1B1 and BCRP on statin use and safety addresses the area well (Generaux et al., 2011).

As drug is measured only in the blood (and sometimes the urine), little information is obtained from these studies on drug tissue distribution. *In vivo* imaging techniques are available, but are complex and expensive, and not generally practical for larger scale clinical trials required for drug development. Although *ex vivo* drug tissue measurement technologies (e.g. MALDI) are developing, their application will be limited by supply of suitable samples and assay sensitivity (Menger et al., 2012; Peukert et al., 2012). Direct imaging techniques can also be applied to measure exposure of the CNS and the impact of efflux transporter inhibitors (de Klerk et al., 2010; Syvanen et al., 2011). These studies can very elegantly demonstrate the impact of a drug transporter on CNS exposure, and rely on using short lived radioisotope (^{11}C), and are therefore not routinely applied in drug clinical trials (Potschka, 2011).

D. Quantitative Extrapolation and Physiologically Based Pharmacokinetic Modeling

Physiologically based pharmacokinetic (PBPK) and other computational/mathematical approaches to model and predict DME interactions are now widely and successfully used to predict PK and DDI in the pharmaceutical industry. A number of commercial packages are available for this purpose (e.g. SimCyp, Gastroplus) (Bhattachar et al., 2011; Jamei et al., 2009; Motta et al., 2011; Okumu et al., 2009; Rakhit et al., 2008). Transporter modeling is very much a developing field, and there are a number of significant challenges, which industry and academic scientists are working hard to overcome. Robust *in vitro* to *in vivo* scaling factors, improved understanding of the nature of transporter substrate/inhibition kinetics, reliable measures of relative tissue abundance of functional transporter proteins in tissues (Ohtsuki et al., 2012; Shawahna et al., 2011; Tucker et al., 2012), the free fraction of drug in blood and cells, and ability to incorporate permeability factors are amongst these challenges (Hallifax et al., 2011; Reis et al., 2010; Webborn et al., 2007). The large number of diverse transporters, and the need to understand their impact in different tissues and cellular locations (particularly GIT, liver and kidney), make this a much more complex area to investigate when compared to modeling of DME interactions. A number of investigators have published modeling approaches for transporters (Chiba et al., 2009; Paine et al., 2011; Poirier et al., 2008; Poirier et al., 2009a; Poirier et al., 2009b; Watanabe et al., 2010). As these are areas of significant investigation in the field, as transporter knowledge grows, we can expect that reliable PBPK modeling approaches will follow allowing a more in-depth understanding of transporter-DME interplay.

In vitro tools offer the most reliable methodologies to explore individual transporter mechanisms, and multiple tissues and transporters (as well as DMEs) are involved in describing the overall ADME of drug molecules. Computational modeling approaches can combine the data from many different sources, offering the most realistic way forward to understand the true contribution of transporters to *in vivo* drug behavior.

The ITC whitepaper, and more recently the EMA and FDA have outlined some quantitative *in vitro* to *in vivo* extrapolation approaches for some transporters (e.g. OATPs), but these cannot currently be extended to cover all the clinically relevant transporters, or for that matter all the relevant drugs which interact with them (Giacomini et al., 2010). As previously discussed, the quality of some of the *in vitro* outputs can be questionable. Although quantitative extrapolation is the best way forward for transporter integration, significant improvements are needed.

VI. Conclusion

Knowledge and awareness of drug transporters and their impact on drug ADME and safety has grown rapidly across the pharmaceutical industry, the scientific community, and in the clinic. Transporter drug interactions have been demonstrated clinically, and are now accepted as significant risk factors for drug development and therapeutic use. Regulatory expectations are high, and pharmaceutical companies are currently expected to provide interaction information for at least nine drug transporters for drug registration purposes. This list is likely to grow over the coming years, but we can also expect some refinement in expectation as the science develops.

It is now evident that multiple transporters and/or DMEs are implicated in the ADME of some important drugs. Integrating these different mechanisms together to understand their relative contributions to overall human ADME is a key challenge to the industry, although there is no consensus in the industry on standard experimental approaches to help achieve this.

Preclinical evidence of the potential for transporter proteins as mediators of drug toxicity is growing, particularly in hepatotoxicity and DILI. Discovering and contextualizing the role of membrane transporters in the already complex mechanisms underlying drug toxicity is a significant new challenge to transportology. Integrating transporters into metabolic schemes is only just beginning to happen, but will be of great benefit in to the toxicology field, facilitating a more complete appreciation of their involvement in endogenous processes, which may be adversely impacted by drugs.

Although there is evidence for efflux and uptake membrane transporter modulation of tissue and intracellular concentrations of therapeutic agents, with the exception of CNS therapies, their role in drug disposition is not routinely considered in mainstream drug discovery or drug development. In a clinical context this is not too surprising, as the technology required for routine, real-time measurement of tissue drug concentrations *in vivo* is challenging, and still in development. We have a limited appreciation of the cellular localization, tissue distribution, expression levels, and functionality of transporters in humans. However, as the analytical technologies improve, it is reasonable to expect that its application to measurement of drug disposition will follow, and with it our understanding of the impact of drug transporters in these tissues, opening the possibility of utilizing drug target transporters as delivery agents.

Computational modeling approaches, notably physiology-based/pharmacokinetic (PB/PK) modeling, will permit the exploration of not only transporter interactions at a number of different body sites, but also the impact of multiple mechanisms on drug ADME. Reliable transporter *in vitro* to *in vivo* scaling factors to enable the application of these approaches are required. This area is developing very rapidly, and values for some key transporters in key tissues are already available. Although empirical approaches are being successfully applied, given the range of tissues and transporters of interest, it is likely that absolute quantitation of transporter proteins will be required to facilitate the generation of robust *in vitro–in vivo* scaling factors.

In conclusion, membrane transporter science (transportology) is here to stay and will continue to develop. Although highly advanced, there is still a great deal to learn and understand about the functional significance of membrane transporters on drug ADME, action and toxicity.

Acknowledgments

The author would like to acknowledge former colleagues at GlaxoSmithKline R&D Ltd. for their many stimulating and knowledgeable discussions on membrane transporter mechanisms, their investigation and understanding, particularly Joseph Polli, Harma Ellens, Kathryn Kenworthy, Joan Humphreys, Grant Generaux, James Clarke, Catherine Cartwright, Michael Hobbs and Catherine Booth-Genthe.

Conflict of Interest: The author is an independent DMPK consultant, and is a former employee of GlaxoSmithKline R&D Ltd., a drug discovery and development company.

Abbreviations

ABC	ATP-binding cassette
SLC	solute carrier
ADME	absorption, distribution, metabolism, elimination
DME	drug metabolising enzyme
Pgp	P-glycoprotein
MRP	multi-drug resistance associated protein
MDR	multi-drug resistance transporter
OCT	organic cation transporter
OAT	organic anion transporter
OATP	organic anion transporter protein
BSEP	bile salt export pump
ASBT	apical sodium-dependent bile transporter
NTCP	sodium-taurocholate co-transporting polypeptide
OST	organic solute and steroid transporter
BCRP	breast cancer resistance protein
MATE	multi-drug and toxic-compound extrusion transporter
OCTN	organic cation/l-carnitine transporter
PEPT	peptide transporter
GLUT	facilitated glucose transporter
SGLT	sodium-glucose co-transporter
ENT	equilibrative nucleoside transporter
CYP	cytochrome P450
GIT	gastrointestinal tract

CNS	central nervous system
BBB	blood–brain barrier
SNP	single nucleotide polymorphism
PK	pharmacokinetic
PB	physiology-based
PD	pharmacodynamic
DDI	drug–drug interaction
DILI	drug induced liver injury
NTI	narrow therapeutic index
NCE	new chemical entity
ITC	International Transporter Consortium
EMA	European Medicines Agency
FDA	Food and Drug Administration
MDCK	Madin–Darby canine kidney cell line
Caco2	colon-carcinoma cell line
MALDI	matrix-assisted laser desorption/ionization

References

Acharya, P., O'Connor, M. P., Polli, J. W., Ayrton, A., Ellens, H., & Bentz, J. (2008). Kinetic identification of membrane transporters that assist P-glycoprotein-mediated transport of digoxin and loperamide through a confluent monolayer of MDCKII-hMDR1 cells. *Drug Metabolism and Disposition*, *36*(2), 452–460.

Adkison, K. K., Vaidya, S. S., Lee, D. Y., Koo, S. H., Li, L., Mehta, A. A., et al. (2010). Oral sulfasalazine as a clinical BCRP probe substrate: pharmacokinetic effects of genetic variation (C421A) and pantoprazole coadministration. *Journal of Pharmaceutical Sciences*, *99*(2), 1046–1062.

Agarwal, S., Sane, R., Ohlfest, J., & Elmquist, W. (2011). The role of the breast cancer resistance protein (ABCG2) in the distribution of sorafenib to the brain. *Journal of Pharmacology and Experimental Therapeutics*, *336*(1), 223–233.

Agnani, D., Acharya, P., Martinez, E., Tran, T. T., Abraham, F., Tobin, F., et al. (2011). Fitting the elementary rate constants of the P-gp transporter network in the hMDR1-MDCK confluent cell monolayer using a particle swarm algorithm. *PLoS One*, *6*(10), e25086.

Akamine, Y., Miura, M., Yasai-Furukori, N., Kojima, M., & Uno, T. (2011). Carbamazepine Differentially Affects the Pharmacokinetics of Fexofenadine Enantiomers.

Ayrton, A., & Morgan, P. (2008). Role of transport proteins in drug discovery and development: a pharmaceutical perspective. *Xenobiotica*, *38*(7, 8), 676–708.

Benet, L. Z., Amidon, G. L., Barends, D. M., Lennernas, H., Polli, J. E., Shah, V. P., et al. (2008). The use of BDDCS in classifying the permeability of marketed drugs. *Pharmaceutical Research*, *25*(3), 483–488.

Bhattachar, S. N., Perkins, E. J., Tan, J. S., & Burns, L. J. (2011). Effect of gastric pH on the pharmacokinetics of a BCS class II compound in dogs: utilization of an artificial stomach and duodenum dissolution model and GastroPlus, simulations to predict absorption. *Journal of Pharmaceutical Sciences*, *100*(11), 4756–4765.

Biermann, J., Lang, D., Gorboulev, V., Koepsell, H., Sindic, A., Schroter, R. , et al. (2006). Characterization of regulatory mechanisms and states of human organic cation transporter 2. *Am. J. Physiol Cell Physiol*, *290*,(6), C1521–C1531.

Brown, C., Sayer, C., Windass, A., Haslam, I., De Broe, M., D'Haese, P., et al. (2008). Characterisation of human tubular cell monolayers as a model of proximal tubular xenobiotic handling. *Toxicology and Applied Pharmacology*, *233*(3), 428–438.

Burnell, J. M., & Kirby, W. M. (1951). Effectiveness of a new compound, benemid, in elevating serum penicillin concentrations. *Journal of Clinical Investigation*, *30*(7), 697–700.

Chiba, M., Ishii, Y., & Sugiyama, Y. (2009). Prediction of hepatic clearance in human from in vitro data for successful drug development. *AAPS Journal*, *11*(2), 262–276.

Dawson, P., Hubbert, M. L., & Rao, A. (2010). Getting the mOST from OST: Role of organic solute transporter, OSTalpha-OSTbeta, in bile acid and steroid metabolism. *Biochimica et Biophysica Acta*, *1801*(9), 994–1004.

Dawson, S., Stahl, S., Paul, N., Barber, J., & Kenna, J. G. (2012). In vitro inhibition of the bile salt export pump correlates with risk of cholestatic drug-induced liver injury in humans. *Drug Metabolism and Disposition*, *40*(1), 130–138.

de Klerk, O. L., Willemsen, A. T., Bosker, F. J., Bartels, A. L., Hendrikse, N. H., den Boer, J. A., et al. (2010). Regional increase in P-glycoprotein function in the blood–brain barrier of patients with chronic schizophrenia: a PET study with [(11)C]verapamil as a probe for P-glycoprotein function. *Psychiatry Research*, *183*(2), 151–156.

European Medicines Agency (2010). *Guideline on The Investigation of Drug Interactions*: http://www.ema.europa.eu/docs/en_GB/document_library/Scientific_guideline/2010/05/WC500090112.pdf2010. (February 21, 2012).

Food and Drugs Administration (2012). *Drug Development and Drug Interactions: Possible Models for Decision-Making*. http://www.fda.gov/Drugs/DevelopmentApprovalProcess/DevelopmentResources/DrugInteractionsLabeling/ucm093583.htm2012. (February 21, 2012).

Food and Drugs Administration (2006). *Guidance for Industry Drug Interaction Studies – Study Design, Data Analysis, and Implications for Dosing and Labeling*. http://www.fda.gov/downloads/Drugs/GuidanceComplianceRegulatoryInformation/Guidances/UCM072101.pdf2006. (February 20, 2012).

Foti, R. S., Rock, D. A., Wienkers, L. C., & Wahlstrom, J. L. (2010). Selection of alternative CYP3A4 probe substrates for clinical drug interaction studies using in vitro data and in vivo simulation. *Drug Metabolism and Disposition*, *38*(6), 981–987.

Generaux, G. T., Bonomo, F. M., Johnson, M., & Doan, K. M. (2011). Impact of SLCO1B1 (OATP1B1) and ABCG2 (BCRP) genetic polymorphisms and inhibition on LDL-C lowering and myopathy of statins. *Xenobiotica*, *41*(8), 639–651.

Giacomini, K. M., Huang, S. M., Tweedie, D. J., Benet, L. Z., Brouwer, K. L., Chu, X., et al. (2010). Membrane transporters in drug development. *Nature Reviews Drug Discovery*, *9*(3), 215–236.

Gutman, A. B., & Yu, T. F. (1957). Renal function in gout; with a commentary on the renal regulation of urate excretion, and the role of the kidney in the pathogenesis of gout. *American Journal of Medicine*, *23*(4), 600–622.

Gutman, A. B., & Yu, T. F. (1958). Renal regulation of uric acid excretion in normal and gouty man; modification by uricosuric agents. *Bulletin of the New York Academy of Medicine*, *34*(5), 287–296.

Hallifax, D., Turlizzi, E., Zanelli, U., & Houston, J.B. (2011). Clearance-dependent underprediction of in vivo intrinsic clearance from human hepatocytes: comparison with permeabilities from artificial membrane (PAMPA) assay, in silico and caco-2 assay, for 65 drugs. PM:22214813 (February 23, 2012).

Heddiger, M. A. (2010). SLC tables. Available from: http://www.bioparadigms.org/, February 21, 2012.

Ho, R. H., Tirona, R. G., Leake, B. F., Glaeser, H., Lee, W., Lemke, C. J., et al. (2006). Drug and bile acid transporters in rosuvastatin hepatic uptake: function, expression, and pharmacogenetics. *Gastroenterology*, *130*(6), 1793–1806.

Hobbs, M., Parker, C., Birch, H., & Kenworthy, K. E.. (2011). Understanding the interplay of drug transporters involved in the disposition of rosuvastatin in the isolated perfused rat liver using a physiologically-based pharmacokinetic model.

Ieiri, I., Higuchi, S., & Sugiyama, Y. (2009). Genetic polymorphisms of uptake (OATP1B1, 1B3) and efflux (MRP2, BCRP) transporters: implications for inter-individual differences in the pharmacokinetics and pharmacodynamics of statins and other clinically relevant drugs. *Expert Opinion on Drug Metabolism & Toxicology*, *5*(7), 703–729.

Jamei, M., Marciniak, S., Feng, K., Barnett, A., Tucker, G., & Rostami-Hodjegan, A. (2009). The Simcyp population-based ADME simulator. *Expert Opinion on Drug Metabolism & Toxicology*, *5*(2), 211–223.

Jeffrey, S., & Summerfield, S. (2010). Assessment of the blood-brain barrier in CNS drug discovery. *Neurobiology of Disease*, *37*(1), 33–37.

Jemnitz, K., Veres, Z., Tugyi, R., & Vereczkey, L. (2010). Biliary efflux transporters involved in the clearance of rosuvastatin in sandwich culture of primary rat hepatocytes. *Toxicology In Vitro*, *24*(2), 605–610.

Johnson, B. M., Zhang, P., Schuetz, J. D., & Brouwer, K. L. (2006). Characterization of transport protein expression in multidrug resistance-associated protein (Mrp) 2-deficient rats. *Drug Metabolism and Disposition*, *34*(4), 556–562.

Kajosaari, L. I., Niemi, M., Neuvonen, M., Laitila, J., Neuvonen, P. J., & Backman, J. T. (2005). Cyclosporine markedly raises the plasma concentrations of repaglinide. *Clinical Pharmacology & Therapeutics*, *78*(4), 388–399.

Kell, D. B., Dobson, P. D., & Oliver, S. G. (2011). Pharmaceutical drug transport: the issues and the implications that it is essentially carrier-mediated only. *Drug Discovery Today*, *16*(15, 16), 704–714.

Kelly, R., Draper, D., Chen, C. C., Robey, R. W., Figg, W. D., Piekarz, R. L., et al. (2011). A pharmacodynamic study of docetaxel in combination with the P-glycoprotein antagonist tariquidar (XR9576) in patients with lung, ovarian, and cervical cancer. *Clinical Cancer Research*, *17*(3), 569–580.

Keppler, D. (2011). Cholestasis and the role of basolateral efflux pumps. *Zeitschrift fur Gastroenterologie*, *49*(12), 1553–1557.

Kharasch, E. D., Bedynek, P. S., Walker, A., Whittington, D., & Hoffer, C. (2008). Mechanism of ritonavir changes in methadone pharmacokinetics and pharmacodynamics: II. Ritonavir effects on CYP3A and P-glycoprotein activities. *Clinical Pharmacology & Therapeutics*, *84*(4), 506–512.

Kitamura, S., Maeda, K., & Sugiyama, Y. (2008). Recent progresses in the experimental methods and evaluation strategies of transporter functions for the prediction of the pharmacokinetics in humans. *Naunyn-Schmiedebergs Archives of Pharmacology*, *377*(4–6), 617–628.

Knut and Alice Wallenberg Foundation (2011). The Human Protein Atlas. Available from: http://www.proteinatlas.org/ (February 20, 2012).

Kolhatkar, V., & Polli, J. E. (2010). Reliability of inhibition models to correctly identify type of inhibition. *Pharmaceutical Research*, *27*(11), 2433–2445.

Kotani, N., Maeda, K., Watanabe, T., Hiramatsu, M., Gong, L. K., Bi, Y. A., et al. (2011). Culture period-dependent changes in the uptake of transporter substrates in sandwich-cultured rat and human hepatocytes. *Drug Metabolism and Disposition*, *39*(9), 1503–1510.

Kusuhara, H., & Sugiyama, Y. (2009). In vitro–in vivo extrapolation of transporter-mediated clearance in the liver and kidney. *Drug Metabolism and Pharmacokinetics*, *24*(1), 37–52.

Lankas, G. R., Cartwright, M. E., & Umbenhauer, D. (1997). P-glycoprotein deficiency in a subpopulation of CF-1 mice enhances avermectin-induced neurotoxicity. *Toxicology and Applied Pharmacology*, *143*(2), 357–365.

Lee, C. A. (2011). S8-Application of P-gp decision tree: what have we learned? *Drug Metabolism Reviews*, *43*(S2), 8.

Lee, E. W., Lai, Y., Zhang, H., & Unadkat, J. D. (2006). Identification of the mitochondrial targeting signal of the human equilibrative nucleoside transporter 1 (hENT1): implications for interspecies differences in mitochondrial toxicity of fialuridine. *Journal of Biological Chemistry*, *281*(24), 16700–16706.

Lee, W. K., Reichold, M., Edemir, B., Ciarimboli, G., Warth, R., Koepsell, H., et al. (2009). Organic cation transporters OCT1, 2, and 3 mediate high-affinity transport of the mutagenic vital dye ethidium in the kidney proximal tubule. *Am. J. Physiol Renal Physiol*, *296*,(6), F1504–F1513.

Link, E., Parish, S., Armitage, J., Bowman, L., Heath, S., Matsuda, F., et al. (2008). SLCO1B1 variants and statin-induced myopathy–a genomewide study. *New England Journal of Medicine*, *359*(8), 789–799.

Lippmann, E., Weidenfeller, C., Svendsen, C., & Shusta, E. (2011). Blood-brain barrier modeling with co-cultured neural progenitor cell-derived astrocytes and neurons. *Journal of Neurochemistry*, *119*(3), 507–520.

Maeda, K., & Sugiyama, Y. (2010). The use of hepatocytes to investigate drug uptake transporters. *Methods in Molecular Biology*, *640*, 327–353.

Marion, T. L., Perry, C. H., St Claire, R. L., Yue, W., & Brouwer, K. L. (2011). Differential disposition of chenodeoxycholic acid versus taurocholic acid in response to acute troglitazone exposure in rat hepatocytes. *Toxicological Sciences*, *120*(2), 371–380.

Menger, R. F., Stutts, W. L., Anbukumar, D. S., Bowden, J. A., Ford, D. A., & Yost, R. A. (2012). MALDI mass spectrometric imaging of cardiac tissue following myocardial infarction in a rat coronary artery ligation model. *Analytical Chemistry*, *84*(2), 1117–1125.

Morjani, H., & Madoulet, C. (2010). Immunosuppressors as multidrug resistance reversal agents. *Methods in Molecular Biology*, *596*, 433–446.

Motta, P., Pons, N., Pagliarusco, S., Pellegatti, M., & Bonomo, F. (2011). Casopitant: in vitro data and SimCyp simulation to predict in vivo metabolic interactions involving cytochrome P450 3A4. *Drug Metabolism and Disposition*, *39*(3), 363–372.

Muller, M. (2006). Human ABC-Transporters. Available from: http://nutrigene.4t.com/humanabc.htm (February 20, 2012).

Nakanishi, T., Shibue, Y., Fukuyama, Y., Yoshida, K., Fukuda, H., Shirasaka, Y., et al. (2011). Quantitative time-lapse imaging-based analysis of drug-drug interaction mediated by hepatobiliary transporter, multidrug resistance-associated protein 2, in sandwich-cultured rat hepatocytes. *Drug Metabolism and Disposition*, *39*(6), 984–991.

Niemi, M., Pasanen, M. K., & Neuvonen, P. J. (2011). Organic anion transporting polypeptide 1B1: a genetically polymorphic transporter of major importance for hepatic drug uptake. *Pharmacological Reviews*, *63*(1), 157–181.

Nies, A. T., Koepsell, H., Damme, K., & Schwab, M. (2011). Organic cation transporters (OCTs, MATEs), in vitro and in vivo evidence for the importance in drug therapy. *Handbook of Experimental Pharmacology*, *201*, 105–167.

Ohtsuki, S., Schaefer, O., Kawakami, H., Inoue, T., Liehner, S., Saito, A., et al. (2012). Simultaneous absolute protein quantification of transporters, cytochromes P450, and UDP-glucuronosyltransferases as a novel approach for the characterization of individual human liver: comparison with mRNA levels and activities. *Drug Metabolism and Disposition*, *40*(1), 83–92.

Okumu, A., DiMaso, M., & Lobenberg, R. (2009). Computer simulations using GastroPlus to justify a biowaiver for etoricoxib solid oral drug products. *European Journal of Pharmaceutics and Biopharmaceutics*, *72*(1), 91–98.

Paine, S. W., Menochet, K., Denton, R., McGinnity, D. F., & Riley, R. J. (2011). Prediction of human renal clearance from preclinical species for a diverse set of drugs that exhibit both active secretion and net reabsorption. *Drug Metabolism and Disposition*, *39*(6), 1008–1013.

Paine, S. W., Parker, A. J., Gardiner, P., Webborn, P. J., & Riley, R. J. (2008). Prediction of the pharmacokinetics of atorvastatin, cerivastatin, and indomethacin using kinetic models applied to isolated rat hepatocytes. *Drug Metabolism and Disposition*, *36*(7), 1365–1374.

Peukert, M., Matros, A., Lattanzio, G., Kaspar, S., Abadia, J., & Mock, H. P. (2012). Spatially resolved analysis of small molecules by matrix-assisted laser desorption/ionization mass spectrometric imaging (MALDI-MSI). *New Phytology*, *193*(3), 806–815.

Poirier, A., Cascais, A. C., Funk, C., & Lave, T. (2009a). Prediction of pharmacokinetic profile of valsartan in humans based on in vitro uptake-transport data. *Chemistry & Biodiversity*, *6*(11), 1975–1987.

Poirier, A., Funk, C., Scherrmann, J. M., & Lave, T. (2009b). Mechanistic modeling of hepatic transport from cells to whole body: application to napsagatran and fexofenadine. *Molecular Pharmacology*, *6*(6), 1716–1733.

Poirier, A., Lave, T., Portmann, R., Brun, M. E., Senner, F., Kansy, M., et al. (2008). Design, data analysis, and simulation of in vitro drug transport kinetic experiments using a mechanistic in vitro model. *Drug Metabolism and Disposition*, *36*(12), 2434–2444.

Polli, J. W., Olson, K. L., Chism, J. P., John-Williams, L. S., Yeager, R. L., Woodard, S. M., et al. (2009). An unexpected synergist role of P-glycoprotein and breast cancer resistance protein on the central nervous system penetration of the tyrosine kinase inhibitor lapatinib (N-{3-chloro-4-[(3-fluorobenzyl)oxy]phenyl}-6-[5-({[2-(methylsulfonyl)ethyl]amino} methyl)-2-furyl]-4-quinazolinamine; GW572016). *Drug Metabolism and Disposition*, *37*(2), 439–442.

Potschka, H. (2011). Role of CNS efflux drug transporters in antiepileptic drug delivery: overcoming CNS efflux drug transport, PM:22210135 (February 23, 2012).

Rakhit, A., Pantze, M. P., Fettner, S., Jones, H. M., Charoin, J. E., Riek, M., et al. (2008). The effects of CYP3A4 inhibition on erlotinib pharmacokinetics: computer-based simulation (SimCYP) predicts in vivo metabolic inhibition. *European Journal of Clinical Pharmacology*, *64*(1), 31–41.

Reis, J. M., Sinko, B., & Serra, C. H. (2010). Parallel artificial membrane permeability assay (PAMPA) - Is it better than Caco-2 for human passive permeability prediction? *Mini-Reviews in Medicinal Chemistry*, *10*(11), 1071–1076.

Schaefer, O., Ohtsuki, S., Kawakami, H., Inoue, T., Liehner, S., Saito, A., et al. (2012). Absolute quantification and differential expression of drug transporters, cytochrome P450 enzymes, and UDP-glucuronosyltransferases in cultured primary human hepatocytes. *Drug Metabolism and Disposition*, *40*(1), 93–103.

Shawahna, R., Uchida, Y., Decleves, X., Ohtsuki, S., Yousif, S., Dauchy, S., et al. (2011). Transcriptomic and quantitative proteomic analysis of transporters and drug metabolizing enzymes in freshly isolated human brain microvessels. *Molecular Pharmacology*, *8*(4), 1332–1341.

Shirasaka, Y., Suzuki, K., Nakanishi, T., & Tamai, I. (2011). Differential effect of grapefruit juice on intestinal absorption of statins due to inhibition of organic anion transporting polypeptide and/or P-glycoprotein. *Journal of Pharmaceutical Sciences*, *100*(9), 3843–3853.

Shitara, Y., & Sugiyama, Y. (2006). Pharmacokinetic and pharmacodynamic alterations of 3-hydroxy-3-methylglutaryl coenzyme A (HMG-CoA) reductase inhibitors: drug-drug interactions and interindividual differences in transporter and metabolic enzyme functions. *Pharmacology & Therapeutics*, *112*(1), 71–105.

Sugano, K., Kansy, M., Artursson, P., Avdeef, A., Bendels, S., Di, L., et al. (2010). Coexistence of passive and carrier-mediated processes in drug transport. *Nature Reviews Drug Discovery*, *9*(8), 597–614.

Summerfield, S., Lucas, A., Porter, R., Jeffrey, P., Gunn, R., Read, K., et al. (2008). Toward an improved prediction of human in vivo brain penetration. *Xenobiotica*, *38*(12), 1518–1535.

Svoboda, M. (2011). Organic anion transporting polypeptides (OATPs): regulation of expression and function. *Current Drug Metabolism*, *12*(2), 139–153.

Syvanen, S., Luurtsema, G., Molthoff, C. F., Windhorst, A. D., Huisman, M. C., Lammertsma, A. A., et al. (2011). (R)-[11C]verapamil PET studies to assess changes in P-glycoprotein expression and functionality in rat blood-brain barrier after exposure to kainate-induced status epilepticus. *BMC Medical Imaging*, *11*, 1.

Takane, H. (2011). [Genetic polymorphisms of SLCO1B1 for drug pharmacokinetics and its clinical implications]. *Yakugaku Zasshi*, *131*(11), 1589–1594.

Tamaki, A., Ierano, C., Szakacs, G., Robey, R. W., & Bates, S. E. (2011). The controversial role of ABC transporters in clinical oncology. *Essays in Biochemistry*, *50*(1), 209–232.

Tamhane, M., Chakilam, A., Jayaraj, A., Thakkar, V., & Taft, D. (2010). Comparative renal excretion of VX-702, a novel p38 MAPK inhibitor, and methotrexate in the perfused rat kidney model. *Drug Development and Industrial Pharmacy*, *36*(3), 315–322.

Taub, M. E., Mease, K., Sane, R. S., Watson, C. A., Chen, L., Ellens, H., et al. (2011). Digoxin is not a substrate for organic anion-transporting polypeptide transporters OATP1A2, OATP1B1, OATP1B3, and OATP2B1 but is a substrate for a sodium-dependent transporter expressed in HEK293 cells. *Drug Metabolism and Disposition*, *39*(11), 2093–2102.

Tirona, R. (2011). Molecular mechanisms of drug transporter regulation. *Handbook of Experimental Pharmacology*, *201*, 372–402.

Tucker, T. G., Milne, A. M., Fournel-Gigleux, S., Fenner, K. S., & Coughtrie, M. W. (2012). Absolute immunoquantification of the expression of ABC transporters P-glycoprotein, breast cancer resistance protein and multidrug resistance-associated protein 2 in human liver and duodenum. *Biochemical Pharmacology*, *83*(2), 729–785.

Tzvetkov, M. V., Saadatmand, A. R., Bokelmann, K., Meineke, I., Kaiser, R., & Brockmoller, J. (2012). Effects of OCT1 polymorphisms on the cellular uptake, plasma concentrations and efficacy of the 5-HT(3) antagonists tropisetron and ondansetron. *Pharmacogenomics Journal*, *12*(1), 22–29.

Tzvetkov, M. V., Saadatmand, A. R., Lotsch, J., Tegeder, I., Stingl, J. C., & Brockmoller, J. (2011). Genetically polymorphic OCT1: another piece in the puzzle of the variable pharmacokinetics and pharmacodynamics of the opioidergic drug tramadol. *Clinical Pharmacology & Therapeutics*, *90*(1), 143–150.

Tzvetkov, M. V., Vormfelde, S. V., Balen, D., Meineke, I., Schmidt, T., Sehrt, D., et al. (2009). The effects of genetic polymorphisms in the organic cation transporters OCT1, OCT2, and OCT3 on the renal clearance of metformin. *Clinical Pharmacology & Therapeutics*, *86*(3), 299–306.

Umehara, K. I., Iwatsubo, T., Noguchi, K., & Kamimura, H. (2007). Comparison of the kinetic characteristics of inhibitory effects exerted by biguanides and H2-blockers on human and rat organic cation transporter-mediated transport: Insight into the development of drug candidates. *Xenobiotica*, *37*,(6), 618–634.

Urakami, Y., Kimura, N., Okuda, M., & Inui, K. (2004). Creatinine transport by basolateral organic cation transporter hOCT2 in the human kidney. *Pharm. Res.*, *21*,(6), 976–981.

van de Steeg, E., Wagenaar, E., van der Kruijssen, C. M., Burggraaff, J. E., de Waart, D. R., et al. (2010). Organic anion transporting polypeptide 1a/1b-knockout mice provide insights into hepatic handling of bilirubin, bile acids, and drugs. *The Journal of Clinical Investigation*, *120*(8), 2942–2952.

Van Waterschoot, R. A., Lagas, J. S., Wagenaar, E., Rosing, H., Beijnen, J. H., & Schinkel, A. H. (2010). Individual and combined roles of CYP3A, P-glycoprotein (MDR1/ABCB1) and MRP2 (ABCC2) in the pharmacokinetics of docetaxel. *International Journal of Cancer*, *127*(12), 2959–2964.

Vladutiu, G., & Isackson, P. (2008). SLCO1B1 variants and statin-induced myopathy. *New England Journal of Medicine*, *359*(8), 789–799.

Vlaming, M. L., van, E. A., Pala, Z., Wagenaar, E., van de Wetering, K., van, T. O., et al. (2009). Abcc2 (Mrp2), Abcc3 (Mrp3), and Abcg2 (Bcrp1) are the main determinants for rapid elimination of methotrexate and its toxic metabolite 7-hydroxymethotrexate in vivo. *Molecular Cancer Therapeutics*, *8*(12), 3350–3359.

Vlaming, M. L., van, E. A., van de Steeg, E., Pala, Z., Wagenaar, E., van, T. O., et al. (2011). Impact of abcc2 [multidrug resistance-associated protein (MRP) 2], abcc3 (MRP3), and abcg2 (breast cancer resistance protein) on the oral pharmacokinetics of methotrexate and its main metabolite 7-hydroxymethotrexate. *Drug Metabolism and Disposition*, *39*(8), 1338–1344.

Wang, Z., Zhou, Q., Kruh, G. D., & Gallo, J. M. (2011). Dose-dependent disposition of methotrexate in abcc2 and abcc3 gene knockout murine models. *Drug Metabolism and Disposition*, *39*(11), 2155–2161.

Wang, Z. J., Yin, O. Q., Tomlinson, B., & Chow, M. S. (2008). OCT2 polymorphisms and in-vivo renal functional consequence: studies with metformin and cimetidine. *Pharmacogenetics and Genomics*, *18*(7), 637–645.

Watanabe, T., Kusuhara, H., & Sugiyama, Y. (2010). Application of physiologically based pharmacokinetic modeling and clearance concept to drugs showing transporter-mediated distribution and clearance in humans. *J.Pharmacokinet.Pharmacodyn.*, *37*(6), 575–590.

Watanabe, T., Kusuhara, H., Watanabe, T., Debori, Y., Maeda, K., Kondo, T., et al. (2011). Prediction of the overall renal tubular secretion and hepatic clearance of anionic drugs and a renal drug-drug interaction involving organic anion transporter 3 in humans by in vitro uptake experiments. *Drug Metabolism and Disposition*, *39*(6), 1031–1038.

Webborn, P. J., Parker, A. J., Denton, R. L., & Riley, R. J. (2007). In vitro-in vivo extrapolation of hepatic clearance involving active uptake: theoretical and experimental aspects. *Xenobiotica*, *37*(10-11), 1090–1109.

Wen, J., & Xiong, Y. (2010). OATP1B1 388A>G polymorphism and pharmacokinetics of pitavastatin in Chinese healthy volunteers. *Journal of Clinical Pharmacy and Therapeutics*, *35*(1), 99–104.

Wilby, A. J., Maeda, K., Courtney, P. F., Debori, Y., Webborn, P. J., Kitamura, Y., et al. (2011). Hepatic uptake in the dog: comparison of uptake in hepatocytes and human embryonic kidney cells expressing dog organic anion-transporting polypeptide 1B4. *Drug Metabolism and Disposition*, *39*(12), 2361–2369.

Wolf, K. K., Vora, S., Webster, L. O., Generaux, G. T., Polli, J. W., & Brouwer, K. L. (2010). Use of cassette dosing in sandwich-cultured rat and human hepatocytes to identify drugs that inhibit bile acid transport. *Toxicology In Vitro*, *24*(1), 297–309.

Yamada, A., Maeda, K., Ishiguro, N., Tsuda, Y., Igarashi, T., Ebner, T., et al. (2011). The impact of pharmacogenetics of metabolic enzymes and transporters on the pharmacokinetics of telmisartan in healthy volunteers. *Pharmacogenetics and Genomics*, *21*(9), 523–530.

Yang, J., Milton, M., Yu, S., Liao, M., Liu, N., Wu, J., et al. (2010). P-glycoprotein and breast cancer resistance protein affect disposition of tandutinib, a tyrosine kinase inhibitor. *Drug Metabolism Letters*, *4*(4), 201–212.

Yonezawa, A., & Inui, K. (2011). Importance of the multidrug and toxin extrusion MATE/SLC47A family to pharmacokinetics, pharmacodynamics/toxicodynamics and pharmacogenomics. *British Journal of Pharmacology*, *164*(7), 1817–1825.

Zhang, L., Zhang, Y., Strong, J., Reynolds, K., & Huang, S. (2008). A regulatory viewpoint on transporter-based drug interactions. *Xenobiotica*, *37*(7, 8), 709–724.

Zolk, O., Solbach, T. F., Konig, J., & Fromm, M. F. (2009). Functional characterization of the human organic cation transporter 2 variant p.270Ala>Ser. *Drug Metabolism and Disposition*, *37*(6), 1312–1318.

Zolk, O., Solbach, T. F., Konig, J., & Fromm, M. F. (2009). Structural determinants of inhibitor interaction with the human organic cation transporter OCT2 (SLC22A2). *Naunyn Schmiedebergs Arch. Pharmacol*, *379*,(4), 337–348.

Ian M. Copple

The University of Liverpool, MRC Centre for Drug Safety Science,
Department of Molecular & Clinical Pharmacology, Liverpool,
United Kingdom

The Keap1–Nrf2 Cell Defense Pathway – A Promising Therapeutic Target?

Abstract

By regulating the basal and inducible expression of an abundance of detoxification enzymes, antioxidant proteins, xenobiotic transporters and other stress response proteins, the Keap1–Nrf2 pathway plays a crucial role in determining the sensitivity of mammalian cells to chemical and oxidative insults that have the capacity to provoke cellular harm. This review highlights historical and recent advances in our understanding of the molecular mechanisms that regulate the activity of the Keap1–Nrf2 pathway. The important role of Nrf2 in protecting against the onset of specific diseases and drug-induced toxicities is also examined, alongside the emerging role of Nrf2 in promoting oncogenesis and chemotherapeutic drug resistance. A particular emphasis is placed on the potential for translation of this mechanistic understanding into clinical strategies that can improve human health, with consideration of the potential applications of targeting Nrf2 therapeutically.

I. Introduction

Mammalian cells are frequently exposed to intrinsically and extrinsically generated chemical and oxidative insults that pose a risk of disrupting the normal function of nucleic acids, proteins and membrane lipids, and ultimately perturbing host function. In order to combat such insults, cells possess multi-faceted and highly regulated defense systems that serve to detoxify and/or remove the stressor in order to maintain optimal cellular

Advances in Pharmacology, Volume 63 1054-3589/12 $35.00

http://dx.doi.org/10.1016/B978-0-12-398339-8.00002-1

conditions and function. The most basic tier of cell defense comprises non-protein antioxidants such as glutathione, vitamins C and E, β-carotene and bilirubin. In general, the scavenging actions of these molecules are 'suicidal' in nature; by donating an electron to a radical or other reactive entity, and thus generating a non-reactive species, the antioxidant is inactivated, but, in doing so, provides an alternative target to critical cellular macromolecules (Davies, 2000). Our appreciation of the beneficial actions of these and other antioxidants has prompted a surge of commercially available dietary supplements which provide supra-physiological levels of substances that have been shown to inhibit oxidation reactions, although evidence for the actual health benefits of such products is generally lacking (Bjelakovic et al., 2008).

At the protein level, a host of detoxification enzymes and xenobiotic transporters serve to nullify and remove potentially harmful chemical entities, and therefore provide the cell with a degree of basal protection against low-level chemical/oxidative stressors. For example, the superoxide dismutase family catalyze the dismutation of two superoxide anion radicals ($O_2^{\cdot -}$) to hydrogen peroxide (H_2O_2) and oxygen (O_2) (Nordberg et al., 2001). As a cytotoxic entity itself, H_2O_2 is detoxified via reduction to water (H_2O) and O_2 by glutathione peroxidases, catalases and/or peroxiredoxins (Nordberg et al., 2001). In addition to the action of these and other detoxification enzymes, protein-based cell defense also comprises numerous xenobiotic transporters, which actively convey chemicals across the cell membrane, regulating their intracellular concentration and therefore the degree of cellular exposure. For a comprehensive review on the role of xenobiotic transporters in cell defense, see Klaassen (2002). The true elegance of this intermediate layer of cell defense is its capacity to adjust to increasing levels of stress through the upregulated expression of its individual subcomponents. This adaptive response is driven by the activity of a group of transcription factors, and an increasing body of evidence indicates that nuclear factor erythroid 2 (NF-E2)-related factor 2 (Nrf2) is the primary transcriptional regulator of this inducible cell defense.

Should initial efforts to detoxify and eliminate a cellular stressor prove futile, a last-ditch attempt is made to halt the spread of damage to neighboring cells, through the induction of programmed cell death (apoptosis). Characteristic membrane blebbing, cell shrinkage, chromatin condensation and DNA fragmentation culminate in the damaged cell being engulfed by macrophages (Edinger et al., 2004). In this sense, apoptosis is distinct from necrosis, which can be regarded simply as a failure of cellular homeostasis, resulting from a sudden, lethal insult that ultimately promotes an inflammatory response via the uncontrollable release of cellular contents into the local environment, leading to the damage of nearby cells (Edinger et al., 2004). The overall aim of the above cell defense processes is to minimize the deleterious effects of internal and external stressors and to maintain normal cellular function. The remainder of this review will focus on the contribution of Nrf2 to these goals, and the potential benefits of targeting this important protein therapeutically.

II. The Keap1–Nrf2 Cell Defense Pathway

Nrf2 is expressed in many tissues, particularly the liver, kidney, skin, lung and gastrointestinal tract, i.e. tissues that are frequently exposed to environmental insults (Motohashi et al., 2002). The Nrf2 protein comprises six highly conserved Neh domains. Of these, the N-terminal Neh2 domain facilitates interaction with the negative regulator Kelch-like erythroid cell-derived protein with CNC homology (ECH)-associated protein 1 (Keap1), the Neh1 domain mediates nuclear localization and DNA binding, and the Neh4 and Neh5 domains enable transactivation of target genes (Taguchi et al., 2011). Nrf2 normally resides in the cytosol of unstressed cells, via a physical interaction with Keap1 (for details see part A1 of this section). Keap1 limits the activity of Nrf2 by promoting its proteasomal degradation (Cullinan et al., 2004; Kobayashi et al., 2004; Zhang et al., 2004; Furukawa et al., 2005), yet, in response to a diverse array of stimuli, Nrf2 evades Keap1-mediated repression and accumulates within the nucleus, where it dimerises with members of the small Maf family (Itoh et al., 1997) and binds with high affinity to antioxidant response elements (AREs) located within the promoter regions of an array of cell defense genes.

The ARE is a *cis*-acting DNA enhancer motif with a consensus sequence defined as 5′-gagTcACa**GTgAGtCggC**Aaaatt-3′ (where essential nucleotides are in capitals and the core is in bold) (Nioi et al., 2003). Once bound to the ARE, the Nrf2–Maf heterodimer recruits transcriptional co-activators that promote transcription via intrinsic histone acetyltransferase activity and by bridging to components of the general transcriptional machinery (Katoh et al., 2001; Zhu et al., 2001; Kalkhoven, 2004). AREs have been identified in numerous Nrf2 target genes, including those involved in regulating the synthesis and conjugation of glutathione (for example, glutamate-cysteine ligase catalytic subunit (Mulcahy et al., 1997)), antioxidant proteins specializing in the detoxification of certain reactive species (heme oxygenase 1 (Reichard et al., 2007)), drug metabolizing enzymes (UDP-glucuronosyltransferase 1A1 (Yueh et al., 2007)), xenobiotic transporters (multidrug resistance protein 1 (Kurz et al., 2001)) and numerous other stress response proteins. A detailed overview of the Nrf2-regulated gene battery is provided in an excellent review by Hayes et al. (2010). By inducing the elevated expression of this battery of genes, Nrf2 is able to augment a wide range of cell defense processes, thereby enhancing the overall capacity to detoxify and expunge potentially harmful entities. As such, the Keap1–Nrf2 pathway in general represents a negative feedback loop; elevated levels of a chemical stressor trigger the upregulated expression of genes that ultimately serve to eliminate the stressor from the cell, upon which the system returns to a resting state (Fig. 1).

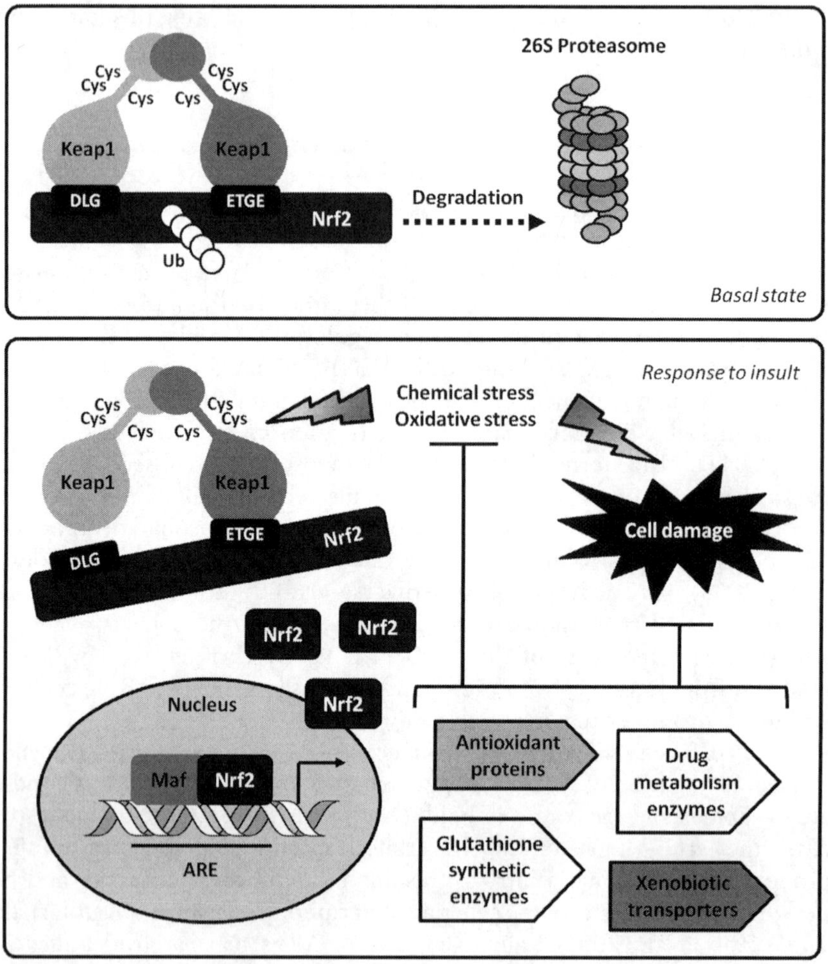

FIGURE 1 **The canonical Keap1–Nrf2 pathway response to cellular stress.** In the absence of chemical and oxidative stress (upper panel), the basal activity of Nrf2 is limited by its physical and functional association with a Keap1 homodimer, which directs the transcription factor for ubiquitination and degradation by the 26S proteasome. Under conditions of cellular stress (lower panel), the association between Keap1 and Nrf2 through the lower-affinity DLG motif of the latter is disrupted, most probably via a conformational change in the structure of Keap1 brought about via modification of one or more of its highly reactive cysteine residues. Although binding via the higher-affinity ETGE motif is maintained, Keap1 can no longer efficiently direct Nrf2 for ubiquitination and proteasomal degradation. Following the saturation of Keap1, newly synthesized Nrf2 accumulates within the cell and translocates to the nucleus, where it binds to antioxidant reponse elements (AREs) within cytoprotective target genes and promotes their enhanced expression. The products of these genes bolster the cellular capacity to detoxify and eliminate the original insult, thereby returning the system to homoestasis.

A. Mechanisms of Nrf2 Regulation

The chemical and molecular mechanisms that control the activity of Nrf2 have been reviewed in detail previously (Baird et al., 2011; Taguchi et al., 2011), and so only fundamental aspects of its regulation by Keap1, in addition to more recently described Keap1-independent mechanisms, will be described here.

1. Keap1-Dependent Nrf2 Regulation

In the absence of chemical and oxidative stress, the activity of Nrf2 is repressed due to its interaction with Keap1, first characterized in 1999 by Itoh et al. (1999). Scrutiny of the role of Keap1 in regulating Nrf2 *in vivo* was initially hampered due to the discovery that genetic deficiency of Keap1 (Keap1$^{-/-}$) is lethal in newborn mice, due to an Nrf2-dependent accumulation of hyper-keratotic lesions in the esophagus and fore-stomach that occlude the upper digestive tract and result in malnutrition, growth retardation and death (Wakabayashi et al., 2003; Taguchi et al., 2010). This problem has been overcome by the engineering of mice in which the Keap1 gene is deleted specifically within the liver (Okawa et al., 2006). Hepatocyte-specific Keap1-null mice exhibit elevated levels of expression of Nrf2-regulated genes in the liver, and a reduced sensitivity to acetaminophen-induced liver toxicity (Okawa et al., 2006), demonstrating the critical role of Keap1 in regulating the cytoprotective activity of Nrf2.

Keap1 is principally a cytosolic protein (Watai et al., 2007) that associates with the actin cytoskeleton (Kang et al., 2004). As such, the binding of Nrf2 by Keap1 physically restricts the transcription factor's subcellular localization, and therefore limits its basal activity. However, it is well established that the expression of Nrf2 target genes is diminished in the tissues of Nrf2 knockout (Nrf2$^{-/-}$) animals (Chan et al., 2000; Ramos-Gomez et al., 2001; Lee et al., 2003) and in cells depleted of Nrf2 by RNA interference (RNAi) (Dhakshinamoorthy et al., 2004; Cao et al., 2005; Copple et al., 2008a, b). Therefore, at least a small proportion of the total cellular complement of Nrf2 must evade Keap1 repression under basal conditions. This may be due to the regulation of Keap1 expression by Nrf2 itself (Lee et al., 2007), or may represent a low-intensity stimulation of the Keap1–Nrf2 pathway by background levels of oxidative stress, such as that caused by the generation of reactive oxygen species (ROS) as byproducts of mitochondrial aerobic respiration. In any case, this ambiguity in the current model of Nrf2 regulation has yet to be fully resolved. In addition to its role in controlling the basal activity of Nrf2, Keap1 also serves as a central node in the adaptive response to cellular stress, through its ability to 'sense' chemical and oxidative insults. The following sections describe in more detail these fundamental mechanisms of Nrf2 regulation by Keap1.

1.1. Ubiquitination and Proteasomal Degradation of Nrf2

In addition to physically restricting the subcellular localization of Nrf2, Keap1 limits the basal activity of Nrf2 by directing its ubiquitination and proteasomal degradation. It was first demonstrated that pharmacological inhibitors of proteasome activity caused the stabilization of Nrf2 and consequent upregulated expression of Nrf2 target genes (Sekhar et al., 2000; Alam et al., 2003; Itoh et al., 2003; McMahon et al., 2003; Nguyen et al., 2003; Stewart et al., 2003). Keap1 drives the ubiquitination of Nrf2 by acting as a substrate adaptor for a Cullin 3 (Cul3)-dependent E3 ubiquitin ligase complex, bridging Nrf2 and the ring-box protein ROC1/RBX1; the latter recruits a ubiquitin charged E2 molecule which is then conjugated on at least one of seven lysine residues located within the Neh2 domain of Nrf2 (Cullinan et al., 2004; Kobayashi et al., 2004; Zhang et al., 2004; Furukawa et al., 2005). Indeed, compound mutation of these lysines increases the steady-state level of Nrf2 by inhibiting its Keap1-dependent ubiquitination, whereas reversion of individual mutant residues back to lysine re-establishes Keap1-mediated repression of Nrf2 (Zhang et al., 2004). Polyubiquitination of Nrf2 targets the transcription factor for degradation by the 26S proteasome (Cullinan et al., 2004; Kobayashi et al., 2004; Zhang et al., 2004; Furukawa et al., 2005). As a result, the constant cycle of Nrf2 production and decomposition limits the basal expression of cell defense genes (Fig. 1). These factors may at least partly explain the relatively short half-life of Nrf2 (10–30min) in the absence of cellular stress (Alam et al., 2003; Itoh et al., 2003), and may also account for the difficulties associated with its detection under these conditions in some cell types.

The dissociation of Keap1 and Cul3 has been proposed as a mechanism by which some chemical inducers stabilize Nrf2 (Zhang et al., 2004; Gao et al., 2007; Rachakonda et al., 2008). Additionally, a switch from ubiquitination of Nrf2 to that of Keap1 under certain conditions of chemical and oxidative stress has been described (Hong et al., 2005b; Zhang et al., 2005). The central intervening region (IVR) of Keap1 appears to represent a target for ubiquitination induced by the Nrf2 inducer *tert*-butylhydroquinone (Zhang et al., 2005), and conjugation of ubiquitin onto Lys-298 within this domain has been demonstrated by tandem mass spectrometry following exposure of Keap1-V5 expressing cells to this compound or a modified iodoacetamide molecule (Hong et al., 2005b). However, not all Nrf2 inducers appear to promote the ubiquitination of Keap1 (Hong et al., 2005a; Zhang et al., 2005; Sakurai et al., 2006). It is plausible that this mechanism, along with the dissociation of Keap1 and Cul3, underlies the ability of only selected molecules to activate Nrf2, and that distinct triggering mechanisms are utilized by different inducers.

1.2. Keap1 as a Sensor of Chemical and Oxidative Stress

Keap1 is a relatively cysteine-rich protein; the human protein comprises 27 cysteines out of 624 total amino acids. This is double the average cysteine frequency of all human proteins (Miseta et al., 2000). Many of the cysteine residues in Keap1 are flanked by one or more basic amino acid that lowers the predicted pK_a value and increases the relative reactivity of the cysteine thiol (Snyder et al., 1981). Furthermore, many Nrf2-activating molecules are electrophilic and capable of reacting with nucleophilic thiols including cysteine sulfhydryl groups (Talalay et al., 1988; Prestera et al., 1993; Dinkova-Kostova et al., 2002). Taken together, these observations prompted a concerted effort to explore the potential role of Keap1 as a sensor of chemical and oxidative stress.

Initially, the importance of selected cysteine residues for the function of Keap1 was examined through site-directed mutagenesis experiments. Located within the IVR domain of Keap1, Cys-273 and Cys-288 were the first to be shown to have a critical role in determining the ability of Keap1 to repress Nrf2 under basal conditions. Mutation of one or both of these residues renders Keap1 unable to direct the ubiquitination, and thus inhibit the stabilization and nuclear accumulation, of Nrf2 (Zhang et al., 2003; Levonen et al., 2004; Wakabayashi et al., 2004; Kobayashi et al., 2006). Additionally, mutation of Cys-273 and/or Cys-288 perturbs the ability of Nrf2 to respond to model inducers (Zhang et al., 2003; Levonen et al., 2004). Using a similar experimental approach, Cys-151 has been established as a critical mediator in Keap1's ability to transduce the onset of chemical stress into the activation of Nrf2 (Zhang et al., 2003, 2004).

The validity of these observations has been demonstrated more recently *in vivo* using a transgenic complementation rescue model, in which the elevated tissue levels of Nrf2 in mice that are deficient in the innate Keap1 gene are diminished by the transgenic expression of wild type Keap1, but not Cys-273 and/or Cys-288 mutant Keap1 (Yamamoto et al., 2008). Moreover, the transgenic expression of Keap1 Cys-273 and/or Cys-288 mutants, in contrast to wild type Keap1, fails to reverse the ultimate lethality of Keap1 gene deletion, further indicating that an inability to repress Nrf2 underlies the compromised viability of Keap1-null animals (Yamamoto et al., 2008). Although the transgenic expression of a Keap1 Cys-151 mutant was able to repress Nrf2 and rescue Keap1-null mice from lethality, embryonic fibroblasts derived from these mice demonstrated decreased expression of Nrf2-regulated genes in the presence of a model Nrf2 inducer (Yamamoto et al., 2008), emphasizing the important role of Keap1 Cys-151 in mediating the adaptive response to chemical stress. The hitherto undefined crystal structures of the Bric-a-brac, tram-track, broad complex (BTB) and IVR domains of Keap1 will shed further light on the molecular basis of the apparent importance of Cys-151, Cys-273 and Cys-288 for the functional integrity of Keap1.

In addition to the above molecular genetic investigations, a number of independent groups have also employed mass spectrometry to identify the specific patterns of Keap1 cysteine modification associated with different inducers of Nrf2. The pioneering work of Dinkova-Kostova and colleagues first demonstrated that the thiol-reactive steroid dexamethasone 21-mesylate was able to activate Nrf2 and selectively modify five cysteine residues (Cys-257, Cys-273, Cys-288, Cys-297, Cys-613) in recombinantly expressed Keap1 protein (Dinkova-Kostova et al., 2002). Work in this author's laboratory has further validated this observation in a cellular model, as well as providing the first evidence for the modification of Keap1, under conditions of Nrf2 activation, by the metabolite (*N*-acetyl-*p*-benzoquinoneimine) of a therapeutic drug (acetaminophen) associated with clinical toxicity (Copple et al., 2008a). A number of other studies have provided evidence for the modification of Keap1 by Nrf2-activating molecules, both *in vitro* (Eggler et al., 2005; Hong et al., 2005a, b; Luo et al., 2007; Rachakonda et al., 2008; Sumi et al., 2009; Abiko et al., 2011; Hu et al., 2011) and in a cellular context (Itoh et al., 2004; Levonen et al., 2004; Hong et al., 2005b; Ahn et al., 2010; McMahon et al., 2010; Abiko et al., 2011). For a concise review of this aspect of Keap1–Nrf2 pathway biology, see Sekhar et al. (2010).

Although no single cysteine appears to be a universal target for all Nrf2 inducers that have been shown to modify Keap1, the targeting of one or more cysteine(s) within the IVR domain is a common feature of those molecules tested to date (Holland et al., 2008; Hayes et al., 2010). It is possible that such non-specific modification within this region is sufficient to disrupt the ability of Keap1 to repress Nrf2. Notably, 1-biotinamido-4-(4′-[maleimidoethyl-cyclohexane]carboxamido)-butane, which does not activate Nrf2, modifies human Keap1 *in vitro*, but only at cysteine residues outside of the IVR domain (Hong et al., 2005b). As well as undergoing modification by Nrf2-activating xenobiotics, Keap1 is also able to sense the endogenously generated stress markers nitric oxide, zinc and the alkenals 4-hydroxy-2-nonenal and acrolein using distinct subsets of cysteines (McMahon et al., 2010). These studies further emphasize the important role of Keap1 in perceiving the onset of discrete forms of cellular damage.

The unique modification patterns reported for different Nrf2 inducers has coined the notion of a 'cysteine code', whereby inducers of a similar chemical class will provoke a similar biological response through targeting a particular subset of cysteine residues within Keap1 (Kobayashi et al., 2009). Although this concept has yet to be fully validated, such a phenomenon may underlie the capacity of the Keap1–Nrf2 pathway to respond to such a diverse array of chemical and oxidative insults. Further support for the role of Keap1 cysteine modification in the activation of Nrf2 has been provided by an elegant zebrafish study (Li et al., 2008). It was demonstrated that only one of the two zebrafish Keap1 gene products was able to transduce a signal for the activation of Nrf2 in response to a model electrophile (Li et al., 2008). Importantly, the cysteine residue of the responsive Keap1 variant that corresponds to Cys-151 of human Keap1 is flanked by a basic lysine residue that increases its reactivity, whereas the equivalent cysteine residue of the unresponsive Keap1 variant is flanked by a neutral threonine, which does not have such an effect on reactivity of the thiol (Li et al., 2008). Notably, it has yet to be determined exactly how modification of cysteine residues in Keap1 leads to its inactivation, and such information will provide a vital insight into this important aspect of Nrf2 regulation.

1.3. The Hinge and Latch Model of Nrf2 Regulation

Although additional models have been proposed (for details see the reviews by (Hayes et al., 2009; Baird et al., 2011)), the most compelling mechanism for the overall regulation of Nrf2 by Keap1 to date is the 'hinge and latch' model (Tong et al., 2006). Keap1 exists as a homodimer in cells (McMahon et al., 2006), and recent single particle electron microscopy data indicates that the overall structure of this dimer bears a resemblance to a cherry-bob structure, with two globular units (the double glycine repeat and C-terminal, or DC, domains) connected to a stem (the homodimerising BTB domains) (Ogura et al., 2010). The Keap1 homodimer binds to a single molecule of Nrf2 using two distinct binding sites within the Neh2 domain of the latter (Lo et al., 2006b; McMahon et al., 2006; Padmanabhan et al., 2006; Tong et al., 2006). The conserved ETGE and DLG motifs of Nrf2 bind to a single overlapping site, comprising arginine, serine and asparagines residues, in the DC domain of Keap1 (Lo et al., 2006b; McMahon et al., 2006; Padmanabhan et al., 2006; Tong et al., 2006). These distinct interaction motifs have affinities for Keap1 differing by two orders of magnitude, with binding via the high-affinity ETGE motif providing the 'hinge' through which Nrf2 can move in space relatively freely (McMahon et al., 2006; Tong et al., 2006, 2007; Padmanabhan et al., 2008b). Simultaneous binding of Keap1 via the lower-affinity DLG motif of Nrf2 provides the 'latch' which facilitates the optimal positioning of lysine residues located between the ETGE and DLG motifs for conjugation with ubiquitin (McMahon et al., 2006; Tong et al., 2006, 2007; Padmanabhan et al., 2008b). As a result, Keap1 is able to efficiently target Nrf2 for proteasomal degradation.

The stabilization and nuclear accumulation of Nrf2 does not appear to depend upon its physical release from Keap1, as Nrf2 induction by diverse stimuli is abrogated following inhibition of *de novo* protein synthesis (Itoh et al., 2003; Kobayashi et al., 2006). This implies that the adaptive response to cellular stress is mediated by newly synthesized Nrf2 protein, rather than that which is physically liberated from Keap1 repression. Indeed, the 'hinge and latch' model proposes that Nrf2 stabilization occurs as a result of a disruption in the binding of the lower-affinity DLG motif to Keap1, leading to the improper spatial positioning of lysine residues in the Neh2 domain of Nrf2, and a consequent interruption of the efficient ubiquitination and proteasomal degradation of the transcription factor (Tong et al., 2006). In a sense, Nrf2-activating molecules prompt the uncoupling of the 'latch' whilst the 'hinge' remains in operation.

Whilst the precise mechanism(s) is yet to be defined, the destabilization of the Keap1–Nrf2 interaction may occur through a conformational change in the IVR domain of Keap1, brought about through modification of cysteine residues by Nrf2-activating molecules. In support of this notion, evidence does indicate that Nrf2-activating molecules can bind to and induce changes in the structural conformation of Keap1 (Dinkova-Kostova et al., 2005; Gao et al., 2007; Rachakonda et al., 2008; Ohnuma et al., 2010). Destabilization of the Keap1–Nrf2 interaction may also occur through the competitive binding of Keap1 by other protein partners (see Section II.A.2.1). As noted earlier, the dissociation of Keap1 and Cul3 may further contribute to the inhibition of Nrf2 recycling under certain conditions of chemical and oxidative stress (Zhang et al., 2004; Gao et al., 2007; Rachakonda et al., 2008). As a result of the destabilization of the Nrf2–Keap1–Cul3 complex, Nrf2 remains associated with Keap1 via the high-affinity ETGE motif, but is no longer directed for proteasomal degradation (Tong et al., 2006). Additional molecules of Nrf2 bind to the vacant sites on the Keap1 dimer, and as a result Keap1 becomes saturated due to its inability to direct the ubiquitination of bound Nrf2 (Tong et al., 2006). Consequently, newly synthesized Nrf2 evades Keap1 repression and accumulates within the nucleus, where a plethora of ARE-containing genes are transactivated (Tong et al., 2006). The basal state may be restored via the elimination of the cellular stressor and/or the Nrf2-dependent upregulated expression of Keap1 (Lee et al., 2007) and Cul3 (Kaspar et al., 2010). An overview of the 'hinge and latch' model is provided in Fig. 1.

2. *Novel Mechanisms of Nrf2 Regulation*

Many years of research have consolidated our understanding of the role played by Keap1 in controlling the activity of Nrf2 in mammalian cells. Recently, however, innovative studies have shed light on novel, Keap1-independent mechanisms of Nrf2 regulation that may point to roles for Nrf2 in the pathogenesis of specific diseases. A better understanding of these alternative mechanisms of regulation is vital to support the ultimate aim of targeting Nrf2 therapeutically.

2.1. *Regulation of Nrf2 via Interaction with Novel Protein Partners*

In addition to its well-characterized ability to sense and respond to changes in the intracellular concentration for a variety of structurally diverse chemical entities, numerous studies have also revealed that assorted protein partners can also activate or repress the Nrf2 cell defense response. For example, by competing with Nrf2 for binding to Keap1, fetal Alz-50 clone (Strachan et al., 2004) and prothymosin alpha (Karapetian et al., 2005; Padmanabhan et al., 2008a) can promote the stabilization of Nrf2 and upregulation of Nrf2-dependent cell defense processes. In addition, the Parkinson's disease-associated protein DJ-1 inhibits the ubiquitination and promotes the stabilization of Nrf2 through a mechanism that does not involve its direct binding to Nrf2 or Keap1 (Clements et al., 2006). Although loss of DJ-1 sensitizes cells to toxic insult *in vitro* and *in vivo* (Yokota et al., 2003; Taira et al., 2004; Kim et al., 2005), and there is evidence that DJ-1 can at least partly control the basal and inducible activity of Nrf2 (Clements et al., 2006; Yang et al., 2007; Malhotra et al., 2008; Gan et al., 2010), these effects are limited to certain cell types, and so DJ-1 does not appear to represent a universal regulator of the Keap1–Nrf2 pathway.

Similarly to Nrf2, the transcription factor nuclear factor κB (NF-κB) plays an important role in maintaining cellular homeostasis, particularly through its ability to modulate apoptotic, immune and inflammatory responses to a diverse range of stimuli (Oeckinghaus et al., 2011). Recent studies have revealed a degree of cross-talk between Nrf2 and NF-κB. For example, the p65 subunit of NF-κB has been shown to bind to Keap1 and inhibit the basal and inducible activity of Nrf2 in mammalian cells, by enhancing the ubiquitination and decreasing the ARE-binding activity of Nrf2 (Liu et al., 2008). Furthermore, activation of the NF-κB pathway appears to antagonize both the basal and inducible activity of Nrf2 (Liu et al., 2008). The NF-κB regulator inhibitor of κB kinase β (IKKβ) is also a binding partner of Keap1, and this interaction favors the ubiquitination and degradation of IKKβ, such that alterations in the level of Keap1 affect the activity of the NF-κB pathway (Lee et al., 2009; Kim et al., 2010a). Although the capacity for alterations in the level of IKKβ to impinge on the activity of Nrf2 has yet to be established, taken together these findings imply that the integrated response of the Keap1–Nrf2, NF-κB and perhaps other pathways underlies a holistic reaction to a wide variety of cellular stresses. The molecular mechanisms that govern these inter-relationships certainly warrant further examination, particularly in light of the current interest in Nrf2 as a potential drug target.

Another potential link between Nrf2 and NF-κB is the polyubiquitin-binding protein p62/Sequestosome 1, which can regulate the activity of both pathways (Liu et al., 2007; Moscat et al., 2009). Recently, the molecular mechanisms underlying p62's ability to activate Nrf2 were delineated in five independent papers published within the space of four months. It was shown that p62 binds to Keap1 in mammalian cells (Copple et al., 2010b; Fan et al., 2010; Jain et al., 2010; Komatsu et al., 2010; Lau et al., 2010), at the bottom side of the six-bladed β-propeller structure formed by the DC domain of the latter (Komatsu et al., 2010). Notably, as with Nrf2 (Tong et al., 2006), IKKβ (Lee et al., 2009; Kim et al., 2010a) and the phosphoglycerate mutase PGAM5 (Lo et al., 2006a; Lo et al., 2008), the Keap1-interacting motif in p62 (Jain et al., 2010; Komatsu et al., 2010; Lau et al., 2010) conforms to the consensus sequence (D/N)X(E/S)(T/S)GE, indicating a common binding mechanism amongst these molecular activators of Nrf2. p62 appears to regulate the activity of the Keap1–Nrf2 pathway by

(a) competing with Nrf2 for binding to Keap1, and thus disrupting the normal ubiquitination and proteasomal degradation of the transcription factor (Komatsu et al., 2010), and (b) promoting the degradation of Keap1 (Copple et al., 2010b; Bui et al., 2011), most probably via autophagy (Jain et al., 2010), a process in which p62 directs substrates for lysosomal degradation. Importantly, the expression of p62 itself is subject to regulation by Nrf2, due to the presence of an ARE in the promoter region of the p62 gene (Jain et al., 2010). Therefore, the net result of an increase in cellular p62 level is an induction of Nrf2-dependent defense processes, via a positive feedback loop, that enhance the capacity to survive chemical and environmental insult. p62 levels are typically elevated in response to a disruption of autophagy, and this appears to represent an additional cellular stress condition under which Nrf2 is activated (Komatsu et al., 2010).

Chen et al. have demonstrated that the basal and inducible activity of Nrf2 is subject to positive regulation by the cyclin-dependent kinase inhibitor p21 (Chen et al., 2009b). Nrf2 is stabilized in response to p21 elevation, through the latter's capacity to disrupt the ability of Keap1 to bind and direct the ubiquitination and consequent proteasomal degradation of Nrf2 (Chen et al., 2009b). Conversely, the basal and inducible expression of Nrf2-regulated genes is disrupted *in vitro* and *in vivo* in the absence of p21 (Chen et al., 2009b). In this regard, it is notable that p21 and Nrf2 transgenic knockout mice each display similar phenotypes in terms of perturbed adaptive response and enhanced sensitivity to numerous toxic insults (Gartel et al., 2002; Lloberas et al., 2009). The above findings, taken together with the assertion that the ability of p21 to promote cellular survival under conditions of oxidative stress is dependent upon the activity of Nrf2 (Chen et al., 2009b), indicates that the interaction between these two proteins has an important influence on the regulation of cell defense processes.

2.2. *Epigenetic Regulation of Nrf2 and Keap1 Expression*

The molecular detail of Nrf2's ability to regulate the expression of numerous cell defense genes is well established, yet our understanding of the mechanisms that control the expression of Nrf2 itself is relatively inferior. Micro-RNAs (miRNAs) are 21–23 nucleotide-long, single-stranded, non-coding RNAs (Filipowicz et al., 2008). Following processing to their mature form, miRNAs are incorporated into the RNA-induced silencing complex that binds to complimentary sequences in the 3′ untranslated regions of target messenger RNA molecules and prompts the degradation and/or inhibited translation of the transcript (Filipowicz et al., 2008). Many hundreds of miRNAs are predicted to be expressed in human cells. miR-144 was the first miRNA to be fully characterized as a negative regulator of Nrf2 expression (Sangokoya et al., 2010). By targeting two distinct sites at positions 265–271 and 370–377 of the 3′ untranslated region of the Nrf2 gene, miR-144 represses the expression of Nrf2 and ARE-containing cell defense genes (Sangokoya et al., 2010). By regulating the activity of Nrf2, miR-144 may play an important role in determining the oxidative stress tolerance of erythroid cells in sickle cell anemia (Sangokoya et al., 2010). Nrf2 expression has also been shown to be negatively regulated by miR-28 (Yang et al., 2011). Indeed, a substantial decrease in the level of Nrf2 messenger RNA and protein has been demonstrated in human MCF-7 breast cancer cells upon ectopic expression of miR-28 (Yang et al., 2011). Importantly, these effects have been shown to be independent of changes in the level and/or binding activity of Keap1 (Yang et al., 2011).

During the preparation of this chapter, Eades et al. (2011) provided the first evidence for miRNA regulation of Keap1 expression. miR-200a negatively regulates the stability of Keap1 mRNA and level of Keap1 protein in breast cancer cell lines, and thus promotes the nuclear accumulation of Nrf2 and increased expression of Nrf2-regulated cell defense genes (Eades et al., 2011). As well as unveiling an additional layer of regulatory control within the Keap1–Nrf2 pathway, the demonstration that Nrf2 and Keap1 levels are controlled by specific miRNAs also provides additional research tools with which to manipulate pathway activity in the laboratory. Clarifying the inter-relationship between Nrf2, Keap1 and miRNAs, and the latter's role in determining susceptibility to disease, will be an important avenue of future research.

The differential expression of Nrf2 and/or Keap1 has been described in various cancers, and has been postulated to underlie the processes of cancer progression and chemotherapy resistance (discussed in more detail in Section IV of this chapter). The methylation of specific CpG sites within the promoter region of genes is known to affect expression by physically restricting the ability of the transcriptional machinery to bind to the necessary DNA sequences, and by inducing local chromatin remodeling (Klose et al., 2006). Methylation of specific CpG sites within the Nrf2 and Keap1 genes has been shown to contribute to their differential expression in tumor versus non-tumor cells. Yu et al. (2010) have recently demonstrated that differential methylation within a CpG island encompassing the promoter, first exon and part of the first intron of the mouse Nrf2 gene underlies its perturbed expression and transcriptional activity in prostate adenocarcinoma cells.

Hypermethylation of CpG islands around the transcriptional start site of the Keap1 gene has also been demonstrated in human lung (Wang et al., 2008a) and prostate (Zhang et al., 2010a) cancer cell lines, as well as in malignant gliomas (Muscarella et al., 2011a) and primary non-small cell lung cancer tissue (Muscarella et al., 2011b). In the latter study, the presence of epigenetic abnormalities in the Keap1 gene was associated with an increased risk of lung cancer progression in patients (Muscarella et al., 2011b). The repressive action of DNA methyltransferases on Nrf2 and Keap1 expression has been demonstrated *in vitro* through the alleviating effect of the DNA methyltransferase inhibitor 5-azacytidine (Wang et al., 2008a; Yu et al., 2010; Zhang et al., 2010a), whilst the Nrf2-inducing action of curcumin has at least partly been ascribed to its ability to inhibit DNA methyltransferase activity and Nrf2 promoter methylation (Khor et al., 2011).

III. Activation of Nrf2 as a Potential Therapeutic Strategy

The disclosure of fundamental mechanisms underlying the regulation of the Keap1–Nrf2 pathway has led, in recent years, to the search for circumstances in which the pathway can be pharmacologically manipulated in order to derive therapeutic benefit. Apart from the age-related development of vacuolar leukoencephalopathy (Hubbs et al., 2007), retinopathy (Zhao et al., 2011) and lupus-like autoimmune symptoms (Yoh et al., 2001; Ma et al., 2006), Nrf2 deficiency in mice does not appear to result in any significant perturbation of gross phenotype in the absence of environmental stress. However, unsurprisingly Nrf2 knockout (Nrf2$^{-/-}$) mice do exhibit markedly lower basal and inducible levels of important cell defense genes in a variety of tissues. As a result, these mice are inherently more susceptible to certain diseases and drug-induced toxicities affecting a variety of organs (reviewed in more detail in Copple et al. (2008b)). Perhaps more significantly, the targeted induction of Nrf2-regulated cell defense processes can afford protection against these conditions. The investigations highlighted here are intended to provide a broad overview of the potential for inducing Nrf2 in different organs as a means of reducing the risk of disease and drug-induced toxicity (Fig. 2).

A. Liver

Goldring et al. (2004) have previously demonstrated that Nrf2 is activated in the mouse liver following administration of non-toxic and toxic doses of the model hepatotoxin acetaminophen. This induction of Nrf2-dependent cell defense, which can also be triggered directly by the reactive and toxic metabolite of acetaminophen (Copple et al., 2008a), may serve as a critical determinant of the threshold for acetaminophen toxicity, in light of the fact that Nrf2$^{-/-}$ mice are more sensitive to acetaminophen-induced liver injury (Chan et al., 2001; Enomoto et al., 2001). The differential sensitivity to acetaminophen toxicity resulting from loss of Nrf2 is likely due to the distorted basal and inducible activities of critical cell defense processes in these animals, together with an apparent alteration in the metabolism and disposition of the drug (Reisman et al., 2009b). Conversely, as a result of the decreased bioactivation and enhanced detoxification of acetaminophen in the liver, hepatocyte-specific Keap1-null mice are highly resistant to acetaminophen hepatotoxicity (Okawa et al., 2006). In keeping with this

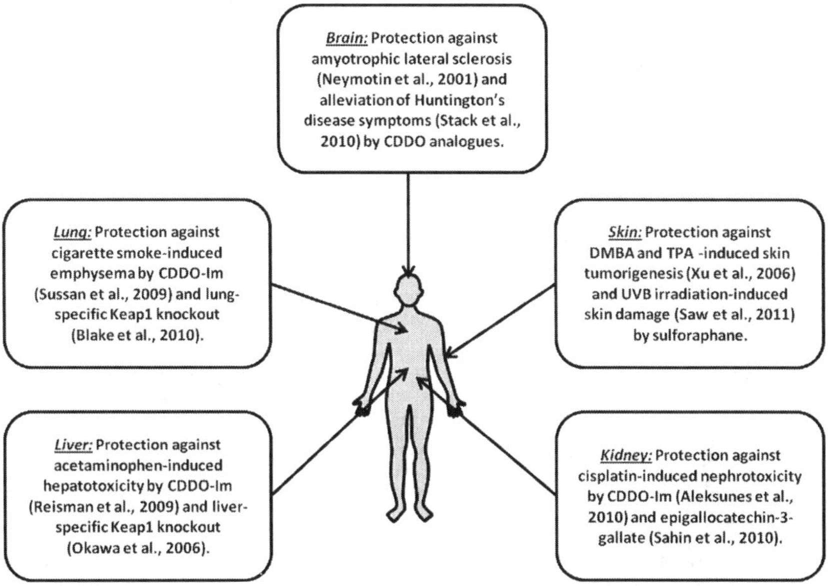

FIGURE 2 **Nrf2 activation affords protection against diseases and drug-induced toxicities in multiple organs.** Selected examples of some of the protective effects elicited in the indicated organs by pharmacological or genetic activation of Nrf2. See the main text (Section III.B.) for further details. CDDO-Im, 2-cyano-3,12-dioxooleana-1,9(11)-dien-28-oic acid imidazolide; DMBA, 7,12-dimethylbenz(a)anthracene; TPA, 12-O-teradecanoylphorbol-13-acetate.

notion, pre-treatment of wild type mice with the Nrf2 activator 2-cyano-3,12-dioxooleana-1,9(11)-dien-28-oic acid imidazolide (CDDO-Im) reduces sensitivity to acetaminophen liver injury (Reisman et al., 2009a). This phenomenon is dependent on Nrf2, as the protection afforded by CDDO-Im is lost in Nrf2$^{-/-}$ mice (Reisman et al., 2009a). An analogous effect has also been reported following pre-treatment of mice with the antioxidant lignan sauchinone (Kay et al., 2011). Such observations raise the possibility of administering a selective Nrf2-activating compound as an adjuvant therapy alongside drugs that are known to cause liver toxicity, which remains the major cause of acute liver failure (Ostapowicz et al., 2002) and a key factor in the attrition of novel and existing medicines (Park et al., 2011).

Exposure of mice to concanavalin A induces T-cell-mediated acute inflammatory liver injury, due to a sustained influx of inflammatory cells provoked by hepatocyte necrosis (Tiegs et al., 1992). However, activation of Nrf2 by hepatocyte-specific knockout of Keap1 or pharmacological stimulation by CDDO-Im lessens this pro-inflammatory response and thus affords substantial protection against concanavalin A liver injury (Osburn et al., 2008). The beneficial effect of CDDO-Im is lost in Nrf2$^{-/-}$ mice, indicating a dependence on the cytoprotective action of Nrf2 (Osburn et al., 2008). Therefore, the targeting of Nrf2 may represent a strategy for the prevention of liver diseases associated with inflammation. For additional details on the role of Nrf2 in protecting against various forms of liver disorder, see the recent review by Klaassen et al. (2010).

B. Skin

Nrf2 appears to confer a protective effect against ultraviolet A (UVA)- and ultraviolet B (UVB)-induced inflammation and damage in the skin, and may therefore represent a promising therapeutic target for such disorders. Indeed, Nrf2$^{-/-}$ mice display enhanced skin photoageing and damage, including epidermal thickening and a loss of skin flexibility, following exposure to UVB irradiation (Hirota et al., 2011; Saw et al., 2011). Furthermore, loss of Nrf2 increases UVB-induced skin inflammation, and prolongs the time required for its resolution (Saw et al., 2011). The tissue-specific over-expression of Nrf2 in keratinocytes *in vivo* reduces the severity of UVB-induced skin damage, at least partly via the enhanced detoxification of ROS (Schafer et al., 2010). Nrf2 also protects against the damaging effects of UVA irradiation, as RNAi depletion of Nrf2 in human HaCaT keratinocytes enhances UVA-induced cell damage (Tian et al., 2011). The constitutive activation of Nrf2 in dermal fibroblasts derived from newborn Keap1$^{-/-}$ mice causes a 50% decrease in the number of apoptotic cells detected following exposure to UVA irradiation *ex vivo* (Hirota et al., 2005). Additionally, it has been demonstrated that the polyphenolic antioxidant quercetin minimizes the cytolethal effect of UVA irradiation toward HaCaT cells (Kimura et al., 2009). Importantly, this effect is abrogated by RNAi depletion of the Nrf2 gene (Kimura et al., 2009). The above observations, together with the fact that sulforaphane protects against UVB-induced skin inflammation and sunburn response in wild type, but not Nrf2$^{-/-}$, mice (Saw et al., 2011), indicates that Nrf2 is an attractive target for the prevention of sunburn and alleviation of its symptoms.

Following exposure to the carcinogens 7,12-dimethylbenz(a)anthracene and 12-O-teradecanoylphorbol-13-acetate, a greater number of skin tumors are developed by Nrf2$^{-/-}$ mice than wild type controls (Xu et al., 2006). However, topical application of the Nrf2 inducer sulforaphane prior to carcinogen exposure provides protection against tumor development, in an Nrf2-dependent manner (Xu et al., 2006). Sulforaphane has also been shown to alleviate the skin blistering caused by a keratin 14 gene mutation in a mouse model of the inherited condition epidermolysis bullosa simplex (Kerns et al., 2007), although the exact role of Nrf2 in this process is unresolved.

C. Brain and Nervous System

The absence of Nrf2 in mice exacerbates the neurological deficit, neuronal apoptosis and brain swelling that characterizes traumatic brain injury following an impact to the head (Jin et al., 2009). Loss of Nrf2 also enhances the motor dysfunction, neuronal death and tissue swelling associated with spinal cord compression injury (Mao et al., 2011a,b). In both cases, the enhanced severity of injury in Nrf2$^{-/-}$ mice appears to be related to an imbalance in the levels of inflammatory cytokines and antioxidant/detoxification enzymes in affected tissues (Jin et al., 2009; Mao et al., 2011a, b). Furthermore, whilst spinal cord injury can be eased in wild type mice by subsequent administration of the Nrf2 activator sulforaphane, such an effect is not observed in Nrf2$^{-/-}$ mice (Mao et al., 2011a, b). These and other findings indicate that Nrf2 has an important protective role within the brain and nervous system. In keeping with this concept, there is extensive evidence that Nrf2 activation protects against diseases and toxicities affecting the brain and nervous system, and this specific facet of Nrf2's activity is reviewed in more detail by Calkins et al. (2009) and van Muiswinkel et al. (2005).

Some of the most convincing data verifying Nrf2 as a promising drug target in the brain has come from studies on neurodegenerative disorders. Notably, a number of such disorders are associated with protein misfolding (Matus et al., 2011), and Nrf2 has been shown to coordinate cytoprotection against endoplasmic reticulum stress triggered by agents that induce the unfolded protein response (Cullinan et al., 2003). Nrf2$^{-/-}$ mice are more susceptible to the nigrostriatal cell damage induced by the mitochondrial complex I inhibitor 1-methyl-4-phenyl-1,2,3,6-tetrahydropyridine (MPTP), an established model of Parkinson's disease-like neuronal cell death (Burton et al., 2006; Chen et al., 2009a; Jazwa et al., 2011). Importantly, astrocyte-specific over-expression of Nrf2 protects against MPTP toxicity in wild type mice and Nrf2$^{-/-}$ mice (in which Nrf2 expression is limited to astrocytes) (Chen et al., 2009a). In the same model, a similar, Nrf2-dependent protective effect is afforded by intraperitoneal injection of sulforaphane (Jazwa et al., 2011). The protective role of Nrf2 in Parkinson's disease has also been demonstrated in a *Drosophila melanogaster* model in which the ectopic expression of Nrf2 or RNAi depletion of Keap1 prevents the progressive decline in locomotor activity and loss of neurons caused by expression of the α-synuclein gene in dopaminergic neurons (Barone et al., 2011).

It is known that haplotype variants of the Nrf2 gene can affect progression of Alzheimer's disease, without affecting disease susceptibility *per se* (von Otter et al., 2010). Using an innovative approach, Kanninen et al. (2009) have shown that a single intrahippocampal injection of an Nrf2-encoding lentivirus leads to improvements in spatial learning and cognitive ability in a mouse model of Alzheimer's disease when assessed six months later. Furthermore, analogs of the potent Nrf2 inducer CDDO have been shown to afford protection against the oxidative stress, neural tissue destruction and motor impairment typically observed in mouse models of Huntington's disease (Stack et al., 2010) and amyotrophic lateral sclerosis (Neymotin et al., 2011). Therefore, activation of Nrf2 represents a promising strategy for protection against a variety of neurological disorders.

C. Lung

Nrf2 appears to play an important role in the defense against various pulmonary disorders (for a review, see Cho et al. (2010)). For instance, there is a notable decline in the activity of Nrf2 in the lungs of patients suffering from chronic obstructive pulmonary disorder (Suzuki et al., 2008; Singh et al., 2009) and emphysema (Goven et al., 2008). Exposure of mice to cigarette smoke triggers emphysema due to inflammatory cell recruitment and an imbalance in the processes of tissue damage and repair, leading to the enlargement of alveolar and other airway spaces (Shapiro, 2000). $Nrf2^{-/-}$ mice are more susceptible to cigarette smoke-induced emphysema (Rangasamy et al., 2004; Iizuka et al., 2005; Sussan et al., 2009), indicating a role for Nrf2-regulated processes in protecting against this disease. Consistent with this concept, activation of Nrf2 by pharmacological (pre-treatment with CDDO-Im) or genetic (lung-specific knockdown of Keap1) strategies diminishes the oxidative stress and alveolar cell death induced in the lungs of mice following chronic exposure to cigarette smoke (Sussan et al., 2009; Blake et al., 2010). This demonstrates that the overall severity of cigarette smoke-induced emphysema can be reduced through the targeting of Nrf2 (Sussan et al., 2009; Blake et al., 2010).

D. Kidney

Nrf2 has been shown to afford protection against the nephrotoxicity that can limit the optimal clinical utilization of the chemotherapeutic agent cisplatin. $Nrf2^{-/-}$ mice develop more severe kidney injury than wild type mice following exposure to this drug, due in part to heightened levels of inflammatory mediators in affected renal tissue (Aleksunes et al., 2010). Importantly, treatment of wild type, but not $Nrf2^{-/-}$, mice with CDDO-Im enhances Nrf2-regulated cytoprotective responses in the kidney and protects against cisplatin toxicity (Aleksunes et al., 2010). A similar protective effect is also induced by epigallocatechin-3-gallate, which also stimulates renal Nrf2 signaling (Sahin et al., 2010). Therefore, pharmacological activation of Nrf2 may represent a novel strategy for the prevention of cisplatin-induced kidney injury.

E. Obesity

Fascinatingly, Nrf2 appears to play an important role in the regulation of lipogenesis. Using a proteomics strategy, Kitteringham et al. (2010) have recently demonstrated that proteins involved in the synthesis and metabolism of fatty acids and other lipids are significantly upregulated in the livers of Nrf2$^{-/-}$ mice, indicating that their expression is subject to negative regulation by Nrf2. The downregulation of these and related genes in Nrf2$^{-/-}$ mice has also been reported by independent groups (Tanaka et al., 2008; Yates et al., 2009; Chowdhry et al., 2010; Zhang et al., 2010b). In keeping with these observations, Nrf2$^{-/-}$ mice fed a high-fat or methionine and choline-free diet accumulate total hepatic lipids and polyunsaturated fatty acids (Chowdhry et al., 2010) and gain body weight and adipose mass (Shin et al., 2009) much more readily than wild type counterparts. Conversely, induction of Nrf2 by oltipraz, CDDO-Im or liver-specific knockout of the Keap1 gene has been shown to downregulate the hepatic expression of lipogenic genes (Shin et al., 2009; Chowdhry et al., 2010), and prevent diet-associated obesity (Shin et al., 2009; Yu et al., 2011), in wild type, but not Nrf2$^{-/-}$, mice. Therefore, Nrf2 represents a novel regulator of cellular lipid synthesis and disposition in the liver and other organs, and may therefore be a promising therapeutic target for the treatment of obesity and other lipid-related diseases.

F. Malaria

An emerging and exciting aspect of Nrf2 biology is its apparent role in the defense against malaria. It is well known that individuals who are heterozygous for a specific mutation affecting the β-chain of hemoglobin have a degree of resistance to malaria (Williams, 2006). Using a mouse model of cerebral malaria, it has recently been demonstrated that the survival advantage provided by this 'sickle' hemoglobin at least partly involves the upregulated expression of heme oxygenase 1, an established Nrf2 target gene, in bone marrow and peripheral blood cells (Ferreira et al., 2011). Heme oxygenase 1 catabolises heme to yield carbon monoxide, which in turn prevents further release and oxidation of free heme from red blood cells, an underlying factor in the pathogenesis of cerebral malaria (Pamplona et al., 2007). Genetic inhibition of Nrf2 in mice carrying a sickle hemoglobin mutation causes the downregulation of heme oxygenase 1 to levels observed in mice expressing wild type hemoglobin, such that protection against cerebral malaria is lost (Ferreira et al., 2011). In addition, a very recent study has demonstrated that, via its ability to regulate CD36 expression on macrophages, Nrf2 can promote the phagocytosis of *Plasmodium falciparum*-infected red blood cells (Olagnier et al., 2011). As a result, exposure of malaria-infected mice to the Nrf2 inducer sulforaphane reduces disease severity and improves survival by enhancing parasite clearance (Olagnier et al., 2011). Nrf2 may therefore represent a novel drug target in the continuing fight against malaria.

G. Small Molecule Inducers of Nrf2

In light of the above evidence, and the many other studies that have demonstrated an important role for Nrf2 in protecting against various diseases and toxicities, there is a substantial interest in the identification and development for therapeutic use of small molecules capable of activating Nrf2-dependent cell defense processes in a potent and specific manner. Notably, the naturally occurring Nrf2 activators sulforaphane, resveratrol and curcumin have all entered clinical trials for various diseases based in part on their known abilities to induce cytoprotective responses via Nrf2 signaling.

To date, some of the most promising small molecule Nrf2 inducers to emerge are a series of triterpenoids derived from oleanolic acid, which itself has antioxidant and anti-cancer properties (Sporn et al., 2011). As the result of a laudable medicinal chemistry effort, focussed on enhancing anti-inflammatory action, CDDO was shown to be almost 400,000 times more potent than the oleanolic acid template in blocking inducible nitric oxide synthase activation by interferon γ (Suh et al., 1999). It was subsequently demonstrated that CDDO and its analogs were potent inducers of Nrf2 (Dinkova-Kostova et al., 2005; Liby et al., 2005). Indeed, the methyl ester derivative (CDDO-Me) remains one of the most potent small molecule inducers of Nrf2 reported to date, with low nanomolar concentrations invoking a robust stimulation of Nrf2-dependent cytoprotective processes in cell-based experiments (Dinkova-Kostova et al., 2005). Even greater potencies have recently been achieved through further structural revisions (Dinkova-Kostova et al., 2010). At higher (micromolar) concentrations, CDDO and its derivatives induce apoptosis in sensitive cancer cells (Konopleva et al., 2002; Deeb et al., 2007; Ryu et al., 2010). CDDO-Me has recently entered clinical trials, under the generic name bardoxolone methyl, to assess its potential for the treatment of a variety of disorders, including chronic kidney disease, type 2 diabetes, liver dysfunction and certain cancers. Whilst early results appear promising (Pergola et al., 2011a,b), the true test of the potential therapeutic usefulness of bardoxolone methyl and other small molecule inducers of Nrf2 will come in much larger patient exposures, such as the BEACON trial (NCT01351675) that aims to assess the efficacy of bardoxolone methyl in delaying the need for chronic dialysis or renal transplantation in patients with chronic kidney disease and type 2 diabetes. Nevertheless, the story of these molecules provides an excellent example of the potential for translation of academic knowledge into the generation of urgently needed, novel drug candidates that may provide important human health benefits.

The search for novel Nrf2-inducing molecules will be aided by the development of high-throughput screening assays that provide an indication of Nrf2 activation and/or Keap1 modification. Examples of such assays include a recently described β-galactosidase reporter fused to the Neh2 domain-containing N-terminus of Nrf2, which is highly responsive to molecules that activate Nrf2 (Hirotsu et al., 2011). Leung et al. (2011) have also described an imaging screen for modulators of oxidative stress based on the quantifiable response of a GFP transgenic reporter for *gst-4*, a glutathione s-transferase gene targeted by the transcription factor SKN-1, which is the *Caenorhabditis elegans* homologue of Nrf2. In addition, *in vitro* (Liu et al., 2005) and *in silico* (Wu et al., 2010) screens for compounds capable of modifying Keap1, and thus likely to activate Nrf2, have been proposed. Although such approaches would certainly be aided by the determination of the full crystal structure of Keap1, they may provide a blueprint for high-throughput identification of novel small molecule activators of Nrf2 with therapeutic potential.

IV. Inhibition of Nrf2 as a Potential Therapeutic Strategy

Due to the ever-increasing body of evidence indicating that induction of Nrf2 protects against, whilst disruption of Nrf2 signaling increases vulnerability to, various diseases and toxicities, it has been assumed that the greatest potential for therapeutic benefit to be gained from manipulation of the Keap1–Nrf2 pathway was via its stimulation. However, although tissue-specific knockout of Keap1 function does not appear to lead to alterations in gross phenotype (Okawa et al., 2006; Osburn et al., 2008; Yates et al., 2009; Cheng et al., 2011; Kong et al., 2011), the lethality of non-specific Keap1 gene disruption in newborn mice indicates that chronic elevation of Nrf2 activity throughout the body is not without its physiological caveats (Wakabayashi et al., 2003; Taguchi et al., 2010). In recent years a number of independent studies have demonstrated a link between the process of oncogenesis and mutations in the Keap1 and/or Nrf2 genes that result in the constitutive activation of Nrf2. In addition, the resistance of certain cancer cell lines and tissues to different chemotherapies has been attributed to an exacerbation of Nrf2 signaling. As such, there is now much interest in adding to our chemopreventive and chemotherapeutic arsenal through the development of molecules that can specifically inhibit Nrf2.

A. Role of Nrf2 in Oncogenesis

There is mounting evidence that the acute cytoprotective benefit of Nrf2 activation must be juxtaposed with a degree of chronic liability in terms of enhancing the promotion and/or progression of certain cancers. Elevated Nrf2 levels have been detected in various cancer tissues, including those from the lung (Padmanabhan et al., 2006; Singh et al., 2006; Ohta et al., 2008; Shibata et al., 2008b; Takahashi et al., 2010), pancreas (DeNicola et al., 2011; Lister et al., 2011) and endometrium (Chen et al., 2010; Jiang et al., 2010). Padmanabhan et al. (2006) were the first to identify functionally important genetic variants of the Keap1 gene, in two lung adenocarcinoma cell lines and in a lung cancer patient. These discrete missence mutations, affecting the DC domain of Keap1, alter the conformation of the protein such that its ability to repress Nrf2 is diminished, and as a result Nrf2 is constitutively stabilized under these conditions (Padmanabhan et al., 2006).

Additional, somatic Keap1 gene mutations, insertions and deletions have been identified in the tumor tissue of lung cancer patients (Singh et al., 2006; Ohta et al., 2008; Takahashi et al., 2010). These mutations are also associated with the stabilization of Nrf2 (Singh et al., 2006; Takahashi et al., 2010). Mutations in the Keap1 gene have also been recognized in breast (Sjoblom et al., 2006; Nioi et al., 2007), gallbladder (Shibata et al., 2008a), liver (Shibata et al., 2008a), ovarian (Konstantinopoulos et al., 2011), endometrial (Wong et al., 2011) and papillary (Li et al., 2011) cancers. Mutations in the Nrf2 gene have been reported in head and neck, lung, airway and skin cancer biopsies (Shibata et al., 2008b; Kim et al., 2010b). These mutations are also associated with elevated levels and activity of Nrf2 in cancer cells (Shibata et al., 2008b; Kim et al., 2010b). For a comprehensive list of mutations identified in the human genes encoding Keap1 and Nrf2, see the recent review by Taguchi et al. (2011).

Importantly, it has been shown that mutations in the Keap1 gene affecting amino acids in or around the point of interaction with Nrf2 lead to the latter's upregulation (Padmanabhan et al., 2006; Ohta et al., 2008). Furthermore, so far the only mutations identified within the Nrf2 gene affect the DLG or ETGE motifs within the Neh2 domain of the protein, and disrupt its ability to interact with Keap1 (Shibata et al., 2008b; Kim et al., 2010b). This adds further support to the concept of the 'hinge and latch' mechanism of Keap1–Nrf2 pathway regulation. Taken together, the above observations indicate that mutations within the Keap1 and Nrf2 genes that disrupt the normal regulation of the Keap1–Nrf2 pathway are associated with various types of cancer.

The selective advantage afforded to cancer cells through the constitutive activation of Nrf2 could be due to the enhanced ability to detoxify heightened levels of ROS associated with their recurrent division and growth. Indeed, disruption of Nrf2 signaling affects the cell cycle progression and proliferation of cancer cell lines *in vitro* (Reddy et al., 2008; Homma et al., 2009; Lister et al., 2011; Ma et al., 2011). Such an effect may at least partly be underpinned by the ability of Nrf2 to regulate the expression of Notch1, which serves as a central node in the control of differentiation, proliferation and programmed cell death (Wakabayashi et al., 2010). It has recently been demonstrated that the oncogenes K-Ras, B-Raf and Myc can stimulate Nrf2 transcription and activation in mouse fibroblasts and in an *in vivo* model of pancreatic cancer, leading to an overall reduction in the cellular burden of ROS (DeNicola et al., 2011). The authors of this important study highlighted the potential for targeting Nrf2 in certain cancers by providing evidence that oncogene-induced tumourigenesis is inhibited in Nrf2$^{-/-}$ mice (DeNicola et al., 2011). As such, the process of oncogenesis may at least partly depend on the enhanced activity of Nrf2 facilitating unencumbered proliferation in an otherwise highly oxidative environment. This exciting area of Nrf2 biology certainly warrants further exploration.

B. Role of Nrf2 in Resistance to Chemotherapy

Besides the growing association between constitutive activation of Nrf2 and the development of cancer, such conditions also appear to enhance the resistance of cancerous cells to various forms of chemotherapy (for a review, see Slocum et al. (2011)). At least in terms of the cytotoxic properties of these agents, and ability of Nrf2 to control the expression of detoxification enzymes, antioxidant proteins and xenobiotic transporters, this concept appears rational. The elevated level and activity of Nrf2 in cancer cells has been shown to decrease their sensitivity to the common chemotherapeutic agents etoposide, carboplatin, cisplatin, 5-fluorouracil and doxorubicin (Singh et al., 2006; Ohta et al., 2008; Shibata et al., 2008a; Wang et al., 2008b; Homma et al., 2009; Jiang et al., 2010; Lister et al., 2011). Consistent with this notion, RNAi-mediated inhibition of Nrf2 signaling has been shown to reverse drug resistance (Shibata et al., 2008a; Wang et al., 2008b; Homma et al., 2009; Jiang et al., 2010; Lister et al., 2011). Repression of Nrf2 also enhances the cytotoxic action of γ-irradiation toward lung (Singh et al., 2010) and pancreatic (Lister et al., 2011) cancer cell lines.

Nrf2 signaling appears to be tightly repressed in a number of cancer cells which retain sensitivity to cytotoxic agents. For example, the doxorubicin-sensitive human ovarian carcinoma cell line A2780 exhibits lower Nrf2 signaling activity than drug-resistant counterparts, and RNAi depletion of Nrf2 in the former cells does not affect sensitivity to doxorubicin (Shim et al., 2009). However, the pharmacological induction of doxorubicin resistance in A2780 cells is accompanied by an increase in Nrf2 activity, and under these conditions depletion of Nrf2 does restore drug sensitivity (Shim et al., 2009). Consistent with this observation, an elevated level of Cul3 in drug-sensitive breast cancer tissue samples and cell lines is associated with the constitutive repression of Nrf2 (Loignon et al., 2009), presumably through its enhanced ubiquitination and proteasomal degradation.

Knockdown of Cul3 in these cells leads to the upregulated expression of cytoprotective Nrf2 target genes and the development of a drug-resistant phenotype (Loignon et al., 2009). Overall, these findings indicate a key role for Nrf2 in the development of drug resistance in cancer cells, and that the selective targeting of Nrf2 may hold promise as an adjuvant strategy in patients receiving chemotherapy.

C. Small Molecule Inhibitors of Nrf2

In the context of the apparent role of Nrf2 in driving oncogenesis and resistance to cancer therapy, the pharmacological inhibition of Nrf2 signaling represents a promising strategy to improve the clinical management of this disease. Retinoic acid receptor α agonists have been shown to rapidly inhibit the basal and inducible activity of Nrf2, independent of effects on Nrf2 protein stability and subcellular localization (Wang et al., 2007). Indeed, the negative regulation of Nrf2 activity by retinoic acid appears to involve the formation of complexes between retinoic acid receptor α and Nrf2 that prevent the latter from binding to the ARE and transactivating target genes (Wang et al., 2007). Recently, brusatol, a component of the *Brucea javanica* shrub, emerged from a screen of natural compounds as an potent inhibitor of Nrf2 activity through its ability to provoke a sustained, but reversible, reduction in Nrf2 protein level across a panel of mammalian cell lines (Ren et al., 2011). The inhibitory action of brusatol was shown to be independent of changes in the level of Keap1 mRNA or protein, but was attributed to the enhanced ubiquitination and degradation of Nrf2, leading to a 2.5-fold decrease in its protein half-life (Ren et al., 2011). Importantly, through inhibiting the activity of Nrf2, brusatol enhances the growth-limiting action of, and reduces resistance to, various chemotherapeutic drugs in both cancer cell lines *in vitro* and xenografts in an *in vivo* mouse model (Ren et al., 2011). Although additional research is needed to fully establish the specificity and mechanism of action of these and other putative Nrf2 inhibitors, such molecules may prove to be useful therapeutic tools in the management of cancer and other diseases.

V. Conclusion

Since its discovery in 1994 (Moi et al., 1994), there have been significant advances in our understanding of the function and mechanisms of regulation of Nrf2. In particular, the generation of transgenic Nrf2 knockout mice (Chan et al., 1996; Itoh et al., 1997) has provided invaluable insights into the important contribution of this transcription factor in maintaining cellular homeostasis and resisting xenobiotic insult. In demonstrating the progressive transition from elegant mechanistic research to translatable applications, this review has highlighted the potential benefits of targeting Nrf2 for therapeutic means. Although a wide body of evidence indicates that activation of Nrf2 protects cells and animals against a variety of diseases and toxicities (Copple et al., 2010a), the sustained activation of Nrf2 appears to favor the progression of certain cancers (Taguchi et al., 2011). As such, the recent emergence of commercially available dietary supplements marketed as 'Nrf2 activators' causes some unease, particularly in light of the apparent lack of health benefits afforded by other antioxidant interventions (Bjelakovic et al., 2008) and our relatively poor appreciation of the importance of the Keap1–Nrf2 pathway in humans, compared to cell or animal models. A better appreciation of the most desirable balance between the protective and deleterious effects of Nrf2 activation, in acute and chronic settings, is needed before we can fully determine the likely value of targeting Nrf2 for therapeutic benefit in humans.

The potential utility of our increasing understanding of the Keap1–Nrf2 pathway may extend beyond direct clinical intervention. In 2007, the U.S. National Research Council published a report aimed at advancing future strategy for testing the toxicity of environmental agents and xenobiotics (N.R.C., 2007). The key focus was to take advantage of our detailed understanding of stress response pathways to enable cell-based *in vitro* models to take a front-line role in the toxicity screening process, and as a result further reduce the reliance on animal testing. An excellent recent review of the implications of this report highlighted the potential of using the activation of Nrf2 as one component of a novel toxicity testing strategy (Krewski et al., 2011). By defining the sensitivity of Nrf2 and other stress response pathways to certain forms of toxic insult, it may be possible to identify drug candidates, xenobiotics and environmental agents that are likely to induce certain forms of cellular stress, based on known patterns of pathway perturbations (Krewski et al., 2011). The value of such an approach in detecting skin sensitizing chemicals has been demonstrated in a keratinocyte model (Emter et al., 2010; Delaine et al., 2011). Again, the human relevance of the activation of Nrf2 and other stress response pathways in cell or animal models needs to be clarified if such applications are to be fully realized. As with most biological research, the translation of detailed mechanistic understanding of the Keap1–Nrf2 pathway into strategies for improving human health represents a critical challenge, but one that appears likely to bring numerous benefits.

Acknowledgments

The author acknowledges the many excellent studies that have furthered our understanding of the Keap1–Nrf2 pathway that could not be cited due to the space constraints and scope of this article. The author also acknowledges the valuable support of colleagues at the MRC

Centre for Drug Safety Science at The University of Liverpool. Within the Centre, work on the Keap1–Nrf2 pathway is facilitated by generous funding from the Biotechnology and Biological Sciences Research Council, the Medical Research Council, the Paget's Association and the Wellcome Trust.

Conflict of Interest: The author has no conflicts of interest to declare.

Abbreviations

ARE	antioxidant response element
BTB	bric-a-brac, tram-track, broad complex
CDDO	2-cyano-3,12-dioxooleana-1,9(11)-dien-28-oic acid
Cul3	Cullin 3
DC	double glycine repeat and C-terminal
IKKβ	inhibitor of κB kinase β
IVR	intervening region
Keap1	Kelch-like erythroid cell-derived protein with CNC homology (ECH)-associated protein 1
miRNA	micro-RNA
MPTP	1-methyl-4-phenyl-1,2,3,6-tetrahydropyridine
NF-κB	nuclear factor κB
Nrf2	nuclear factor erythroid 2 (NF-E2) -related factor 2
RNAi	RNA interference
ROS	reactive oxygen species
UV	ultraviolet

References

Abiko, Y., et al. (2011). Participation of covalent modification of Keap1 in the activation of Nrf2 by tert-butylbenzoquinone, an electrophilic metabolite of butylated hydroxyanisole. *Toxicology and Applied Pharmacology*, *255*(1), 32–39.

Ahn, Y. H., et al. (2010). Electrophilic tuning of the chemoprotective natural product sulforaphane. *Proceedings of the National Academy of Sciences of the United States of America*, *107*(21), 9590–9595.

Alam, J., et al. (2003). Heme activates the heme oxygenase-1 gene in renal epithelial cells by stabilizing Nrf2. *American Journal of Physiology – Renal Physiology*, *284*(4), F743–F752.

Aleksunes, L. M., et al. (2010). Transcriptional regulation of renal cytoprotective genes by Nrf2 and its potential use as a therapeutic target to mitigate cisplatin-induced nephrotoxicity. *Journal of Pharmacology and Experimental Therapeutics*, *335*(1), 2–12.

Baird, L., et al. (2011). The cytoprotective role of the Keap1–Nrf2 pathway. *Archives of Toxicology*, *85*(4), 241–272.

Barone, M. C., et al. (2011). Genetic activation of Nrf2 signaling is sufficient to ameliorate neurodegenerative phenotypes in a Drosophila model of Parkinson's disease. *Disease Models & Mechanisms*, *4*(5), 701–707.

Bjelakovic, G., et al. (2008). Antioxidant supplements for prevention of mortality in healthy participants and patients with various diseases. *Cochrane Database of Systematic Reviews*, 2, CD007176.

Blake, D. J., et al. (2010). Deletion of Keap1 in the lung attenuates acute cigarette smoke-induced oxidative stress and inflammation. *American Journal of Respiratory Cell and Molecular Biology*, *42*(5), 524–536.

Bui, C. B., et al. (2011). Persistent expression of Nqo1 by p62-mediated Nrf2 activation facilitates p53-dependent mitotic catastrophe. *Biochemical and Biophysical Research Communications*, *412*(2), 347–352.

Burton, N. C., et al. (2006). In vivo modulation of the Parkinsonian phenotype by Nrf2. *Neurotoxicology*, *27*(6), 1094–1100.

Calkins, M. J., et al. (2009). The Nrf2/ARE pathway as a potential therapeutic target in neurodegenerative disease. *Antioxidants & Redox Signaling*, *11*(3), 497–508.

Cao, T. T., et al. (2005). Increased nuclear factor-erythroid 2 p45-related factor 2 activity protects SH-SY5Y cells against oxidative damage. *Journal of Neurochemistry*, *95*(2), 406–417.

Chan, J. Y., et al. (2000). Impaired expression of glutathione synthetic enzyme genes in mice with targeted deletion of the Nrf2 basic-leucine zipper protein. *Biochimica et Biophysica Acta*, *1517*(1), 19–26.

Chan, K., et al. (2001). An important function of Nrf2 in combating oxidative stress: detoxification of acetaminophen. *Proceedings of the National Academy of Sciences of the United States of America*, *98*(8), 4611–4616.

Chan, K., et al. (1996). NRF2, a member of the NFE2 family of transcription factors, is not essential for murine erythropoiesis, growth, and development. *Proceedings of the National Academy of Sciences of the United States of America*, *93*(24), 13943–13948.

Chen, N., et al. (2010). Nrf2 expression in endometrial serous carcinomas and its precancers. *International Journal of Clinical and Experimental Pathology*, *4*(1), 85–96.

Chen, P. C., et al. (2009a). Nrf2-mediated neuroprotection in the MPTP mouse model of Parkinson's disease: Critical role for the astrocyte. *Proceedings of the National Academy of Sciences of the United States of America*, *106*(8), 2933–2938.

Chen, W., et al. (2009b). Direct interaction between Nrf2 and p21(Cip1/WAF1) upregulates the Nrf2-mediated antioxidant response. *Molecular Cell*, *34*(6), 663–673.

Cheng, Q., et al. (2011). Constitutive activation of nuclear factor-E2-related factor 2 induces biotransformation enzyme and transporter expression in livers of mice with hepatocyte-specific deletion of Kelch-like ECH-associated protein 1. *Journal of Biochemical and Molecular Toxicology*, *25*(5), 320–329.

Cho, H. Y., et al. (2010). Nrf2 protects against airway disorders. *Toxicology and Applied Pharmacology*, *244*(1), 43–56.

Chowdhry, S., et al. (2010). Loss of Nrf2 markedly exacerbates nonalcoholic steatohepatitis. *Free Radical Biology & Medicine*, *48*(2), 357–371.

Clements, C. M., et al. (2006). DJ-1, a cancer- and Parkinson's disease-associated protein, stabilizes the antioxidant transcriptional master regulator Nrf2. *Proceedings of the National Academy of Sciences of the United States of America*, *103*(41), 15,091–15,096.

Copple, I. M., et al. (2008a). The hepatotoxic metabolite of acetaminophen directly activates the Keap1–Nrf2 cell defense system. *Hepatology*, *48*(4), 1292–1301.

Copple, I. M., et al. (2008b). The Nrf2–Keap1 defence pathway: role in protection against drug-induced toxicity. *Toxicology*, *246*(1), 24–33.

Copple, I. M., et al. (2010a). The Keap1–Nrf2 cellular defense pathway: mechanisms of regulation and role in protection against drug-induced toxicity. *Handbook of Experimental Pharmacology*, *196*, 233–266.

Copple, I. M., et al. (2010b). Physical and functional interaction of sequestosome 1 with Keap1 regulates the Keap1–Nrf2 cell defense pathway. *Journal of Biological Chemistry*, *285*(22), 16,782–16,788.

Cullinan, S. B., et al. (2004). The Keap1-BTB protein is an adaptor that bridges Nrf2 to a Cul3-based E3 ligase: oxidative stress sensing by a Cul3-Keap1 ligase. *Molecular and Cellular Biology*, *24*(19), 8477–8486.

Cullinan, S. B., et al. (2003). Nrf2 is a direct PERK substrate and effector of PERK-dependent cell survival. *Molecular and Cellular Biology*, *23*(20), 7198–7209.

Davies, K. J. (2000). Oxidative stress, antioxidant defenses, and damage removal, repair, and replacement systems. *IUBMB Life*, *50*(4, 5), 279–289.

Deeb, D., et al. (2007). CDDO-me induces apoptosis and inhibits Akt, mTOR and NF-kappaB signaling proteins in prostate cancer cells. *Anticancer Research*, *27*(5A), 3035–3044.

Delaine, T., et al. (2011). Structure–activity relationship between the in vivo skin sensitizing potency of analogues of phenyl glycidyl ether and the induction of Nrf2-dependent luciferase activity in the keratinosens in vitro assay. *Chemical Research in Toxicology*, *24*(8), 1312–1318.

DeNicola, G. M., et al. (2011). Oncogene-induced Nrf2 transcription promotes ROS detoxification and tumorigenesis. *Nature*, *475*(7354), 106–109.

Dhakshinamoorthy, S., et al. (2004). Nitric oxide-induced transcriptional up-regulation of protective genes by Nrf2 via the antioxidant response element counteracts apoptosis of neuroblastoma cells. *Journal of Biological Chemistry*, *279*(19), 20,096–20,107.

Dinkova-Kostova, A. T., et al. (2002). Direct evidence that sulfhydryl groups of Keap1 are the sensors regulating induction of phase 2 enzymes that protect against carcinogens and oxidants. *Proceedings of the National Academy of Sciences of the United States of America*, *99*(18), 11,908–11,913.

Dinkova-Kostova, A. T., et al. (2005). Extremely potent triterpenoid inducers of the phase 2 response: correlations of protection against oxidant and inflammatory stress. *Proceedings of the National Academy of Sciences of the United States of America*, *102*(12), 4584–4589.

Dinkova-Kostova, A. T., et al. (2010). An exceptionally potent inducer of cytoprotective enzymes: elucidation of the structural features that determine inducer potency and reactivity with Keap1. *Journal of Biological Chemistry*, *285*(44), 33,747–33,755.

Eades, G., et al. (2011). miR-200a regulates Nrf2 activation by targeting Keap1 mRNA in breast cancer cells. *Journal of Biological Chemistry*, *286*(47), 40,725–40,733.

Edinger, A. L., et al. (2004). Death by design: apoptosis, necrosis and autophagy. *Current Opinion in Cell Biology*, *16*(6), 663–669.

Eggler, A. L., et al. (2005). Modifying specific cysteines of the electrophile-sensing human Keap1 protein is insufficient to disrupt binding to the Nrf2 domain Neh2. *Proceedings of the National Academy of Sciences of the United States of America*, *102*(29), 10,070–10,075.

Emter, R., et al. (2010). Performance of a novel keratinocyte-based reporter cell line to screen skin sensitizers in vitro. *Toxicology and Applied Pharmacology*, *245*(3), 281–290.

Enomoto, A., et al. (2001). High sensitivity of Nrf2 knockout mice to acetaminophen hepatotoxicity associated with decreased expression of ARE-regulated drug metabolizing enzymes and antioxidant genes. *Toxicological Sciences*, *59*(1), 169–177.

Fan, W., et al. (2010). Keap1 facilitates p62-mediated ubiquitin aggregate clearance via autophagy. *Autophagy*, *6*(5), 614–621.

Ferreira, A., et al. (2011). Sickle hemoglobin confers tolerance to Plasmodium infection. *Cell*, *145*(3), 398–409.

Filipowicz, W., et al. (2008). Mechanisms of post-transcriptional regulation by microRNAs: are the answers in sight? *Nature Reviews Genetics*, *9*(2), 102–114.

Furukawa, M., et al. (2005). BTB protein Keap1 targets antioxidant transcription factor Nrf2 for ubiquitination by the Cullin 3-Roc1 ligase. *Molecular and Cellular Biology*, *25*(1), 162–171.

Gan, L., et al. (2010). Keap1–Nrf2 activation in the presence and absence of DJ-1. *European Journal of Neurosciences*, *31*(6), 967–977.

Gao, L., et al. (2007). Novel n-3 fatty acid oxidation products activate Nrf2 by destabilizing the association between Keap1 and Cullin3. *Journal of Biological Chemistry*, *282*(4), 2529–2537.

Gartel, A. L., et al. (2002). The role of the cyclin-dependent kinase inhibitor p21 in apoptosis. *Molecular Cancer Therapeutics*, *1*(8), 639–649.

Goldring, C. E., et al. (2004). Activation of hepatic Nrf2 in vivo by acetaminophen in CD-1 mice. *Hepatology*, *39*(5), 1267–1276.

Goven, D., et al. (2008). Altered Nrf2/Keap1-Bach1 equilibrium in pulmonary emphysema. *Thorax*, *63*(10), 916–924.

Hayes, J. D., et al. (2009). NRF2 and KEAP1 mutations: permanent activation of an adaptive response in cancer. *Trends in Biochemical Sciences*, *34*(4), 176–188.

Hayes, J. D., et al. (2010). Cancer chemoprevention mechanisms mediated through the Keap1–Nrf2 pathway. *Antioxidants & Redox Signaling*, *13*(11), 1713–1748.

Hirota, A., et al. (2005). Ultraviolet A irradiation induces NF-E2-related factor 2 activation in dermal fibroblasts: protective role in UVA-induced apoptosis. *Journal of Investigative Dermatology*, *124*(4), 825–832.

Hirota, A., et al. (2011). Acceleration of UVB-induced photoageing in nrf2 gene-deficient mice. *Experimental Dermatology*, *20*(8), 664–668.

Hirotsu, Y., et al. (2011). Nrf2 degron-fused reporter system: a new tool for specific evaluation of Nrf2 inducers. *Genes Cells*, *16*(4), 406–415.

Holland, R., et al. (2008). Prospective type 1 and type 2 disulfides of Keap1 protein. *Chemical Research in Toxicology*, *21*(10), 2051–2060.

Homma, S., et al. (2009). Nrf2 enhances cell proliferation and resistance to anticancer drugs in human lung cancer. *Clinical Cancer Research*, *15*(10), 3423–3432.

Hong, F., et al. (2005a). Identification of sensor cysteines in human Keap1 modified by the cancer chemopreventive agent sulforaphane. *Chemical Research in Toxicology*, *18*(12), 1917–1926.

Hong, F., et al. (2005b). Specific patterns of electrophile adduction trigger Keap1 ubiquitination and Nrf2 activation. *Journal of Biological Chemistry*, *280*(36), 31,768–31,775.

Hu, C., et al. (2011). Modification of keap1 cysteine residues by sulforaphane. *Chemical Research in Toxicology*, *24*(4), 515–521.

Hubbs, A. F., et al. (2007). Vacuolar leukoencephalopathy with widespread astrogliosis in mice lacking transcription factor nrf2. *American Journal of Pathology*, *170*(6), 2068–2076.

Iizuka, T., et al. (2005). Nrf2-deficient mice are highly susceptible to cigarette smoke-induced emphysema. *Genes Cells*, *10*(12), 1113–1125.

Itoh, K., et al. (1997). An Nrf2/small Maf heterodimer mediates the induction of phase II detoxifying enzyme genes through antioxidant response elements. *Biochemical and Biophysical Research Communications*, *236*(2), 313–322.

Itoh, K., et al. (2004). Transcription factor Nrf2 regulates inflammation by mediating the effect of 15-deoxy-Delta(12,14)-prostaglandin j(2). *Molecular and Cellular Biology*, *24*(1), 36–45.

Itoh, K., et al. (1999). Keap1 represses nuclear activation of antioxidant responsive elements by Nrf2 through binding to the amino-terminal Neh2 domain. *Genes & Development*, *13*(1), 76–86.

Itoh, K., et al. (2003). Keap1 regulates both cytoplasmic-nuclear shuttling and degradation of Nrf2 in response to electrophiles. *Genes Cells*, *8*(4), 379–391.

Jain, A., et al. (2010). p62/SQSTM1 is a target gene for transcription factor NRF2 and creates a positive feedback loop by inducing antioxidant response element-driven gene transcription. *Journal of Biological Chemistry*, *285*(29), 22,576–22,591.

Jazwa, A., et al. (2011). Pharmacological targeting of the transcription factor Nrf2 at the basal ganglia provides disease modifying therapy for experimental parkinsonism. *Antioxidants & Redox Signaling*, *14*(12), 2347–2360.

Jiang, T., et al. (2010). High levels of Nrf2 determine chemoresistance in type II endometrial cancer. *Cancer Research*, *70*(13), 5486–5496.

Jin, W., et al. (2009). Role of Nrf2 in protection against traumatic brain injury in mice. *Journal of Neurotrauma*, *26*(1), 131–139.

Kalkhoven, E. (2004). CBP and p300: HATs for different occasions. *Biochemical Pharmacology*, *68*(6), 1145–1155.

Kang, M. I., et al. (2004). Scaffolding of Keap1 to the actin cytoskeleton controls the function of Nrf2 as key regulator of cytoprotective phase 2 genes. *Proceedings of the National Academy of Sciences of the United States of America*, *101*(7), 2046–2051.

Kanninen, K., et al. (2009). Intrahippocampal injection of a lentiviral vector expressing Nrf2 improves spatial learning in a mouse model of Alzheimer's disease. *Proceedings of the National Academy of Sciences of the United States of America*, *106*(38), 16,505–16,510.

Karapetian, R. N., et al. (2005). Nuclear oncoprotein prothymosin alpha is a partner of Keap1: implications for expression of oxidative stress-protecting genes. *Molecular and Cellular Biology*, *25*(3), 1089–1099.

Kaspar, J. W., et al. (2010). An autoregulatory loop between Nrf2 and Cul3-Rbx1 controls their cellular abundance. *Journal of Biological Chemistry*, *285*(28), 21,349–21,358.

Katoh, Y., et al. (2001). Two domains of Nrf2 cooperatively bind CBP, a CREB binding protein, and synergistically activate transcription. *Genes Cells*, *6*(10), 857–868.

Kay, H. Y., et al. (2011). Nrf2-mediated liver protection by sauchinone, an antioxidant lignan, from acetaminophen toxicity through the PKCdelta-GSK3beta pathway. *British Journal of Pharmacology*, *163*(8), 1653–1665.

Kerns, M. L., et al. (2007). Reprogramming of keratin biosynthesis by sulforaphane restores skin integrity in epidermolysis bullosa simplex. *Proceedings of the National Academy of Sciences of the United States of America*, *104*(36), 14,460–14,465.

Khor, T. O., et al. (2011). Pharmacodynamics of curcumin as DNA hypomethylation agent in restoring the expression of Nrf2 via promoter CpGs demethylation. *Biochemical Pharmacology*, *82*(9), 1073–1078.

Kim, J. E., et al. (2010a). Suppression of NF-kappaB signaling by KEAP1 regulation of IKK-beta activity through autophagic degradation and inhibition of phosphorylation. *Cellular Signalling*, *22*(11), 1645–1654.

Kim, R. H., et al. (2005). Hypersensitivity of DJ-1-deficient mice to 1-methyl-4-phenyl-1,2,3,6-tetrahydropyrindine (MPTP) and oxidative stress. *Proceedings of the National Academy of Sciences of the United States of America*, *102*(14), 5215–5220.

Kim, Y. R., et al. (2010b). Oncogenic NRF2 mutations in squamous cell carcinomas of oesophagus and skin. *Journal of Pathology*, *220*(4), 446–451.

Kimura, S., et al. (2009). Essential role of Nrf2 in keratinocyte protection from UVA by quercetin. *Biochemical and Biophysical Research Communications*, *387*(1), 109–114.

Kitteringham, N. R., et al. (2010). Proteomic analysis of Nrf2 deficient transgenic mice reveals cellular defence and lipid metabolism as primary Nrf2-dependent pathways in the liver. *Journal of Proteomics*, *73*(8), 1612–1631.

Klaassen, C. D. (2002). Xenobiotic transporters: another protective mechanism for chemicals. *International Journal of Toxicology*, *21*(1), 7–12.

Klaassen, C. D., et al. (2010). Nrf2 the rescue: effects of the antioxidative/electrophilic response on the liver. *Toxicology and Applied Pharmacology*, *244*(1), 57–65.

Klose, R. J., et al. (2006). Genomic DNA methylation: the mark and its mediators. *Trends in Biochemical Sciences*, *31*(2), 89–97.

Kobayashi, A., et al. (2004). Oxidative stress sensor Keap1 functions as an adaptor for Cul3-based E3 ligase to regulate proteasomal degradation of Nrf2. *Molecular and Cellular Biology*, *24*(16), 7130–7139.

Kobayashi, A., et al. (2006). Oxidative and electrophilic stresses activate Nrf2 through inhibition of ubiquitination activity of Keap1. *Molecular and Cellular Biology*, *26*(1), 221–229.

Kobayashi, M., et al. (2009). The antioxidant defense system Keap1–Nrf2 comprises a multiple sensing mechanism for responding to a wide range of chemical compounds. *Molecular and Cellular Biology*, *29*(2), 493–502.

Komatsu, M., et al. (2010). The selective autophagy substrate p62 activates the stress responsive transcription factor Nrf2 through inactivation of Keap1. *Nature Cell Biology*, *12*(3), 213–223.

Kong, X., et al. (2011). Enhancing Nrf2 pathway by disruption of keap1 in myeloid leukocytes protects against sepsis. *American Journal of Respiratory and Critical Care Medicine*, *184*(8), 928–938.

Konopleva, M., et al. (2002). Novel triterpenoid CDDO-Me is a potent inducer of apoptosis and differentiation in acute myelogenous leukemia. *Blood*, *99*(1), 326–335.

Konstantinopoulos, P. A., et al. (2011). Keap1 mutations and Nrf2 pathway activation in epithelial ovarian cancer. *Cancer Research*, *71*(15), 5081–5089.

Krewski, D., et al. (2011). New directions in toxicity testing. *Annual Review of Public Health*, *32*, 161–178.

Kurz, E. U., et al. (2001). Identification of DNA-protein interactions in the 5' flanking and 5' untranslated regions of the human multidrug resistance protein (MRP1) gene: evaluation of a putative antioxidant response element/AP-1 binding site. *Biochemical and Biophysical Research Communications*, *285*(4), 981–990.

Lau, A., et al. (2010). A noncanonical mechanism of Nrf2 activation by autophagy deficiency: direct interaction between Keap1 and p62. *Molecular and Cellular Biology*, *30*(13), 3275–3285.

Lee, D. F., et al. (2009). KEAP1 E3 ligase-mediated downregulation of NF-kappaB signaling by targeting IKKbeta. *Molecular Cell*, *36*(1), 131–140.

Lee, J. M., et al. (2003). Identification of the NF-E2-related factor-2-dependent genes conferring protection against oxidative stress in primary cortical astrocytes using oligonucleotide microarray analysis. *Journal of Biological Chemistry*, *278*(14), 12,029–12,038.

Lee, O. H., et al. (2007). An auto-regulatory loop between stress sensors INrf2 and Nrf2 controls their cellular abundance. *Journal of Biological Chemistry*, *282*(50), 36,412–36,420.

Leung, C. K., et al. (2011). High-throughput screening and biosensing with fluorescent *C. elegans* strains. *Journal of Visualized Experiments*, *51*, pii 2745.

Levonen, A. L., et al. (2004). Cellular mechanisms of redox cell signalling: role of cysteine modification in controlling antioxidant defences in response to electrophilic lipid oxidation products. *Biochemical Journal*, *378*(Pt 2), 373–382.

Li, L., et al. (2008). Molecular evolution of Keap1. Two Keap1 molecules with distinctive intervening region structures are conserved among fish. *Journal of Biological Chemistry*, *283*(6), 3248–3255.

Li, Q. K., et al. (2011). KEAP1 gene mutations and NRF2 activation are common in pulmonary papillary adenocarcinoma. *Journal of Human Genetics*, *56*(3), 230–234.

Liby, K., et al. (2005). The synthetic triterpenoids, CDDO and CDDO-imidazolide, are potent inducers of heme oxygenase-1 and Nrf2/ARE signaling. *Cancer Research*, *65*(11), 4789–4798.

Lister, A., et al. (2011). Nrf2 is overexpressed in pancreatic cancer: implications for cell proliferation and therapy. *Molecular Cancer*, *10*, 37.

Liu, G., et al. (2005). Screening method for the discovery of potential cancer chemoprevention agents based on mass spectrometric detection of alkylated Keap1. *Analytical Chemistry*, *77*(19), 6407–6414.

Liu, G. H., et al. (2008). NF-kappaB/p65 antagonizes Nrf2-ARE pathway by depriving CBP from Nrf2 and facilitating recruitment of HDAC3 to MafK. *Biochimica et Biophysica Acta*, *1783*(5), 713–727.

Liu, Y., et al. (2007). A genomic screen for activators of the antioxidant response element. *Proceedings of the National Academy of Sciences of the United States of America*, *104*(12), 5205–5210.

Lloberas, J., et al. (2009). p21(waf1/CIP1), a CDK inhibitor and a negative feedback system that controls macrophage activation. *European Journal of Immunology*, *39*(3), 691–694.

Lo, S. C., et al. (2006a). PGAM5, a Bcl-XL-interacting protein, is a novel substrate for the redox-regulated Keap1-dependent ubiquitin ligase complex. *Journal of Biological Chemistry*, *281*(49), 37,893–37,903.

Lo, S. C., et al. (2008). PGAM5 tethers a ternary complex containing Keap1 and Nrf2 to mitochondria. *Experimental Cell Research*, *314*(8), 1789–1803.

Lo, S. C., et al. (2006b). Structure of the Keap1:Nrf2 interface provides mechanistic insight into Nrf2 signaling. *EMBO Journal*, *25*(15), 3605–3617.

Loignon, M., et al. (2009). Cul3 overexpression depletes Nrf2 in breast cancer and is associated with sensitivity to carcinogens, to oxidative stress, and to chemotherapy. *Molecular Cancer Therapeutics*, *8*(8), 2432–2440.

Luo, Y., et al. (2007). Sites of alkylation of human Keap1 by natural chemoprevention agents. *Journal of The American Society for Mass Spectrometry*, *18*(12), 2226–2232.

Ma, Q., et al. (2006). Multiorgan autoimmune inflammation, enhanced lymphoproliferation, and impaired homeostasis of reactive oxygen species in mice lacking the antioxidant-activated transcription factor Nrf2. *American Journal of Pathology*, *168*(6), 1960–1974.

Ma, X., et al. (2011). Nrf2 knockdown by shRNA inhibits tumor growth and increases efficacy of chemotherapy in cervical cancer. *Cancer Chemotherapy and Pharmacology*.

Malhotra, D., et al. (2008). Decline in NRF2-regulated antioxidants in chronic obstructive pulmonary disease lungs due to loss of its positive regulator, DJ-1. *American Journal of Respiratory and Critical Care Medicine*, *178*(6), 592–604.

Mao, L., et al. (2011a). Transcription factor Nrf2 protects the spinal cord from inflammation produced by spinal cord injury. *Journal of Surgical Research*, *170*(1), e105–e115.

Mao, L., et al. (2011b). Disruption of Nrf2 exacerbated the damage after spinal cord injury in mice. *Journal of Trauma*, *72*(1), 189–198.

Matus, S., et al. (2011). Protein folding stress in neurodegenerative diseases: a glimpse into the ER. *Current Opinion in Cell Biology*, *23*(2), 239–252.

McMahon, M., et al. (2003). Keap1-dependent proteasomal degradation of transcription factor Nrf2 contributes to the negative regulation of antioxidant response element-driven gene expression. *Journal of Biological Chemistry*, *278*(24), 21,592–21,600.

McMahon, M., et al. (2010). Keap1 perceives stress via three sensors for the endogenous signaling molecules nitric oxide, zinc, and alkenals. *Proceedings of the National Academy of Sciences of the United States of America*, *107*(44), 18,838–18,843.

McMahon, M., et al. (2006). Dimerization of substrate adaptors can facilitate cullin-mediated ubiquitylation of proteins by a "tethering" mechanism: a two-site interaction model for the Nrf2–Keap1 complex. *Journal of Biological Chemistry*, *281*(34), 24,756–24,768.

Miseta, A., et al. (2000). Relationship between the occurrence of cysteine in proteins and the complexity of organisms. *Molecular Biology and Evolution*, *17*(8), 1232–1239.

Moi, P., et al. (1994). Isolation of NF-E2-related factor 2 (Nrf2), a NF-E2-like basic leucine zipper transcriptional activator that binds to the tandem NF-E2/AP1 repeat of the beta-globin locus control region. *Proceedings of the National Academy of Sciences of the United States of America*, *91*(21), 9926–9930.

Moscat, J., et al. (2009). p62 at the crossroads of autophagy, apoptosis, and cancer. *Cell*, *137*(6), 1001–1004.

Motohashi, H., et al. (2002). Integration and diversity of the regulatory network composed of Maf and CNC families of transcription factors. *Gene*, *294*(1, 2), 1–12.

Mulcahy, R. T., et al. (1997). Constitutive and beta-naphthoflavone-induced expression of the human gamma-glutamylcysteine synthetase heavy subunit gene is regulated by a distal antioxidant response element/TRE sequence. *Journal of Biological Chemistry*, *272*(11), 7445–7454.

Muscarella, L. A., et al. (2011a). Regulation of KEAP1 expression by promoter methylation in malignant gliomas and association with patient's outcome. *Epigenetics*, *6*(3), 317–325.

Muscarella, L. A., et al. (2011b). Frequent epigenetics inactivation of KEAP1 gene in non-small cell lung cancer. *Epigenetics*, *6*(6), 710–719.

N.R.C. (2007). *Toxicity Testing in the 21st Century: A Vision and A Strategy*. Washington, DC: National Research Council.

Neymotin, A., et al. (2011). Neuroprotective effect of Nrf2/ARE activators, CDDO ethylamide and CDDO trifluoroethylamide, in a mouse model of amyotrophic lateral sclerosis. *Free Radical Biology and Medicine*, *51*(1), 88–96.

Nguyen, T., et al. (2003). Increased protein stability as a mechanism that enhances Nrf2-mediated transcriptional activation of the antioxidant response element. Degradation of Nrf2 by the 26 S proteasome. *Journal of Biological Chemistry*, *278*(7), 4536–4541.

Nioi, P., et al. (2003). Identification of a novel Nrf2-regulated antioxidant response element (ARE) in the mouse NAD(P)H:quinone oxidoreductase 1 gene: reassessment of the ARE consensus sequence. *Biochemical Journal*, *374*(Pt 2), 337–348.

Nioi, P., et al. (2007). A mutation of Keap1 found in breast cancer impairs its ability to repress Nrf2 activity. *Biochemical and Biophysical Research Communications*, *362*(4), 816–821.

Nordberg, J., et al. (2001). Reactive oxygen species, antioxidants, and the mammalian thioredoxin system. *Free Radical Biology and Medicine*, *31*(11), 1287–1312.

Oeckinghaus, A., et al. (2011). Crosstalk in NF-kappaB signaling pathways. *Nature Immunology*, *12*(8), 695–708.

Ogura, T., et al. (2010). Keap1 is a forked-stem dimer structure with two large spheres enclosing the intervening, double glycine repeat, and C-terminal domains. *Proceedings of the National Academy of Sciences of the United States of America*, *107*(7), 2842–2847.

Ohnuma, T., et al. (2010). Activation of the Nrf2/ARE pathway via S-alkylation of cysteine 151 in the chemopreventive agent-sensor Keap1 protein by falcarindiol, a conjugated diacetylene compound. *Toxicology and Applied Pharmacology*, *244*(1), 27–36.

Ohta, T., et al. (2008). Loss of Keap1 function activates Nrf2 and provides advantages for lung cancer cell growth. *Cancer Research*, *68*(5), 1303–1309.

Okawa, H., et al. (2006). Hepatocyte-specific deletion of the keap1 gene activates Nrf2 and confers potent resistance against acute drug toxicity. *Biochemical and Biophysical Research Communications*, *339*(1), 79–88.

Olagnier, D., et al. (2011). Nrf2, a PPARgamma alternative pathway to promote CD36 expression on inflammatory macrophages: implication for malaria. *PLOS Pathogens*, *7*(9), e1002254.

Osburn, W. O., et al. (2008). Genetic or pharmacologic amplification of nrf2 signaling inhibits acute inflammatory liver injury in mice. *Toxicological Sciences*, *104*(1), 218–227.

Ostapowicz, G., et al. (2002). Results of a prospective study of acute liver failure at 17 tertiary care centers in the United States. *Annals of Internal Medicine*, *137*(12), 947–954.

Padmanabhan, B., et al. (2008a). Structural analysis of the complex of Keap1 with a prothymosin alpha peptide. *Acta Crystallographica Section F – Structural Biology and Crystallization Communications*, *64*(Pt. 4), 233–238.

Padmanabhan, B., et al. (2008b). Structural insights into the similar modes of Nrf2 transcription factor recognition by the cytoplasmic repressor Keap1. *Journal of Synchrotron Radiation*, *15*(Pt. 3), 273–276.

Padmanabhan, B., et al. (2006). Structural basis for defects of Keap1 activity provoked by its point mutations in lung cancer. *Molecular Cell*, *21*(5), 689–700.

Pamplona, A., et al. (2007). Heme oxygenase-1 and carbon monoxide suppress the pathogenesis of experimental cerebral malaria. *Nature Medicine*, *13*(6), 703–710.

Park, B. K., et al. (2011). Drug bioactivation and protein adduct formation in the pathogenesis of drug-induced toxicity. *Chemico-Biological Interactions*, *192*(1, 2), 30–36.

Pergola, P. E., et al. (2011a). Effect of bardoxolone methyl on kidney function in patients with T2D and Stage 3b-4 CKD. *American Journal of Nephrology*, *33*(5), 469–476.

Pergola, P. E., et al. (2011b). Bardoxolone methyl and kidney function in CKD with type 2 diabetes. *New England Journal of Medicine*, *365*(4), 327–336.

Prestera, T., et al. (1993). Chemical and molecular regulation of enzymes that detoxify carcinogens. *Proceedings of the National Academy of Sciences of the United States of America*, *90*(7), 2965–2969.

Rachakonda, G., et al. (2008). Covalent modification at Cys151 dissociates the electrophile sensor Keap1 from the ubiquitin ligase CUL3. *Chemical Research in Toxicology*, *21*(3), 705–710.

Ramos-Gomez, M., et al. (2001). Sensitivity to carcinogenesis is increased and chemoprotective efficacy of enzyme inducers is lost in nrf2 transcription factor-deficient mice. *Proceedings of the National Academy of Sciences of the United States of America*, *98*(6), 3410–3415.

Rangasamy, T:, et al. (2004). Genetic ablation of Nrf2 enhances susceptibility to cigarette smoke-induced emphysema in mice. *Journal of Clinical Investigastions*, *114*(9), 1248–1259.

Reddy, N. M., et al. (2008). Genetic disruption of the Nrf2 compromises cell-cycle progression by impairing GSH-induced redox signaling. *Oncogene*, *27*(44), 5821–5832.

Reichard, J. F., et al. (2007). Heme oxygenase-1 induction by NRF2 requires inactivation of the transcriptional repressor BACH1. *Nucleic Acids Research*, *35*(21), 7074–7086.

Reisman, S. A., et al. (2009a). CDDO-Im protects from acetaminophen hepatotoxicity through induction of Nrf2-dependent genes. *Toxicology and Applied Pharmacology*, *236*(1), 109–114.

Reisman, S. A., et al. (2009b). Altered disposition of acetaminophen in Nrf2-null and Keap1-knockdown mice. *Toxicological Sciences*, *109*(1), 31–40.

Ren, D., et al. (2011). Brusatol enhances the efficacy of chemotherapy by inhibiting the Nrf2-mediated defense mechanism. *Proceedings of the National Academy of Sciences of the United States of America*, *108*(4), 1433–1438.

Ryu, K., et al. (2010). Oleanane triterpenoid CDDO-Me induces apoptosis in multidrug resistant osteosarcoma cells through inhibition of Stat3 pathway. *BMC Cancer*, *10*, 187.

Sahin, K., et al. (2010). Epigallocatechin-3-gallate activates Nrf2/HO-1 signaling pathway in cisplatin-induced nephrotoxicity in rats. *Life Sciences*, *87*(7, 8), 240–245.

Sakurai, T., et al. (2006). Ebselen, a seleno-organic antioxidant, as an electrophile. *Chemical Research in Toxicology*, *19*(9), 1196–1204.

Sangokoya, C., et al. (2010). microRNA miR-144 modulates oxidative stress tolerance and associates with anemia severity in sickle cell disease. *Blood*, *116*(20), 4338–4348.

Saw, C. L., et al. (2011). Impact of Nrf2 on UVB-induced skin inflammation/photoprotection and photoprotective effect of sulforaphane. *Molecular Carcinogenesis*, *50*(6), 479–486.

Schafer, M., et al. (2010). Nrf2 establishes a glutathione-mediated gradient of UVB cytoprotection in the epidermis. *Genes Development*, *24*(10), 1045–1058.

Sekhar, K. R., et al. (2010). Cysteine-based regulation of the CUL3 adaptor protein Keap1. *Toxicology and Applied Pharmacology*, *244*(1), 21–26.

Sekhar, K. R., et al. (2000). Inhibition of the 26S proteasome induces expression of GLCLC, the catalytic subunit for gamma-glutamylcysteine synthetase. *Biochemical and Biophysical Research Communications*, *270*(1), 311–317.

Shapiro, S. D. (2000). Animal models for chronic obstructive pulmonary disease: age of klotho and marlboro mice. *American Journal of Respiratory Cell and Molecular Biology*, *22*(1), 4–7.

Shibata, T., et al. (2008a). Genetic alteration of Keap1 confers constitutive Nrf2 activation and resistance to chemotherapy in gallbladder cancer. *Gastroenterology*, *135*(4), 1358–1368. 1368 e1351–e1354.

Shibata, T., et al. (2008b). Cancer related mutations in NRF2 impair its recognition by Keap1-Cul3 E3 ligase and promote malignancy. *Proceedings of the National Academy of Sciences of the United States of America*, *105*(36), 13,568–13,573.

Shim, G. S., et al. (2009). Acquisition of doxorubicin resistance in ovarian carcinoma cells accompanies activation of the NRF2 pathway. *Free Radical Biology and Medicine*, *47*(11), 1619–1631.

Shin, S., et al. (2009). Role of Nrf2 in prevention of high-fat diet-induced obesity by synthetic triterpenoid CDDO-imidazolide. *European Journal of Pharmacology*, *620*(1–3), 138–144.

Singh, A., et al. (2010). Gain of Nrf2 function in non-small-cell lung cancer cells confers radioresistance. *Antioxidants & Redox Signaling*, *13*(11), 1627–1637.

Singh, A., et al. (2009). Nrf2-dependent sulfiredoxin-1 expression protects against cigarette smoke-induced oxidative stress in lungs. *Free Radical Biology and Medicine*, *46*(3), 376–386.

Singh, A., et al. (2006). Dysfunctional KEAP1–NRF2 interaction in non-small-cell lung cancer. *PLoS Medicine*, *3*(10), e420.

Sjoblom, T., et al. (2006). The consensus coding sequences of human breast and colorectal cancers. *Science*, *314*(5797), 268–274.

Slocum, S. L., et al. (2011). Nrf2: control of sensitivity to carcinogens. *Archives of Toxicology*, *85*(4), 273–284.

Snyder, G. H., et al. (1981). Electrostatic influence of local cysteine environments on disulfide exchange kinetics. *Biochemistry*, *20*(23), 6509–6519.

Sporn, M. B., et al. (2011). New synthetic triterpenoids: potent agents for prevention and treatment of tissue injury caused by inflammatory and oxidative stress. *Journal of Natural Products*, *74*(3), 537–545.

Stack, C., et al. (2010). Triterpenoids CDDO-ethyl amide and CDDO-trifluoroethyl amide improve the behavioral phenotype and brain pathology in a transgenic mouse model of Huntington's disease. *Free Radical Biology and Medicine*, *49*(2), 147–158.

Stewart, D., et al. (2003). Degradation of transcription factor Nrf2 via the ubiquitin-proteasome pathway and stabilization by cadmium. *Journal of Biological Chemistry*, *278*(4), 2396–2402.

Strachan, G. D., et al. (2004). Fetal Alz-50 clone 1 interacts with the human orthologue of the Kelch-like Ech-associated protein. *Biochemistry*, *43*(38), 12,113–12,122.

Suh, N., et al. (1999). A novel synthetic oleanane triterpenoid, 2-cyano-3,12-dioxoolean-1, 9-dien-28-oic acid, with potent differentiating, antiproliferative, and anti-inflammatory activity. *Cancer Research*, *59*(2), 336–341.

Sumi, D., et al. (2009). Catechol estrogens mediated activation of Nrf2 through covalent modification of its quinone metabolite to Keap1. *Journal of Toxicological Sciences*, *34*(6), 627–635.

Sussan, T. E., et al. (2009). Targeting Nrf2 with the triterpenoid CDDO-imidazolide attenuates cigarette smoke-induced emphysema and cardiac dysfunction in mice. *Proceedings of the National Academy of Sciences of the United States of America*, *106*(1), 250–255.

Suzuki, M., et al. (2008). Down-regulated NF-E2-related factor 2 in pulmonary macrophages of aged smokers and patients with chronic obstructive pulmonary disease. *American Journal of Respiratory Cell and Molecular Biology*, *39*(6), 673–682.

Taguchi, K., et al. (2010). Genetic analysis of cytoprotective functions supported by graded expression of Keap1. *Molecular and Cellular Biology*, *30*(12), 3016–3026.

Taguchi, K., et al. (2011). Molecular mechanisms of the Keap1–Nrf2 pathway in stress response and cancer evolution. *Genes Cells*, *16*(2), 123–140.

Taira, T., et al. (2004). DJ-1 has a role in antioxidative stress to prevent cell death. *EMBO Reports*, *5*(2), 213–218.

Takahashi, T., et al. (2010). Mutations in Keap1 are a potential prognostic factor in resected non-small cell lung cancer. *Journal of Surgical Oncology*, *101*(6), 500–506.

Talalay, P., et al. (1988). Identification of a common chemical signal regulating the induction of enzymes that protect against chemical carcinogenesis. *Proceedings of the National Academy of Sciences of the United States of America*, *85*(21), 8261–8265.

Tanaka, Y., et al. (2008). NF-E2-related factor 2 inhibits lipid accumulation and oxidative stress in mice fed a high-fat diet. *Journal of Pharmacology and Experimental Therapeutics*, *325*(2), 655–664.

Tian, F. F., et al. (2011). Nrf2-mediated protection against UVA radiation in human skin keratinocytes. *Bioscience Trends*, *5*(1), 23–29.

Tiegs, G., et al. (1992). A T cell-dependent experimental liver injury in mice inducible by concanavalin A. *Journal of Clinical Investigations*, *90*(1), 196–203.

Tong, K. I., et al. (2006). Keap1 recruits Neh2 through binding to ETGE and DLG motifs: characterization of the two-site molecular recognition model. *Molecular and Cellular Biology*, *26*(8), 2887–2900.

Tong, K. I., et al. (2006). Two-site substrate recognition model for the Keap1–Nrf2 system: a hinge and latch mechanism. *Biological Chemistry*, *387*(10, 11), 1311–1320.

Tong, K. I., et al. (2007). Different electrostatic potentials define ETGE and DLG motifs as hinge and latch in oxidative stress response. *Molecular and Cellular Biology*, *27*(21), 7511–7521.

van Muiswinkel, F. L., et al. (2005). The Nrf2-ARE Signalling pathway: promising drug target to combat oxidative stress in neurodegenerative disorders. *Current Drug Targets CNS & Neurological Disorders*, *4*(3), 267–281.

von Otter, M., et al. (2010). Nrf2-encoding NFE2L2 haplotypes influence disease progression but not risk in Alzheimer's disease and age-related cataract. *Mechanisms of Ageing and Development*, *131*(2), 105–110.

Wakabayashi, N., et al. (2004). Protection against electrophile and oxidant stress by induction of the phase 2 response: fate of cysteines of the Keap1 sensor modified by inducers. *Proceedings of the National Academy of Sciences of the United States of America*, *101*(7), 2040–2045.

Wakabayashi, N., et al. (2003). Keap1-null mutation leads to postnatal lethality due to constitutive Nrf2 activation. *Nature Genetics*, *35*(3), 238–245.

Wakabayashi, N., et al. (2010). Regulation of notch1 signaling by nrf2: implications for tissue regeneration. *Science Signaling*, *3*(130), ra52.

Wang, R., et al. (2008a). Hypermethylation of the Keap1 gene in human lung cancer cell lines and lung cancer tissues. *Biochemical and Biophysical Research Communications*, *373*(1), 151–154.

Wang, X. J., et al. (2007). Identification of retinoic acid as an inhibitor of transcription factor Nrf2 through activation of retinoic acid receptor alpha. *Proceedings of the National Academy of Sciences of the United States of America*, *104*(49), 19,589–19,594.

Wang, X. J., et al. (2008b). Nrf2 enhances resistance of cancer cells to chemotherapeutic drugs, the dark side of Nrf2. *Carcinogenesis*, *29*(6), 1235–1243.

Watai, Y., et al. (2007). Subcellular localization and cytoplasmic complex status of endogenous Keap1. *Genes Cells*, *12*(10), 1163–1178.

Williams, T. N. (2006). Human red blood cell polymorphisms and malaria. *Current Opinion in Microbiology*, *9*(4), 388–394.

Wong, T. F., et al. (2011). Association of Keap1 and Nrf2 genetic mutations and polymorphisms With endometrioid endometrial adenocarcinoma survival. *International Journal of Gynecological Cancer*, *21*(8), 1428–1435.

Wu, J. H., et al. (2010). Identification and characterization of novel Nrf2 inducers designed to target the intervening region of Keap1. *Chemical Biology & Drug Design*, *75*(5), 475–480.

Xu, C., et al. (2006). Inhibition of 7,12-dimethylbenz(a)anthracene-induced skin tumorigenesis in C57BL/6 mice by sulforaphane is mediated by nuclear factor E2-related factor 2. *Cancer Research*, *66*(16), 8293–8296.

Yamamoto, T., et al. (2008). Physiological significance of reactive cysteine residues of Keap1 in determining Nrf2 activity. *Molecular and Cellular Biology*, *28*(8), 2758–2770.

Yang, M., et al. (2011). MiR-28 regulates Nrf2 expression through a Keap1-independent mechanism. *Breast Cancer Research and Treatment*, *129*(3), 983–991.

Yang, W., et al. (2007). Paraquat induces dopaminergic dysfunction and proteasome impairment in DJ-1-deficient mice. *Human Molecular Genetics*, *16*(23), 2900–2910.

Yates, M. S., et al. (2009). Genetic versus chemoprotective activation of Nrf2 signaling: overlapping yet distinct gene expression profiles between Keap1 knockout and triterpenoid-treated mice. *Carcinogenesis*, *30*(6), 1024–1031.

Yoh, K., et al. (2001). Nrf2-deficient female mice develop lupus-like autoimmune nephritis. *Kidney International*, *60*(4), 1343–1353.

Yokota, T., et al. (2003). Down regulation of DJ-1 enhances cell death by oxidative stress, ER stress, and proteasome inhibition. *Biochemical and Biophysical Research Communications*, *312*(4), 1342–1348.

Yu, S., et al. (2010). Nrf2 expression is regulated by epigenetic mechanisms in prostate cancer of TRAMP mice. *PLoS One*, *5*(1), e8579.

Yu, Z., et al. (2011). Oltipraz upregulates the nuclear factor (erythroid-derived 2)-like 2 (NRF2) antioxidant system and prevents insulin resistance and obesity induced by a high-fat diet in C57BL/6J mice. *Diabetologia*, *54*(4), 922–934.

Yueh, M. F., et al. (2007). Nrf2–Keap1 signaling pathway regulates human UGT1A1 expression in vitro and in transgenic UGT1 mice. *Journal of Biological Chemistry*, *282*(12), 8749–8758.

Zhang, D. D., et al. (2003). Distinct cysteine residues in Keap1 are required for Keap1-dependent ubiquitination of Nrf2 and for stabilization of Nrf2 by chemopreventive agents and oxidative stress. *Molecular and Cellular Biology*, *23*(22), 8137–8151.

Zhang, D. D., et al. (2004). Keap1 is a redox-regulated substrate adaptor protein for a Cul3-dependent ubiquitin ligase complex. *Molecular and Cellular Biology*, *24*(24), 10941–10953.

Zhang, D. D., et al. (2005). Ubiquitination of Keap1, a BTB-Kelch substrate adaptor protein for Cul3, targets Keap1 for degradation by a proteasome-independent pathway. *Journal of Biological Chemistry*, *280*(34), 30,091–30,099.

Zhang, P., et al. (2010a). Loss of Kelch-like ECH-associated protein 1 function in prostate cancer cells causes chemoresistance and radioresistance and promotes tumor growth. *Molecular Cancer Therapeutics*, *9*(2), 336–346.

Zhang, Y. K., et al. (2010b). Enhanced expression of Nrf2 in mice attenuates the fatty liver produced by a methionine- and choline-deficient diet. *Toxicology and Applied Pharmacology*, *245*(3), 326–334.

Zhao, Z., et al. (2011). Age-related retinopathy in NRF2-deficient mice. *PLoS One*, *6*(4), e19,456.

Zhu, M., et al. (2001). Functional characterization of transcription regulators that interact with the electrophile response element. *Biochemical and Biophysical Research Communications*, *289*(1), 212–219.

Winnie Ng[1], Alexandra R. M. Lobach[1], Xu Zhu[1], Xin Chen[1], Feng Liu[1], Imir G. Metushi[2], Amy Sharma[1], Jinze Li[1,3], Ping Cai[1], Julia Ip[1], Maria Novalen[1], Marija Popovic[1,4], Xiaochu Zhang[1], Tadatoshi Tanino[1,5], Tetsuya Nakagawa[1,6], Yan Li[7], and Jack Uetrecht[1,2]

[1]Department of Pharmaceutical Sciences, Leslie Dan Faculty of Pharmacy, University of Toronto, Toronto, Ontario, Canada
[2]Department of Pharmacology and Toxicology, Faculty of Medicine, University of Toronto, Toronto, Ontario, Canada
[3]Current address: Department of Immunotoxicology, Drug Safety Evaluation, R&D, Bristol-Myers Squibb Company, New Brunswick, New Jersey, USA
[4]Current address: Non-Clinical Safety Assessment, Eli Lilly & Co., Indianapolis, IN, USA
[5]Current address: Faculty of Pharmacy, Kinki University, Osaka, Japan
[6]Current address: Dainippon Sumitomo Pharma Co., Osaka, Japan
[7]Current address: Therapure Biopharma Inc, Mississauga, Ontario, Canada

Animal Models of Idiosyncratic Drug Reactions

Abstract

If we could predict and prevent idiosyncratic drug reactions (IDRs) it would have a profound effect on drug development and therapy. Given our present lack of mechanistic understanding, this goal remains elusive. Hypothesis testing requires valid animal models with characteristics similar to the idiosyncratic reactions that occur in patients. Although it has not been conclusively demonstrated, it appears that almost all IDRs are immune-mediated, and a dominant characteristic is a delay between starting the drug and the onset of the adverse reaction. In contrast, most animal models are acute and therefore involve a different mechanism than idiosyncratic reactions. There are, however, a few animal models such as the nevirapine-induced skin rash in rats that have characteristics very similar to the idiosyncratic reaction that occurs in humans and presumably have a very similar mechanism. These models have allowed testing hypotheses that would be impossible to test in any other way. In addition there are models in which there is a delayed onset of mild hepatic injury that resolves despite

Advances in Pharmacology, Volume 63
1054-3589/12 $35.00
http://dx.doi.org/10.1016/B978-0-12-398339-8.00003-3

continued treatment similar to the "adaptation" reactions that are more common than severe idiosyncratic hepatotoxicity in humans. This probably represents the development of immune tolerance. However, most attempts to develop animal models by stimulating the immune system have been failures. A specific combination of MHC and T cell receptor may be required, but it is likely more complex. Animal studies that determine the requirements for an immune response would provide vital clues about risk factors for IDRs in patients.

I. Introduction

The use and meaning of the term idiosyncratic drug reaction (IDR) is inconsistent. It will be used in this review to designate adverse drug reactions that do not occur in most patients at any dose and do not involve the therapeutic activity of the drug, but until they are better understood, there is no perfect definition. IDRs represent a significant problem; they are often serious, even life threatening, and their unpredictable nature makes them virtually impossible to prevent. They also represent a major problem for drug development. Other issues that would result in the failure of a drug candidate are usually detected early and before a large amount of resources have been invested, but IDR potential is almost always detected late, either late in phase 3 clinical trials or often after the drug has been marketed. Even after a million patients have been treated with a drug there can be controversy as to whether the drug is associated with a significant incidence of serious IDRs. Legal action against the company is not uncommon, and one "bad" drug can lead to the failure of a major pharmaceutical company. Therefore, there are major efforts to predict or detect IDR risk early, but presently no reliable methods exist. It is likely that progress toward better prediction and early detection will depend on a better mechanistic understanding.

Mechanistic studies of IDRs represent a real challenge. Prospective studies in humans to determine the events that preceded the onset of the adverse reaction would be very valuable, but given their unpredictable nature, this is virtually impossible. Animal models are very important for mechanistic studies in all areas of biomedical research because they allow for control of the variables. In fact, as will be demonstrated in the section on the rat model of nevirapine (NVP)-induced skin rash, an animal model is the only way to test what chemical species is responsible for the IDR and to determine the sequence of events leading up to the IDR. However, although animals can also have IDRs, they are also unpredictable in animals, and this hampers the development of practical models. If we had a clear understanding of why it is difficult to develop animal models we would know a lot more about their mechanisms.

A. Risk Factors and Characteristics of IDRs

The general characteristics of IDRs provide important clues to the mechanism of IDRs although not everyone agrees on the interpretation of these characteristics. A major risk factor for a drug causing a relatively high incidence of IDRs is the formation of reactive metabolites. When corrected for dose, there is a correlation between the amount of reactive metabolite formed and IDR risk (Obach et al., 2008; Usui et al., 2009), but there are drugs that form substantial amounts of reactive metabolite and are not associated with a significant risk of IDRs. There are also drugs such as ximelagatran and allopurinol that do not appear to form reactive metabolites and yet do cause IDRs (Uetrecht, 2007).

Specific patient characteristics such as age, female gender, and concomitant viral infection can increase the risk of IDRs to specific drugs, but the increased risk is usually small (Uetrecht, 2007). The strongest patient risk factor for some IDRs is pharmacogenetic (Pirmohamed, 2010). Specific human leukocyte antigen (HLA) genotypes, either major histocompatibility complex (MHC) I or MHC II, are strongly associated with certain drug IDRs. For example, abacavir-induced hypersensitivity is strongly associated with HLA-B*5701 (Martin et al., 2004), and screening patients for this gene prior to starting abacavir treatment is one example in which an IDR can be prevented.

An important characteristic of IDRs is a delay in onset of the IDR, except when a patient has been previously exposed to the drug. There are a few exceptions such as telithromycin-induced liver failure where there are convincing cases of a very rapid reaction on first exposure (Clay et al., 2006), but this is quite unusual. Different types of IDRs have different typical times to onset: simple rashes, 1–2 weeks; generalized hypersensitivity reactions, 2–3 weeks; hepatotoxicity and agranulocytosis 1–2 months; and autoimmune reactions, usually 1 year or more (Uetrecht, 2007). For an animal model to be useful it must involve the same, or at least a very similar, mechanism as the mechanism of the IDR in humans. This will be a theme of this review. If the mechanism is the same, the characteristics should also be the same. Unfortunately, most animal models have different characteristics. For example, most animal models involve acute toxicity rather than having a delay in onset, and some even have very different histology. Conclusions based on invalid models are likely to be misleading. Even if the characteristics are similar it is not proved that the mechanism is the same, and attempts should always be made to take findings from animal models back to IDRs in humans to make sure that they are consistent.

II. Animal Models of Skin Rash

A. Nevirapine

NVP (Viramune) is a non-nucleoside reverse transcriptase inhibitor used to treat human immunodeficiency virus-1 infections. Soon after being marketed, it was found to cause skin rash, including Stevens–Johnson syndrome and toxic epidermal necrolysis, and liver toxicity (Pollard et al., 1998). In early studies the incidence of skin rash was 16% and that of clinically evident hepatotoxicity was 1% (Pollard et al., 1998). However, the incidence is lower at present because patients are started at a lower dose (200mg once daily) for 2 weeks followed by the full dose (200mg twice daily). Female patients are more susceptible to skin rash than males (Wong et al., 2001; Bersoff-Matcha et al., 2001). We found that NVP also causes a skin rash in female Brown Norway (BN) rats with similar characteristics to those in humans (Table I).

1. Characteristics

NVP-induced skin rash in rats is strain- and sex-dependent (Shenton et al., 2003). When female BN rats are fed a diet containing NVP at the dose of 150mg/kg/day, they develop red ears in about 7 days and skin rash in 14–21 days with an incidence of 100% (Shenton et al., 2003). The incidence in female Sprague Dawley rats was only 20%, whereas none of the male rats of either strain developed a rash. However, the blood levels of NVP and its

TABLE I Similar Characteristics of NVP-induced Skin Rash in Humans and Female BN Rats

Characteristic	*Humans*	*BN Rats*
Time to onset	Less than 6 weeks, usually 1–3 weeks (Pollard et al., 1998)	Develop red ears in 7 days and skin lesions in 2–3 weeks
Dose–response	Incidence increases with dose	Incidence increases with dose
Female sex	Increased susceptibility (Wong et al., 2001; Bersoff-Matcha et al., 2001)	Increased susceptibility (Shenton et al., 2003)
NVP plasma levels	~5μg/mL	~20–40μg/mL
Rechallenge	Earlier onset and more severe rash	Earlier onset of red ears (<24h) and skin rash (1 week)
Lead-in dose treatment	A 2-week low dose (200mg/day) followed by the full dose (200mg twice daily) decreased the incidence of rash	A 2-week low dose (40mg/kg/day) followed by the full dose (150mg/kg/day) prevented the rash (Shenton et al., 2003)
$CD4^+$ T cell count	Low $CD4^+$ T cell count is protective (Patel et al., 2004)	Partial depletion of $CD4^+$ T cells delayed the rash (Shenton et al., 2005)
Response of lymphocytes from patients/rats with a rash	T cells produce IFN-γ when stimulated with NVP (Keane et al., 2007)	T cells proliferate and produce IFN-γ when stimulated with NVP (Chen et al., 2009)

12-hydroxy-metabolite, 12-hydroxy-nevirapine (12-OH-NVP), are also lower in Sprague Dawley rats than in female BNs, and if Sprague Dawley rats are cotreated with aminobenzotriazole to inhibit cytochrome P450 (P450), the incidence of skin rash increases. We were not able to produce a rash in mice treated with NVP or its metabolites. The fact that the characteristics of NVP-induced skin rash in female BN rats are similar to that in humans suggests that the mechanisms are similar; therefore, we have used this as an animal model to study IDRs. However, it should be noted that the skin rash in humans can vary from a mild rash that resolves despite continued treatment, to life-threatening toxic epidermal necrolysis; the rash in rats is intermediate in severity between the two extremes in humans.

2. *Involvement of the Adaptive Immune System*

In patients, the faster onset of the reaction on rechallenge and the presence of drug-specific T cells (see Table I) provide clear evidence of an immune reaction. In addition, NVP-induced skin rash is also reported to be associated with specific HLA genotypes including the MHC II allele HLA-DRB1*01 (Vitezica et al., 2008) and HLA-DRB1*0101 (Martin et al., 2005), as well as the MHC I allele HLA-Cw8 (Gatanaga et al., 2007). These associations suggest involvement of the adaptive immune system. A toxicogenomics study also suggested that the genetic predisposition to NVP-induced IDRs varies between different ethnic groups (Yuan et al., 2011).

Studies in the animal model provide overwhelming evidence of an immune-mediated mechanism. First, histology of skin sections revealed the existence of an inflammatory cell infiltration, primarily T cells and macrophages (Shenton et al., 2003). The rash could be prevented with an antibody to deplete $CD4^+$ T cells, but depletion of $CD8^+$ T cells actually seemed to make it worse. A time course study determined the sequence of these immunological events: before the onset of rash there is an upregulation of adhesion molecules (inter-cellular adhesion molecule-1 and MHC II) and an infiltration of macrophages, with a later appearance of T cells concurrent with the onset of the rash (Popovic et al., 2006). As mentioned above, when rats with a skin rash were allowed to recover by discontinuing NVP treatment, rechallenge with NVP led to a more rapid onset of the reaction, with red ears appearing in less than 24h and skin lesions in about 1 week (Shenton et al., 2003). This suggests an amnestic immune response. Moreover, this sensitivity can be transferred to naïve animals with splenocytes or just splenic $CD4^+$ T cells from rechallenged animals, and the onset of the reaction for these naïve recipients followed the same time course as NVP-rechallenged animals (Shenton et al., 2003). We also found that $CD4^+$ T cells from the auricular lymph nodes of rechallenged animals responded to the parent drug by proliferating and releasing cytokines, such as interferon-gamma (INF-γ) and interleukin-10 (IL-10), and a similar response was found with lymphocytes from patients with a history of NVP-induced skin rash. This further indicates the involvement of the adaptive immune system and $CD4^+$ T cells in mediating the rash as well as the similarity between the rash in rats and humans (Chen et al., 2009). Pretreatment with immunosuppressants, such as cyclosporine and tacrolimus, prevented NVP-induced skin rash in rats and also led to resolution of the rash during NVP treatment, further supporting an immune mechanism (Shenton et al., 2005).

As in humans, 2 weeks of treatment with a lower NVP dose prevented the skin rash; however, cotreatment with aminobenzotriazole, an inhibitor of P450, prevented tolerance. This indicates that this tolerance primarily involved induction of P450 rather than immune tolerance (Shenton et al., 2005). Even though the rash is immune-mediated, pretreatment with poly-inosine-polycytidylic acid (poly (I:C)), a synthetic polymer of inosine and cytosine that strongly stimulates antigen presenting cells through toll-like receptor 3, did not make the animals more sensitive to the rash (the dose–response curve was not shifted to the left) or increase the severity of the rash (Shenton et al., 2005). Although poly (I:C) can inhibit P450 and this could be a confounding factor, it also did not decrease the incidence or severity of the rash.

3. *Chemical Species Responsible*

One fundamental question is whether an IDR is caused by the parent drug or a reactive metabolite. There are several potential reactive metabolites of NVP. A metabolic study in BN rats showed that hydroxylation at the 12 position of NVP to form 12-OH-NVP is required to induce the skin rash (Chen et al., 2008). Specifically, treatment with the 12-OH-NVP metabolite caused a rash at a lower dose. Substitution of the methyl hydrogen atoms at the 12 position of NVP with deuterium decreased the rate of 12-hydroxylation and lead to a decreased incidence of the skin rash; however, paradoxically, it also led to lower levels of NVP. It was discovered that this is because oxidation of the methyl group also leads directly to a reactive quinone methide which inhibits P450. Direct inhibition of P450 by aminobenzotriazole cotreatment lead to a rash at a lower dose of NVP and inhibited most metabolic pathways with the potential to form reactive metabolites except for the production of 12-OH-NVP. Cotreatment of NVP or deuterated NVP with aminobenzotriazole led to similar plasma levels of NVP and the deuterated analog, but the rats treated with deuterated NVP still had lower levels of 12-OH-NVP and a marked decrease in the incidence of rash (Chen et al., 2008). This demonstrates that the 12-OH-NVP pathway is responsible for inducing the rash; however, 12-OH-NVP is not chemically reactive and so it seemed likely that it would not be the species directly responsible for the rash. The quinone methide metabolite is quite reactive, but it cannot be formed by oxidation of 12-OH-NVP because they are at the same oxidation state. On the other hand, 12-OH-NVP can be further metabolized to a benzylic sulfate, which has been detected in the serum of rats treated with NVP.

When the sulfate was injected into rats it was rapidly hydrolyzed back to 12-OH-NVP so its involvement in causing the rash could not be tested in this manner. Although this benzylic sulfate is less reactive than we expected, it does covalently bind to skin proteins *in vitro* (Sharma & Uetrecht, 2011), and covalent binding was detected in the epidermis of NVP-treated animals (Sharma, A., unpublished observation). Cotreatment with salicylamide led to decreased blood levels of the sulfate metabolite, but it did not prevent the rash (Novalen, M., unpublished observation). However, salicylamide works by depleting the cofactor 3′-phosphoadenosine-5′-phosphosulfate, and turnover of salicylamide in the skin is likely to be low; therefore, its effect is probably limited to the liver. Topical treatment with 1-phenyl-1-hexanol, a sulfotransferase inhibitor, prevented the rash where it was applied, which implies that it is local production of the benzylic sulfate in the skin that is responsible for the rash (Sharma, A., unpublished observation). There is a report that 12-mesyloxy-NVP, a synthetic 12-sulfate-NVP surrogate, can form conjugates with glutathione, amino acids, DNA, and hemoglobin (Antunes et al., 2010a,b, 2008). This finding is irrelevant because the mesylate is far more reactive than the sulfate and it is not formed in biological systems.

4. Testing the Danger and Pharmacological Interaction Hypotheses

Another question is how this IDR is initiated, which is virtually impossible to study in humans. There are three major hypotheses explaining the initial steps of IDRs: the hapten hypothesis, the danger hypothesis, and the pharmacological interaction hypothesis. The finding that the sulfate binds to skin proteins is consistent with the hapten hypothesis. We also found that treatment of BN rats led to early changes in gene expression in the skin (at 6 hours) that are consistent with the danger hypothesis, and there were many more gene changes after treatment with 12-OH-NVP than with NVP (442 versus 43 statistically significant changes with an increase of greater than 2-fold), which again points to the involvement of this pathway (Zhang, X., unpublished observation). There were also far more changes in gene expression in the skin than in the liver even though we have detected significantly more covalent binding in the liver than in the skin. As for the pharmacological interaction hypothesis, the fact that T cells from a sensitized animal responded to incubation with NVP with production of cytokines implies that the rash was induced by NVP rather than a metabolite. Although this finding seems consistent with the pharmacological interaction hypothesis, we already know that the induction of rash depends on 12-hydroxylation. Furthermore, T cells from animals in which the rash was induced by treatment with 12-OH-NVP also responded better to NVP than to 12-OH-NVP, even though these animals had never been exposed to NVP. Clearly there is a disconnect between what induces the skin rash and what T cells from the affected animal respond to; therefore, the specificity of the

T cells cannot be used to infer what induced the IDR. The assumption that what causes the immune response is the same as what the T cells respond to forms the basis for the pharmacological interaction hypothesis. This assumption is false and it is only with an animal model that this could be tested.

NVP-induced skin rash in rats, one of the very few animal models with characteristics similar to the IDR that occurs in humans, has allowed testing of several hypotheses that could not be tested in humans. We will continue to use this animal model to study the sequence of events that lead to the immune response that ultimately causes an IDR. It appears that both hapten formation and the induction of a danger signal are involved, but there are probably many factors that make this drug so effective in inducing an immune response and many details remain to be studied.

III. Animal Models of Liver Toxicity

A. Acetaminophen

Acetaminophen (4-hydroxyacetanilide) is widely used as an analgesic/ antipyretic. It is relatively safe when used at therapeutic doses; however, in overdoses it can lead to acute liver failure, which is characterized by centrilobular hepatic necrosis, both in humans and animals (Mitchell et al., 1973). Although the mechanistic details of how acetaminophen leads to drug-induced liver injury (DILI) are incomplete, it does not have the classical characteristics of most idiosyncratic DILI such as a delay of 1 week or more from the initiation of treatment to the onset of liver injury. Despite the fact that acetaminophen-induced DILI in mice is a model of direct hepatotoxicity, but not a good model of idiosyncratic DILI, it has been extensively studied and provides important clues to how drugs can cause liver injury. This is important because there are no good animal models of idiosyncratic DILI, and mild direct liver injury may be one of the first steps in the initiation of idiosyncratic DILI.

The hepatotoxic effects of acetaminophen have been attributed to its electrophilic intermediate N-acetyl-*p*-benzoquinoneimine (Dahlin et al., 1984), which is generated by hepatic P450. At therapeutic doses of acetaminophen, this reactive metabolite is detoxified by conjugation with glutathione, but with an overdose, the formation of the reactive species exceeds the detoxification capacity of glutathione and this results in N-acetyl-*p*-benzoquinoneimine forming protein adducts.

1. Involvement of the Innate Immune System

In early studies, cell death correlated with covalent binding (Jollow et al., 1973); however, it is more complex because covalent binding of the meta isomer (3-hydroxyacetanilide) is similar to that of acetaminophen, but it does not cause acute liver toxicity. The difference in toxicity between the isomers appears to be due to the fact that acetaminophen targets mitochondria (Myers et al., 1995). It also appears that the innate immune system plays a role in the toxicity of acetaminophen. Kupffer cells, natural killer (NK)/natural killer T (NKT) cells, neutrophils, and inflammatory cytokines have all been implicated in acetaminophen-induced liver injury as reviewed elsewhere (Jaeschke et al., 2011). Kupffer cells appear to have a protective role because their depletion exacerbated acetaminophen hepatotoxicity (Ju et al., 2002), and more recently a similar effect was found by depleting dendritic cells (Connolly et al., 2011). In addition, involvement of the immune system is supported by the use of various knockout mice such as interleukin-6 (IL-6) (Masubuchi et al., 2003), IL-10 (Bourdi et al., 2002), and cyclooxygenase-2 (Reilly et al., 2001). The overall conclusion from these studies is that the innate immune system appears to play a protective role in this model of DILI.

B. Halothane

Halothane is a volatile anesthetic that can cause DILI. Up to 20% of patients will have a mild, asymptomatic increase in alanine transaminase (ALT), and from 1 in 6000 to 35,000 develop fulminant liver failure often resulting in death (Kharasch, 2008). Mild halothane-induced liver injury is much more common; it occurs within hours of exposure and presumably represents direct cytotoxicity (Kharasch, 2008). Severe toxicity usually occurs after multiple exposures and is typically delayed. Characteristics include jaundice, markedly elevated serum transaminase levels and fever (Eghtesadi-Araghi, 2008). Histologically, severe halothane liver injury manifests primarily as extensive necrosis, occasionally with a centrilobular pattern and sometimes the cellular infiltrate contains eosinophils (Zimmerman, 1999). The fact that multiple exposures are a major risk factor for halothane hepatitis suggests immune sensitization. In the less common cases in which liver failure occurred after a single exposure to halothane, failure occurred later with an average delay of 12 days, a time when the halothane was long gone but immunogenic protein adducts would likely still be present. Along with the clinical presentation of eosinophilia, fever, and delayed onset, the presence of anti-drug and autoantibodies provide strong evidence that idiosyncratic halothane-induced DILI is immune-mediated (Eghtesadi-Araghi, 2008).

1. Early Animal Models

Early attempts to develop an animal model of halothane-induced DILI led to models with notably different characteristics from that which occurs in humans. Specifically, the toxicity was mild and required hypoxia and pretreatment with P450 inducers such as Aroclor 1254 (Sipes & Brown,

1976; Reynolds & Moslen, 1977). In addition, the toxicity appeared to be due to a reductive pathway with loss of bromide to form a free radical. This is in contrast to oxidation being the major metabolic pathway for halothane, and studies in humans found that the immune response is to the oxidative reactive metabolite.

2. Involvement of the Trifluoroacetyl Chloride Metabolite

Halothane is metabolized extensively in hepatocytes by CYP 2E1 and, to a lesser extent, via CYP 2A6 to form trifluoroacetyl chloride, which is chemically reactive and forms trifluoroacetyl adducts with proteins. Treatment of guinea pigs with halothane leads to hepatic injury, which likely represents a direct cytotoxicity resulting from trifluoroacetyl adduct formation because it occurs early following exposure. Metabolism of halothane to trifluoroacetyl chloride is necessary for hepatotoxicity to occur, and trifluoroacetylated adducts have been identified in liver biopsies from halothane-treated humans and guinea pigs (You et al., 2010). The injury correlated with the levels of trifluoroacetyl protein adducts in outbred guinea pigs, which also implies that covalent binding is responsible for the hepatic injury (Bourdi et al., 2001).

3. Guinea Pig Model

The advantage of the guinea pig model is that no pretreatments or preconditioning of the animals are required and with chronic treatment an adaptive immune response is generated; however, damage to the liver is transient and ALT levels return to normal despite continued treatment. Antibodies in guinea pigs specific to trifluoroacetyl protein adducts have been detected after both primary and secondary exposure to halothane; however, antibody titers upon re-exposure were no greater than primary exposure (Chen & Gandolfi, 1997). Specific antibodies directed against trifluoroacetyl protein adducts were detected in humans that have also been identified in guinea pigs treated with a single dose of halothane (Chen & Gandolfi, 1997). The presence of these antibodies in humans correlates with an increased incidence of liver toxicity, and Bourdi et al. found that trifluoroacetyl protein adducts are released into the blood stream from damaged hepatocytes where they may interact with immune cells and stimulate an immune response (Bourdi et al., 2001). The major interaction with immune cells, particularly at the initial stages of toxicity, likely occurs in the liver, and Furst et al. have shown that halothane-induced liver injury is associated with a cellular immune response in the guinea pig (Furst et al., 1997). It is likely that the innate immune system plays a key role in the early stages of halothane-induced DILI, and it is the individual's ability to develop tolerance to the drug-modified proteins that determines the ultimate degree of toxicity. Therefore, the guinea pig model may represent the initial stages of the immune response in milder or direct halothane hepatotoxicity. Attempts to increase the adaptive immune response by immunization with trifluoroacetylated protein combined with Freund's adjuvant in the guinea pig led to an increase in antibody titers; however, the increase in ALT was mild and did not increase with subsequent exposures (Hastings et al., 1995).

4. *Mouse Models*

Recently, a murine model of halothane liver injury has been developed in BALB/c mice, representing involvement of the innate immune system, where ALT levels can reach up to 1200U/L versus <500U/L for the guinea pig. Using this model You et al. found that all strains tested had similar degrees of covalent binding, and the strain-dependent susceptibility to halothane-induced liver injury appeared to be due to variations in the innate immune response (You et al., 2006). You et al. have shown that halothane-induced hepatic neutrophil infiltration was most pronounced in the BALB/c mouse versus all other species of mice tested, and depletion of neutrophils prevented an increase in ALT by approximately 90% (You et al., 2006). In the same study, it was shown that the number of infiltrating neutrophils in the liver correlated with the degree of liver damage in each of the BALB/c, DBA/1, and C57BL/6 strains of mice tested (You et al., 2006). Yet, histology in the BALB/c mouse model displayed minimal hepatic necrosis and ALT levels resolved quickly. In addition, neutrophils are not prominent in the histology of halothane-induced DILI in humans. Therefore, this model is unlikely to represent the mechanism of halothane-induced DILI in humans. This model has been able to demonstrate involvement of various innate immune cells, but it does not reproduce the severe idiosyncratic toxicity mediated by the adaptive immune system that occurs in humans. It is possible that the adaptive response is initiated by the innate immune system and further work is required to determine if this is true.

CD1d –/– mice are deficient in NKT cells, which play a role in the regulation of neutrophil recruitment to the liver (Diao et al., 2004). Recruitment of neutrophils has been suggested to occur through the release of osteopontin or via production of interleukin-17 (IL-17), a pro-inflammatory cytokine involved in autoimmune responses (Diao et al., 2004; Ruddy et al., 2004). Halothane-treated female CD1d –/– mice on a BALB/c background demonstrated that NKT cells play a role in recruiting neutrophils to the liver in acute halothane-induced liver injury (Cheng et al., 2010). These mice also had 20-fold lower ALT values than their normal BALB/c counterparts when given halothane. It was determined that it is the direct depletion of NKT cells that leads to prevention of halothane-induced DILI rather than loss of cross-talk between NKT cells and other cells of the immune system, a surprising result considering the extensive communication that occurs within the immune system (Cheng et al., 2010). Additional examination of the role of IL-17 in the BALB/c halothane model found that neutralization of IL-17 led to suppression of halothane hepatotoxicity, with significant diminution of ALT and aspartate aminotransferase levels (Kobayashi et al., 2009). Conversely, a single intraperitoneal injection of 1μg of recombinant IL-17 one hour before halothane administration induced significant elevations of these aminotransferases. Differences in IL-17 levels were compared between BALB/c and C57BL/6 mice, and it was found that IL-17 levels were increased upon administration of halothane in BALB/c but not C57BL/6 mice, indicating a role for IL-17 in strain-dependent halothane-induced hepatotoxicity (Kobayashi et al., 2009).

Most recently, immunization of mice with trifluoroacetyl conjugated mouse serum albumin in addition to concurrent administration of the combined CD40/TLR agonist as adjuvant was able to induce trifluoroacetyl-specific and carrier protein independent T cell responses (You et al., 2010). Trifluoroacetyl-specific immune responses were found to occur in the spleen and liver, and BALB/c mice were again shown to be the most sensitive strain. Cells isolated from control mice immunized with albumin combined with complete and/or incomplete Freund's adjuvant did not respond to any form of the antigen upon re-exposure *ex vivo*. It remains to be histologically determined if immunization in addition to halothane exposure results in pronounced liver tissue injury similar to the massive necrosis observed in some humans (You et al., 2010).

While the guinea pig and BALB/c mouse models develop halothane-induced DILI, no animal model has been able to accurately duplicate the characteristics of the DILI that occurs in humans. As with other models such as the amodiaquine model described below, it may be immune tolerance that limits the delayed onset liver damage.

C. Isoniazid

Due to its efficacy, isoniazid (INH) remains a first line drug in the treatment of *Mycobacterium tuberculosis*. INH use is associated with a significant incidence of liver injury that can vary in severity from mild, reversible increases in transaminase levels (up to 20% of patients) to overt hepatic failure (Maddrey & Boitnott, 1973). The mechanism of INH-induced hepatotoxicity has been considered to be metabolic idiosyncrasy; however, this term is vague and there are no examples where polymorphisms in a metabolic pathway that are sufficient to explain the idiosyncratic nature of any idiosyncratic liver toxicity, including that due to INH.

1. The Role of the Adaptive Immune System in INH-induced Hepatotoxicity

The classification of INH-induced DILI as metabolic idiosyncrasy is based in part on the fact that it usually does not occur more rapidly upon rechallenge, which is a typical characteristic of an immune-mediated reaction. Although this is the most common response to rechallenge, there are many cases in which rechallenge in more severe cases of INH-induced hepatotoxicity did lead to a much quicker onset of toxicity, and this was paired with features such as fever, rash and/or eosinophilia that suggest an immune-mediated reaction. In addition, there are several reports in which patients with a history of INH-induced liver toxicity had a positive lymphocyte transformation test, which is another clear indication of an immune-mediated reaction. In particular, Warrington et al. showed that patients who had mild INH-induced DILI had a positive but transient lymphocyte transformation test, and it was only positive when their lymphocytes were incubated with human serum albumin modified with INH, but not with INH itself. In contrast, in patients with more severe INH-induced DILI, the positive lymphocyte transformation test was persistent and was also positive when their lymphocytes were incubated with INH alone (Warrington et al., 1978, 1982). This suggests that INH-induced DILI is caused by an immune response to INH-modified proteins, but in most cases this resolves with immune tolerance, which eliminates memory T cells. In the severe cases, the immune response to INH-modified proteins spreads to the parent drug, a process known as epitope spreading, and it does not resolve with immune tolerance, thereby leaving memory T cells that result in a persistent positive lymphocyte transformation test. This is reminiscent of the response of T cells to NVP in the NVP-induced skin rash in rats discussed earlier. In preliminary experiments we also found a significant increase in peripheral T helper 17 (Th17) cells in patients with a small INH-induced ALT increase, which is additional evidence that INH-induced DILI is immune-mediated (Zhu, X., unpublished observation).

2. *Rat and Rabbit Models: Involvement of Hydrazine and Acetylhydrazine*

Previously, the hepatotoxic effect of INH was attributed to two metabolites: acetylhydrazine (Nelson et al., 1976) and hydrazine (Sarich et al., 1996). As reviewed elsewhere, the characteristics of previous animal models that implicated acetylhydrazine and hydrazine as the hepatotoxic species were very different from those of INH-induced DILI in humans (Metushi et al., 2011). The typical clinical picture of INH-induced DILI includes a long delay in onset (at least 1 week, but more commonly 1–3 months), which in most cases resolves despite continued treatment (Maddrey & Boitnott, 1973). In most previous animal models, rats were treated with high doses of INH leading to acute hepatotoxicity. It was concluded that acetylhydrazine was the hepatotoxin because it covalently bound to liver proteins, while no binding of INH was detected, and the binding of acetylhydrazine correlated with the degree of hepatotoxicity (Mitchell et al., 1976). In contrast, when rabbits were treated with high doses of INH, hydrazine appeared to be the hepatotoxic species (Sarich et al., 1996) because toxicity correlated with hydrazine blood levels but not acetylhydrazine or INH levels. Additionally, pretreatment with an amidase inhibitor, which blocks hydrolysis of

INH to form hydrazine, decreased liver damage (Sarich et al., 1999). However, neither of these animal models displayed the delay in onset that is characteristic of INH-induced DILI in humans, and the pathology in the rabbit model included steatosis, which is uncommon in human cases.

3. *Interference with the ALT Assay by INH*

There are two reports in which treatment of male Wistar rats with relatively low doses of INH (50mg/kg/day) resulted in an increase in ALT by week 2, and this increase in ALT was potentiated by cotreatment with rifampin (Tasduq et al., 2007; Sodhi et al., 1997). We have tried to reproduce these results but have been unsuccessful (Metushi, I. G., and Cai, P., unpublished observation). We also treated rats with INH alone at doses up to three times higher (150mg/kg/day for up to 4 weeks), but ALT did not increase. In addition, we found that the ALT assay is, in fact, inhibited by INH (Fig. 1); therefore, it is surprising that an increase in ALT was detected in the previous studies. The observation that INH-induced depletion of pyridoxal phosphate inhibits the ALT assay had been previously reported (O'Brien et al., 2002). This is less of a problem in humans because the dose per kg is lower, and patients are usually treated with vitamin B6, the precursor to pyridoxal phosphate, to prevent neurotoxicity, which is also caused by depletion of pyridoxal phosphate by INH.

4. *Mouse Model and Direct Bioactivation of INH*

More recently we have shown that INH itself can be bioactivated and covalently bound to liver macromolecules in mice (Metushi et al., 2011). There is significantly more covalent binding in the livers of mice than in rats; therefore, the rat may be a poor choice to develop an animal model (Metushi, I. G., unpublished observation). We have tried to induce an immune response against INH by adapting a similar strategy to that used by Lohse to induce autoimmune hepatitis (Lohse et al., 1990). In this model, mice were immunized with a 100,000*g* supernatant of syngeneic liver homogenate (S-100) in complete Freund's adjuvant. This immunization led to experimental autoimmune hepatitis with a maximum of grade 3 inflammatory lesions, which persisted for up to 6 months. We repeated this procedure by immunizing mice with S-100, and in another set of animals we took it one step further by immunizing mice with S-100 modified with INH, followed by oral treatment with INH. This strategy is also similar to that used by Hastings where he unsuccessfully tried to develop an animal model of halothane-induced hepatitis by prior immunization with protein that had been modified with the reactive metabolite as described in a previous section. Not only did the combination of immunization of animals with INH-modified S-100 protein plus INH treatment not lead to serious DILI, but to our surprise, INH treatment prevented the induction of autoimmune hepatitis (Metushi, I. G., unpublished observation). The mechanism of this

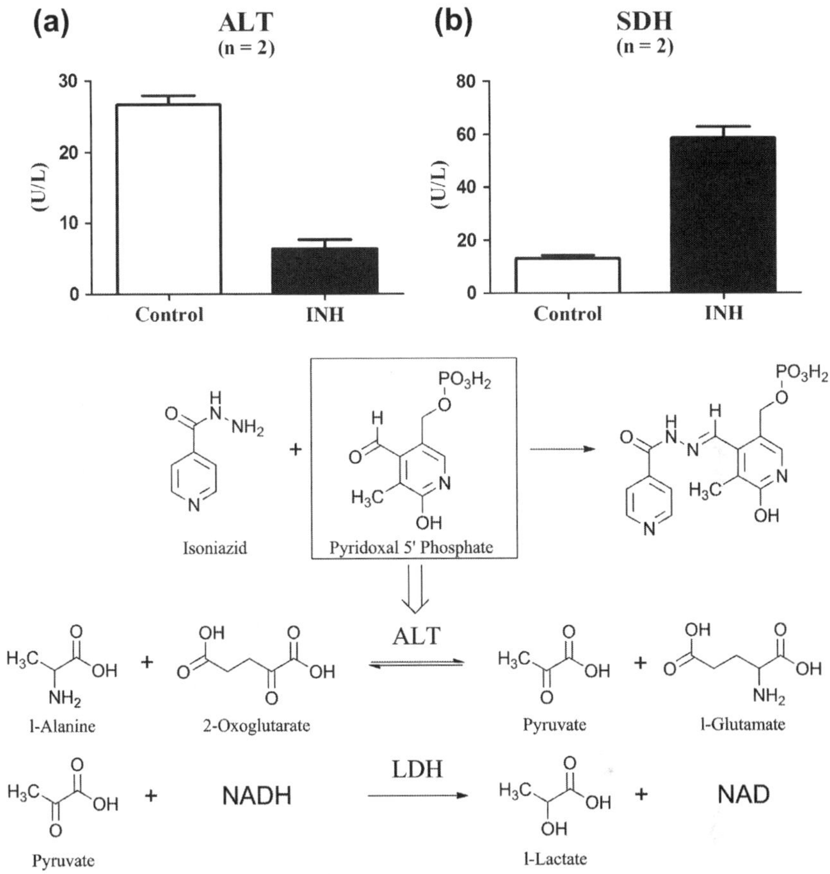

FIGURE 1 **Inhibition of the ALT assay by INH.** Male BN rats were given high doses of INH (400mg/kg/day for up to 7 days) to induce liver injury. The measured ALT was actually decreased by INH treatment when compared to untreated controls (a). In contrast, sorbitol dehydrogenase (SDH), another biomarker of liver injury, was clearly elevated in the same sera (b). The chemistry of the ALT assay and reaction of INH with pyridoxal phosphate, the cofactor for the assay, is illustrated in the lower panel.

inhibition of autoimmunity is unknown, especially because INH can induce a lupus-like autoimmune syndrome, but it again suggests that the dominant response to INH and other drugs that can cause idiosyncratic DILI is immune tolerance.

In animals, we found that chronic treatment of C57BL/6 mice with INH did not result in elevated liver enzyme levels, as measured by the glutamate dehydrogenase assay, but treating the ubiquitin-ligase knockout Cbl-b strain did result in a delayed onset mild increase in glutamate dehydrogenase (Metushi, I. G., unpublished observation). The Cbl-b knockout mice are on a C57BL/6 background and appear phenotypically normal but have impaired immune tolerance. In preliminary experiments we saw that the Cbl-b knockout mouse with the highest glutamate dehydrogenase level had a greater number and activation of cells staining positive for the macrophage marker F4/80 (Fig. 2). This suggests that macrophage activation is important for the induction of liver damage by INH.

Altogether this data suggests, as we have previously argued, that INH-induced DILI is immune-mediated, but the most common response is immune tolerance, and it is only when this fails that severe liver injury results (Metushi et al., 2011). With animals we have also shown that in addition to acetylhydrazine and hydrazine, INH is also bioactivated and covalently binds to liver proteins.

D. Amodiaquine

Amodiaquine, a 4-aminoquinoline derivative used to treat malaria, is associated with agranulocytosis and hepatotoxicity, which led to its withdrawal from the market in the USA. Clinical characteristics of amodiaquine-induced hepatitis include a delay (weeks to months) in the onset of clinical symptoms, and the presence of anti-drug immunoglobulin G (IgG) antibodies. There is usually prompt recovery upon discontinuation of treatment, but a rapid increase in serum ALT on rechallenge with amodiaquine, which is consistent with an immune-mediated reaction (Neftel et al., 1986; Uetrecht, 2005). Intriguingly, many patients simultaneously develop agranulocytosis and hepatitis (Neftel et al., 1986).

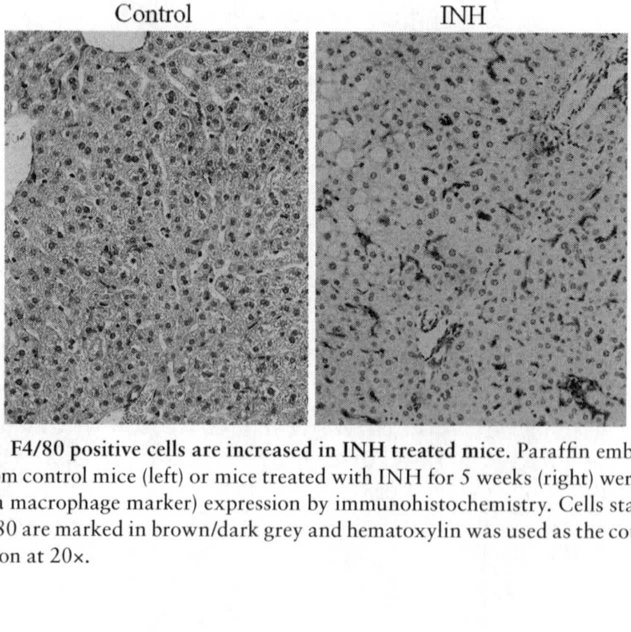

FIGURE 2 **F4/80 positive cells are increased in INH treated mice.** Paraffin embedded liver sections from control mice (left) or mice treated with INH for 5 weeks (right) were evaluated for F4/80 (a macrophage marker) expression by immunohistochemistry. Cells staining positive for F4/80 are marked in brown/dark grey and hematoxylin was used as the counter stain; magnification at 20×.

1. Rodent Models

Amodiaquine is metabolized both in the liver and by neutrophils to a reactive iminoquinone metabolite (Harrison et al., 1992), which can react with endogenous molecules and act as a hapten to trigger an immune response (Christie et al., 1989). A study of amodiaquine in rats found an elevation of serum ALT and anti-amodiaquine antibodies after treatment at a daily dose of 191mg/kg for 4 days; however, there were no histological changes in the liver (Clarke et al., 1990). In another study, a single dose of amodiaquine (180mg/kg) did not cause any liver injury in mice, but cotreatment with a glutathione synthesis inhibitor, L-buthionine-*S*,*R*-sulfoximine, induced centrilobular necrosis 6h post dose (Shimizu et al., 2009). However, this is very different from the delayed onset hepatotoxicity observed in humans. We selected a more clinically relevant dose of 62.5mg/kg/day for rats and 150–200mg/kg/day for mice. We observed a mild elevation (2–3-fold increase) in serum ALT in both mice and rats after 2–3 weeks, which was followed by adaptation during which the serum ALT almost returned to basal levels despite continuation of treatment for up to 6 weeks (Fig. 3; Cai & Uetrecht, 2009). Also, rats tested positive for anti-amodiaquine antibodies by week 1 when serum ALT was still normal, and the antibody titer remained high during continuous treatment and recovery. The liver histology in rats demonstrated individually scattered activated Kupffer cells and Kupffer cell microgranulomas, as well as necrosis and apoptosis of individual hepatocytes,

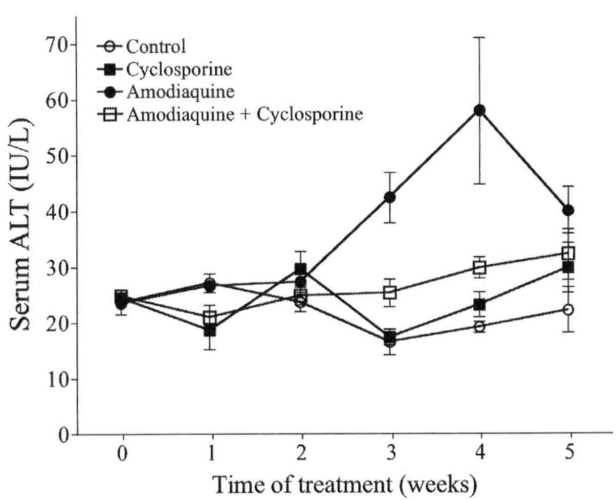

FIGURE 3 **Serum ALT during the treatment of BN rats with amodiaquine** Male BN rats were treated with amodiaquine alone (62.5mg/kg/day, $n=4$) or cyclosporine A alone (20mg/kg/day, $n=3$) or cotreatment ($n=4$) of amodiaquine (62.5mg/kg/day) and cyclosporine A (20mg/kg/day) for 5 weeks. A group of untreated rats acted as the control ($n=3$). The data represent the mean *± standard deviation.

but no frank necrosis, which is consistent with the mild increases in ALT. Paradoxically, in contrast to the acute model described above, buthionine sulfoximine appeared to be protective in this delayed onset model (Cai et al., 2011).

2. *Involvement of the Adaptive Immune System*

The clinical characteristics and the presence of anti-drug antibodies in both humans and animals suggest that amodiaquine-induced DILI is immune-mediated. In addition, cotreatment of rats with cyclosporine A appeared to delay the onset and decrease the magnitude of serum ALT elevation (Cai et al., 2011), which is also consistent with an immune mechanism. Therefore, we performed studies to determine the immune response to amodiaquine in animals that developed an increase in ALT. There were significant phenotypic changes in splenocytes (i.e. increase of relative number of $CD4^+$ T cells, and activation of macrophages and B cells) in rats treated with amodiaquine for 6 weeks. There was also a good correlation between serum levels of ALT and monocyte chemotactic protein-1 (Li et al., 2011b), and a change of immunological environment in the liver as evident in differential expression of genes related to immune functions (i.e. CD3e and CD4; Li et al., 2011a) as well as a mild infiltration of lymphocytes (i.e. total $CD4^+$ T cells, NK cells, and Th17 cells; Liu et al., 2011). This highlights an important role of the immune system in this model.

Although amodiaquine-induced DILI appears to be immune-mediated, amodiaquine also appears to cause direct cytotoxicity that precedes the increase in ALT by weeks, and this may be important for the initiation of an immune response. In particular, there was a significant increase in serum high-mobility group box 1, six hours after the first dose of amodiaquine (Li et al., 2011a). This protein is known to act as a danger signal that is released by cellular damage and activates macrophages via binding to toll-like receptor 4 (Li & Uetrecht, 2010; Scaffidi et al., 2002). This direct cell injury may be involved in the induction of an immune response (Fig. 4).

3. *Immune Tolerance*

The observation that the increase in ALT in both mice and rats treated with amodiaquine resolved despite continued treatment is similar to the pattern observed in humans with drugs that cause idiosyncratic DILI. In humans this is referred to as adaptation and is much more common than severe DILI. If the delayed onset increase in ALT induced by amodiaquine is immune-mediated, then almost certainly this adaptation represents immune tolerance. Consistent with this hypothesis we observed a 3-fold increase in IL-10 liver mRNA 7 days after the start of amodiaquine treatment in rats (Li et al., 2011a). IL-10 is a cytokine produced by T regulatory cells, which play an important role in immune tolerance (Langier et al., 2010; Shevach et al., 2001).

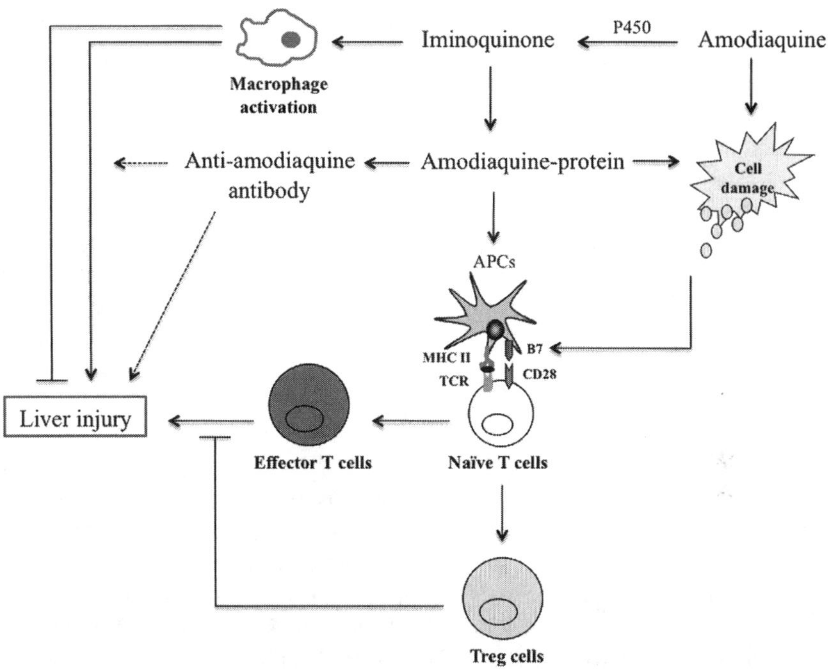

FIGURE 4 Hypothesized mechanism for amodiaquine (AMQ)-induced liver injury.

In short, although we have not yet been able to develop an animal model of severe amodiaquine-induced DILI, we have found that it causes a delayed onset of mild DILI in both rats and mice that appears to be immune-mediated and resolves with what appears to be immune tolerance. Therefore, this may be an excellent model to study the phenomena of adaptation; it is only when adaptation fails that severe liver injury results.

E. Nevirapine

As described in the NVP-induced skin rash section, NVP is a non-nucleoside reverse transcriptase inhibitor used in the treatment of human immunodeficiency virus-1 infections, but it is associated with a relatively high incidence of rash and liver toxicity. The incidence of NVP-induced ALT elevation is 8–18% and usually occurs within the first 6 weeks of treatment (MacGregor & Hall, 2007). Most cases resolve when the drug is stopped, but it can lead to liver failure and death. Clinical characteristics of NVP liver injury include fever, myalgia, fatigue, malaise, nausea, and vomiting (Dieterich et al., 2004), and up to 50% of patients present with concurrent rash (Dieterich et al., 2004). While alcohol, low body mass index, and viral hepatitis co-infection are established risk factors for NVP liver toxicity, female gender and high pre-therapy $CD4^+$ T cell counts (≥250mm^3 for women and ≥400mm^3 for men) appear to be risk factors, but this has not been a consistent finding (Chu et al., 2010). Yuan et al. found an association between the presence of the HLA-DRB*01 allele and NVP hepatotoxicity with ethnicity playing a role due to allelic frequencies (Yuan et al., 2011). Although not universally accepted, these characteristics suggest that this is an immune-mediated IDR.

Our attempts to create a model for NVP-induced liver injury in rats have been unsuccessful. BN rats treated with NVP that developed a skin rash had an increase in liver weight and unusual inclusion bodies, but they did not have an increase in ALT or histologic evidence of hepatic necrosis (Shenton et al., 2003). The observed changes are presumably related to the induction of P450, which also occurs in humans.

1. Liver Injury in Mice

Metabolism of NVP in all mice strains tested was very rapid and plasma levels of the parent drug and metabolites were significantly lower than in rats (Sharma, A., unpublished observation). Studies performed in BALB/c, C57BL/6, and in ubiquitin-ligase knockout Cbl-b mice resulted in an ALT increase to ≥100U/L in C57BL/6 and Cbl-b knockout mice at approximately 2–3 weeks after initiation of NVP treatment; however, the histology in the Cbl-b knockout mice was not typical of the hepatic necrosis observed in humans. Specifically, in Cbl-b knockout mice with the highest ALT levels (200–400U/L), there were isolated areas of complete necrosis surrounded by inflammatory cells, while the rest of the liver looked normal. Where the necrotic areas were close to the surface of the liver there was a thin layer of normal cells and this suggests that the necrosis was caused by ischemia, and the cells near the surface of the liver were preserved because of diffusion of oxygen and nutrients through the liver capsule (Sharma, A., unpublished observation). This does not appear to be a good animal model of idiosyncratic DILI; however, we are continuing to try to develop an animal model of NVP-induced DILI in C57BL/6 mice. This strain shows milder toxicity with an increase in ALT after approximately 3 weeks of treatment, which resolves over time. Areas of focal inflammatory lesions were observed in these mice at the time of peak ALT levels (Sharma, A., unpublished observation). This may be a model of immune tolerance similar to amodiaquine-induced liver injury in rodents, as discussed previously.

F. Penicillamine

As outlined in the section on autoimmunity, treatment with D-penicillamine is associated with a high incidence of a wide variety of adverse effects. The most common adverse effects are various autoimmune syndromes, kidney injury, and skin rash; isolated liver toxicity is uncommon. However, there are reports of liver toxicity including cholestatic hepatitis (Kumar et al., 1985). In another case, a patient developed aplastic anemia and apparent liver failure even though the aspartate aminotransferase was only two times the upper limit of normal (Fishel et al., 1989). It is important to understand that penicillamine reacts with aldehydes including pyridoxal phosphate, which is the cofactor in both the aspartate aminotransferase and ALT assays. Some drugs such as isoniazid have been shown to interfere with these assays by reacting with pyridoxal phosphate as discussed earlier (O'Brien et al., 2002). It is interesting that penicillamine has been found to decrease ALT in patients being treated with the drug and this was ascribed to a hepatoprotective effect (Iorio et al., 2004; Gong et al., 2006); however, it is likely that much of the effect actually involved interference with the ALT assay.

1. Liver Injury in Penicillamine-Induced Autoimmunity

In animal studies, it was found that the liver is involved in penicillamine-induced autoimmunity (Donker et al., 1984). Granulomatous and necrotic lesions were observed in the rats that developed penicillamine-induced autoimmunity. A more recent study was carried out to further characterize the effects of D-penicillamine on the liver (Sayeh & Uetrecht, 2001). In sick animals, histology of the liver showed portal and sinusoidal infiltration of plasma cells, lymphocytes, eosinophils, neutrophils, and macrophages. Also, large aggregates associated with necrosis of the hepatocytes and granulomatous lesions in the liver were demonstrated in these animals. These effects were not observed in the penicillamine-treated non-sick animals, which indicate that these lesions are part of the penicillamine-induced autoimmune syndrome. As with INH, penicillamine-treated animals had ALT levels markedly lower than those in the control animals but the glutamate dehydrogenase levels (another measure of liver injury) were elevated (Zhu, X., unpublished observation).

G. Mitochondrial Superoxide Dismutase-2 Heterozygote Model of DILI

Mitochondria play a central role in controlling cell death by necrosis, apoptosis, and autophagy; therefore, mitochondrial injury is an attractive mechanism for drug-induced liver toxicity (Kass, 2006). There is compelling evidence that the direct hepatotoxicity of agents such as acetaminophen and carbon tetrachloride involve mitochondrial injury (Masubuchi et al., 2005; Padma & Setty, 1999), and this could potentially apply to idiosyncratic DILI. There are also agents such as fialuridine that cause mitochondrial DNA damage, which unlike nuclear DNA cannot be repaired, and lead to serious delayed onset liver toxicity (Horn et al., 1997). Mitochondria are sensitive to oxidative damage because superoxide is formed in the electron transport chain, although it is usually detoxified by enzymes such as superoxide dismutase, glutathione peroxidase, and thioredoxin reductase. Polymorphisms for alanine homozygotes in the mitochondrial targeting sequence of manganese superoxide dismutase-2 (SOD2) were increased in humans with alcoholic liver disease (Degoul et al., 2001) suggesting the involvement of oxidative mitochondrial damage in this liver injury.

1. Underlying Mitochondrial Effects of SOD2 Knockout

Several strains of SOD2 knockout mice were developed to study the effects of mitochondrial oxidative stress; however, none of the SOD2 deficient strains were viable 3 weeks after birth (Boelsterli & Hsiao, 2008). Studies revealed massive mitochondrial injury in the neurons and cardiac myocytes of SOD2 deficient mice (Lebovitz et al., 1996), indicating the importance of this mitochondrial enzyme for survival. In contrast, heterozygous SOD2+/– mice are phenotypically normal, but they display impaired mitochondrial function and increased mitochondrial oxidative stress (Kokoszka et al., 2001), without significant changes in other compensatory antioxidant enzymes such as superoxide dismutase 1, catalase, or glutathione peroxidase (Remmen et al., 1999). The heterozygous SOD2+/– mouse has been used to test drugs associated with idiosyncratic DILI because an underlying mitochondrial dysfunction may contribute to liver injury.

2. SOD2+/– Mouse Model of DILI

Troglitazone incubated with liver mitochondrial fractions from CD1 mice induced mitochondrial swelling and decreased mitochondrial membrane potential which did not occur with less hepatotoxic thiazolidinediones such as rosiglitazone and pioglitazone (Masubuchi et al., 2006). Troglitazone treatment for 4 weeks (30mg/kg/day) in SOD2+/– mice led to increased serum ALT levels and midzonal hepatic necrosis, including changes evident of mitochondrial oxidant stress, that were not apparent in troglitazone-treated wildtype mice (Ong et al., 2007). Furthermore, damage was not observed at 2 weeks and proteomics analysis found an initial adaptive response, manifested as increased levels of stress proteins such as heat shock proteins and catalase, which were eventually depleted at 4 weeks and this was accompanied with mitochondrial injury and decreased ATP synthase levels (Lee et al., 2008). Interestingly, aconitase-2 was decreased throughout troglitazone treatment and was proposed as a potential biomarker to drugs that induce mitochondrial toxicity. Although the pathology manifested in human troglitazone patients with idiosyncratic DILI is similar to what is observed in the SOD2+/– mice (Smith, 2003), these changes were very mild and do not represent a model for idiosyncratic drug-induced liver failure (Jaeschke, 2007). In addition, others have not been able to reproduce this model even at higher doses of troglitazone (Fujimoto et al., 2009). The basis for this discrepancy is unknown; possible causes are a different route of administration (i.e. intraperitoneal versus oral) and solvent (i.e. Solutol HS-15 versus carboxymethylcellulose).

The SOD2+/– mouse has also been used to test other drugs suspected of causing idiosyncratic DILI involving mitochondrial toxicity. Treatment of SOD2+/– mice with flutamide led to hepatocellular necrosis and apoptosis after 4 weeks that did not occur in wildtype-treated mice (Kashimshetty et al., 2009). Likewise, nimesulide treatment for 4 weeks induced hepatocellular apoptosis in SOD2+/– mice (Ong et al., 2006). Increased apoptosis was also observed in wildtype mice upon nimesulide treatment, although to a lesser extent. Exaggerated toxicity to acetaminophen in SOD2+/– mice compared to wildtype was similarly observed, which is consistent with the fact that acetaminophen is known to cause mitochondrial damage (Ramachandran et al., 2011).

Hallmarks of mitochondrial injury include lactic acidosis and microvesicular steatosis, which are presumably due to inhibition of the mitochondria's main function in energy production and lipid metabolism. With the exception of valproate-induced liver injury, these are not hallmarks of idiosyncratic DILI. If idiosyncratic DILI involves a cumulative two stage injury with loss of adaptive responses as proposed, it is difficult to understand why most patients who have significant increases in ALT to drugs that can cause idiosyncratic DILI adapt after the increase in ALT despite continued treatment. In addition, if mitochondrial damage were the sole mediator of idiosyncratic DILI, it would be expected that it would be easier to generate animal models with higher doses of the drug. An alternate hypothesis is that mitochondrial injury represents a relatively common danger signal that can contribute to immune-mediated idiosyncratic DILI. Nevertheless, an underlying mitochondrial dysfunction could partially explain the idiosyncrasy of liver toxicity due to certain drugs, and the SOD2+/– mouse model may be useful in testing this hypothesis.

H. Inflammagen Model

In addition to metabolic and immune idiosyncrasy, inflammatory stress has been proposed by Roth as a mechanism for IDRs. This hypothesis posits that inflammatory events during drug therapy may increase one's susceptibility to drugs that otherwise would not cause adverse reactions, thus explaining the erratic nature of IDRs (Deng et al., 2009). The inflammagen model has focused mainly on idiosyncratic DILI using the endotoxin, lipopolysaccharide, as the stereotypical inflammagen. Co-exposure of drugs such as ranitidine, trovafloxacin, and diclofenac with lipopolysaccharide in rats led to elevated liver aminotransferase enzymes in the serum, and histopathological changes that did not occur with the drug alone (Luyendyk et al., 2003; Waring et al., 2005; Deng et al., 2006). It is known that toll-like receptor agonists such as lipopolysaccharide can increase the toxicity of some hepatotoxins

(Chen & Sun, 2011); therefore, there is some logic to this strategy, but this does not necessarily represent a valid model of idiosyncratic DILI. In virtually every respect, this model is different from the idiosyncratic liver injury observed in humans. Specifically, it occurs acutely (injury in hours) while idiosyncratic DILI almost always occurs after a lag period of more than 1 week of treatment with the drug, and more commonly, it occurs after a month of treatment (Adams et al., 2010). The delay is not random, as would be predicted by a chance coincidence of an inflammatory insult and drug treatment, but rather it has a bell-shaped distribution of the time to onset. Serious clinical idiosyncratic DILI is sustained for a period of weeks, but in the inflammagen model there has been no reported attempt to determine if the injury is sustained, and almost surely it would not be because the response to agents such as lipopolysaccharide is rapidly down-regulated on repeated exposures (Fan & Cook, 2004). In fact, sustained injury is one of the hallmarks of serious idiosyncratic DILI, and it is often possible to differentiate acetaminophen-induced liver injury from idiosyncratic DILI because it characteristically resolves much faster. Moreover, the histology in the inflammagen model is dominated by neutrophils (Deng et al., 2009), which is typical of lipopolysaccharide-induced liver injury, but this is virtually never the histology seen in idiosyncratic DILI, which typically looks like viral hepatitis, dominated by lymphocytes, and sometimes also includes eosinophils (Zimmerman, 1999).

If this were the mechanism of idiosyncratic DILI it would be expected that patients with inflammatory bowel disease would have a very high incidence of idiosyncratic DILI due to the amount of lipopolysaccharide and other inflammatory mediators that reach the liver. However, this has not been observed, and as previously mentioned, the response to agents such as lipopolysaccharide is rapidly down-regulated. We and others have tried to use toll-like receptor agonists such as lipopolysaccharide and poly (I:C) to develop animal models, because these agents would be expected to stimulate an adaptive immune response, but these methods were not successful as discussed elsewhere in this review. For example, others have used poly (I:C) and CD40 agonists to increase the hepatotoxicity of halothane (You et al., 2010), but this did not result in a good model of idiosyncratic DILI. One issue with using such agents is that they decrease P450 levels (Morgan, 2001), which can markedly decrease drug bioactivation. It is interesting that in the inflammagen model, the lipopolysaccharide is given 2h before the drug, while if this were to be a model of idiosyncratic DILI, the only way there could be a delay in the onset is if the inflammatory insult occurred after the drug had been started.

An additional issue is that if this model were used to screen drug candidates, the response to ranitidine should be considered a false positive because ranitidine is a safe, over-the-counter drug, and it would be a mistake to halt its development on the basis of this model. The dose of ranitidine used in these studies (30mg/kg) produces much higher plasma levels of ranitidine than those in humans taking a typical 150mg dose (Grant et al., 1989). No increase in ALT levels was found in rats upon lipopolysaccharide/ranitidine cotreatment at ranitidine doses below 25mg/kg, and doses above 30mg/kg of ranitidine treatment alone were immediately fatal (Luyendyk et al., 2003). Such characteristics are quite problematic.

Although the inflammagen model is not a valid model of idiosyncratic DILI, inflammation may play an important role in the mechanism of IDRs as a source of danger signals to stimulate an adaptive immune response. However, it is difficult to overcome immune tolerance, and as mentioned above, simple cotreatment of a drug with lipopolysaccharide or poly (I:C) is not sufficient to lead to a model of idiosyncratic DILI.

IV. Animal Models of Hematological Toxicity

A. Clozapine

Clozapine is a very effective atypical antipsychotic that causes idiosyncratic agranulocytosis in approximately 1% of patients. Clozapine is metabolized by activated neutrophils to a reactive nitrenium ion, which covalently binds to human neutrophils *in vivo*, independent of the occurrence of agranulocytosis (Liu & Uetrecht, 1995). Similarly, covalent binding to bone marrow protein was detected in clozapine-treated rats (Gardner et al., 1998). This reactive metabolite is presumed to be responsible for clozapine-induced agranulocytosis.

The mechanism of clozapine-induced agranulocytosis is unknown. It has characteristics typical of other IDRs that are likely immune-mediated, but the lack of immune memory (rechallenge of patients with a history of clozapine-induced agranulocytosis did not lead to an immediate recurrence) suggests that it might involve a toxic mechanism (Guest et al., 1998). Consistent with a toxic mechanism, the reactive nitrenium ion was shown to induce neutrophil apoptosis *in vitro* (Williams et al., 2000). Studies designed to detect elevated levels of neutrophil apoptosis in clozapine-treated rats and rabbits were inconclusive, likely due to the rapid intrinsic clearance of apoptotic neutrophils *in vivo* (Iverson et al., 2010).

1. Testing Vitamin C and Selenium Deficiency as Risk Factors

Chronic treatment of mice, rats, guinea pigs, and rabbits with clozapine has not led to an animal model of agranulocytosis (Ip & Uetrecht, 2006). The nitrenium ion is very rapidly reduced back to clozapine by vitamin C, and it was postulated that schizophrenic patients might have a poor diet and be vitamin C deficient, leading to impaired detoxication. This was tested in a guinea pig model because, like humans, they are unable to synthesize vitamin C. However, guinea pigs do not have neutrophils and there was much less covalent binding of clozapine to their analogous cell, the heterophil.

Therefore, this was not an adequate test of the hypothesis. The ODS rat also lacks the ability to synthesize vitamin C, and when they were made vitamin C deficient and treated with clozapine, not only did they not develop agranulocytosis, but there was also no increase in covalent binding to their bone marrow (Ip et al., 2008). Thus, there must be other efficient mechanisms to detoxify the nitrenium ion. There was also a suggestion that clozapine treatment could lead to selenium deficiency, which might also potentiate clozapine toxicity. However, chronic treatment of selenium-deficient rats with clozapine also did not lead to agranulocytosis (Ip & Uetrecht, 2008).

2. *Clozapine-Induced Changes in Neutrophil Kinetics and Cytokine Levels*

Although treatment of animals with clozapine did not result in agranulocytosis, by labeling cells with bromodeoxyuridine, we did find that it decreased the half-life of neutrophils and increased the rate of neutrophil release from the bone marrow in rabbits (Iverson et al., 2010). This was paired with elevated neutrophil counts in the peripheral blood and unchanged total white blood cell counts. This may reflect increased levels of apoptosis in circulating neutrophils, and suggests that an additional insult, such as an immune response, may be required for agranulocytosis to occur. In humans, the delay in onset of the reaction suggests immune involvement, typical of other IDRs, which are clearly immune-mediated. In addition, immune activation is evident from previous studies where increases in inflammatory cytokines such as IL-6, tumor necrosis factor-α, and soluble interleukin receptor-2 were found in almost half of the patients treated with clozapine (Pollmächer et al., 2000). Although these studies have not produced a good animal model of clozapine-induced agranulocytosis, they did provide strong evidence against specific hypotheses such as vitamin C deficiency.

B. Aminopyrine

The analgesic aminopyrine was one of the first drugs associated with drug-induced agranulocytosis, and because of this it is no longer available in most countries (Uetrecht et al., 1995). Several studies have found strong evidence supporting an immune-mediated mechanism, including the detection of drug-dependent anti-neutrophil antibodies in humans that lead to neutrophil destruction (Moeschlin & Wagner, 1952). Aminopyrine is metabolized by activated neutrophils to a reactive dication, and it is likely this reactive species is involved in the induction of neutrophil-specific antibodies (Uetrecht et al., 1995).

1. *Early Rabbit Model*

Although few animal studies have been published recently, some interesting studies were carried out in rabbits in the 1930s (Hoffman et al., 1934). Rabbits were treated chronically with aminopyrine (200–900mg/kg/day), and a consistent leukocytosis, followed a few weeks later by decreases in both white blood cell and neutrophil counts was observed. We attempted to reproduce this model, and although we observed a similar leukocytosis in the treated rabbits at a dose of 200mg/kg/day, the drop in white cell and neutrophil counts did not follow. Increasing the dose of aminopyrine was not feasible because the rabbits would not drink water with higher concentrations of drug and other modes of administration were not practical for chronic administration. Cotreatment with the potent immune stimulator poly (I:C) led to a more pronounced increase in leukocyte count, particularly neutrophils, but this is presumably an effect of poly (I:C) itself, and no hint of agranulocytosis was observed (Ip, 2009).

2. *Attempts to Develop a Rodent Model*

Due to the development of successful models of drug-induced autoimmunity and skin rash with the BN rat, we also pursued an animal model of aminopyrine-induced agranulocytosis with this strain. Chronic treatment with aminopyrine (200mg/kg/day) alone led to a slight downward trend in neutrophil counts, but this was not sustained. Similarly, cotreatment with poly (I:C) did not lead to any significant changes in white cell or neutrophil counts (Ip, 2009). Failure to induce agranulocytosis in both rats and rabbits could be due to immune tolerance because evidence supports that aminopyrine-induced agranulocytosis is immune-mediated. Recent studies in rodents have employed 1-methyl-D-tryptophan to decrease *in vivo* tolerance (Sakurai et al., 2002); however, cotreatment with this agent also did not lead to significant changes in leukocyte levels (Ip, 2009).

Dipyrone is a sodium sulfonate derivative of aminopyrine with a similar metabolic fate, and as a result, is also associated with drug-induced agranulocytosis (Ip & Uetrecht, 2006). In an attempt to induce agranulocytosis in white rats, animals were treated for 8 weeks with high doses of dipyrone (50–100mg/day), but no neutropenia was observed (Ferguson & Novak, 1966). We hypothesized that the chance of inducing agranulocytosis would increase if we could target both reactive metabolite formation and immune stimulation to the neutrophil, the target organ of toxicity. Therefore, we treated BN rats with liposomes containing both dipyrone and poly (I:C), but this also did not lead to an animal model of agranulocytosis. This may be due to the fact that it was difficult to obtain significant aminopyrine doses with this method (Ip, 2009). In short, even though there is strong evidence that aminopyrine-induced agranulocytosis is immune-mediated, attempts to develop a reliable animal model of this IDR by a combination of drug and stimulation of the immune system have failed. This is typical of most attempts to develop valid IDR animal models.

C. Amodiaquine

In addition to idiosyncratic liver injury, amodiaquine is also associated with agranulocytosis in approximately 1 in 2000 patients. Amodiaquine is metabolized by activated human neutrophils to a reactive quinoneimine, which is suspected to be responsible for this adverse reaction (Tingle et al., 1995). Further *in vitro* studies have shown that this reactive metabolite is directly toxic to human neutrophils and can react with cell surface proteins leading to hapten formation (Naisbitt et al., 1997).

An animal model of amodiaquine-induced agranulocytosis was pursued in rats. Animals were cotreated with phorbol myristate acetate, a powerful neutrophil activator, in an attempt to elevate serum levels of the quinoneimine *in vivo*. Paradoxically, neutrophil counts were significantly elevated in both the amodiaquine alone and amodiaquine + phorbol myristate acetate treatment groups, but it is unclear if levels of reactive metabolite were increased by the cotreatment (Ip, 2009).

Human studies suggest that more than direct neutrophil cytotoxicity is responsible for amodiaquine-induced agranulocytosis. In particular, drug-specific antibodies were detected in patients treated prophylactically with amodiaquine (Clarke et al., 1991), and likewise, amodiaquine-treated rats also produced such antibodies (Clarke et al., 1990). In this same study, white blood cell counts were found to drop significantly after the fourth dose; however, this leukopenia was not sustained and was followed by a prolonged leukocytosis. Differential counts were not reported, so it is unclear if there were changes in the number of neutrophils. If amodiaquine-induced agranulocytosis is immune-mediated then failure to produce an animal model could again be due to immune tolerance. In an attempt to prevent immune tolerance, rats were cotreated with amodiaquine and a tolerance suppressor, 1-methyl-D-tryptophan, but this did not lead to a decrease in neutrophil counts (Ip, 2009).

D. Aminoglutethimide

Aminoglutethimide is a first generation aromatase inhibitor used primarily in the past to treat estrogen-dependent breast and prostate cancer. As with most drugs that are primary aromatic amines, aminoglutethimide is associated with a variety of adverse drug reactions ranging from skin rash to more serious hematological toxicities (Cocconi, 1994). Blood dyscrasias, most commonly agranulocytosis, occur in approximately 1% of patients on aminoglutethimide therapy (Harris et al., 1986). This reaction is not due to the pharmacological action of the drug, rendering it idiosyncratic. Clinically the time to onset of agranulocytosis is delayed anywhere from weeks to months after initiation of treatment.

1. *Rodent Models*

To our knowledge there have been no published animal models of true aminoglutethimide-induced agranulocytosis, although leukopenia and thrombocytopenia were reported in female ICI-derived mice (Coleman et al., 2003) and female B6C3F1 hybrids (Ali et al., 1990) treated with aminoglutethimide. Leukopenia was observed as early as 2 weeks in mice given 50mg/kg/day aminoglutethimide orally; however, there was no change in the relative proportions of the white blood cells, indicating an overall decrease in leukocytes rather than a specific effect on the neutrophil/granulocyte population. These findings seem to be strain- and species-dependent as our previous attempts to reproduce these results in CD1 mice failed (Shenton et al., 2004), and no hematological effects were observed in Wistar rats treated with aminoglutethimide (Ali et al., 1990). Siraki et al. at the University of Alberta have recently had greater success in developing an animal model of aminoglutethimide-induced agranulocytosis; a decrease in peripheral blood neutrophil counts was observed after 21 days of 75mg/kg/day aminoglutethimide treatment in female C57BL/6 and B6C3F1 mice (Siraki et al., personal communication). Conversely, in our own experience, male BN rats treated with 125mg/kg/day aminoglutethimide had increased peripheral blood neutrophil counts during the initial 2 weeks of treatment, while the total white blood cell count remained unchanged (Ng, W., unpublished observation). Using bromodeoxyuridine to label cells we also found that aminoglutethimide treatment led to an increased release of newly formed neutrophils from the bone marrow, which suggests a decrease in neutrophil half-life similar to the effect of clozapine (see Section IV.A); however, these studies were performed in rats rather than rabbits so the number of blood samples we could obtain was less, and it was difficult to precisely determine half-life. If all drugs associated with idiosyncratic agranulocytosis induce a similar pattern, i.e. a decrease in neutrophil half-life and neutrophilia, this could be a useful biomarker. This hypothesis is currently being tested with other drugs that cause agranulocytosis such as amodiaquine and aminopyrine.

2. *Reactive Metabolite Formation*

The toxicity of aromatic amines is presumed to be due to their ability to be metabolically activated to reactive hydroxyl and nitroso metabolites (Uetrecht, 2002). The N-acetyl and N-hydroxy-metabolites of aminoglutethimide have been found in the urine of patients (Goss et al., 1985), and mice have been reported to form these metabolites as well (Seago et al., 1985). In contrast, rats have only been reported to form the N-acetyl metabolite and some ring cleavage products (Egger et al., 1982), and the lack of N-hydroxy-aminoglutethimide formation has been used to justify the absence of hematological effects observed in the rat (Ali et al., 1990).

Although most reactive metabolites are formed by P450, reactive metabolite formation by polymorphonuclear cells, mostly neutrophils, may be more relevant for the mechanism of drug-induced agranulocytosis. Neutrophils have been shown to oxidize drugs to reactive intermediates through myeloperoxidase, and this has been shown for clozapine and amodiaquine (Uetrecht, 1992). When aminoglutethimide was incubated with HL-60 cells, myeloperoxidase-protein free radicals were found, and this could be responsible for neutrophil toxicity leading to agranulocytosis (Siraki et al., 2007). Interestingly, glutethimide, a relatively safe sedative hypnotic with the same chemical structure as aminoglutethimide except for the absence of the amino group, does not induce leukopenia in mice nor do structural analogs of aminoglutethimide in which the amine group has been replaced by a nitro group (Coleman et al., 2003).

3. *Production of a Danger Signal*

Given that reactive metabolites have the potential to cause cell stress and damage, immune reactions could arise through mechanisms related to the danger hypothesis. Mice rechallenged with aminoglutethimide developed leukopenia within 7 days, suggesting the involvement of immune memory (Coleman et al., 2003). Yet, as with other drugs, most attempts to produce an animal model have been futile. Again it may be immune tolerance that overrides one's susceptibility to IDRs because some patients that develop reactions to aminoglutethimide recover without discontinuation of the drug (Harris et al., 1986). Our own studies on hepatic gene expression induced by aminoglutethimide in rats have indicated acute signs of cell stress through the upregulation of genes involved with the Nrf2–ARE pathway, while chronic treatment for up to 2 weeks suggests immune suppression with down-regulation of inflammatory cytokines and chemokines (Ng, W., unpublished observation). Interestingly, several genes in the apoptotic and mitochondrial pathways were also found to be upregulated during chronic aminoglutethimide treatment. The cell injury leading to apoptosis could potentially act as a danger signal and activate an immune response. Since aminoglutethimide can also inhibit desmolase (Hughes & Burley, 1970), a mitochondrial enzyme responsible for converting cholesterol to pregnenolone, it is possible that mitochondrial toxicity may contribute to aminoglutethimide-induced IDRs. Despite these results, the liver is not the major target of aminoglutethimide-induced IDRs, and the few reported cases of aminoglutethimide-induced liver toxicity were characterized by cholestasis (Cocconi, 1994). Thus, focusing on direct activation of polymorphonuclear cells leading to toxicity may be a better strategy of studying aminoglutethimide-induced IDRs. Although aminoglutethimide is rarely used because of safer third generation aromatase inhibitors, development of an animal model of aminoglutethimide-induced hematological toxicity may be useful for IDR mechanistic studies.

E. Felbamate

The use of the antiepileptic drug felbamate has been primarily restricted to treating refractory seizures due to its association with hepatotoxicity and aplastic anemia. The incidence of felbamate-induced aplastic anemia is estimated to be approximately 1 in 7800 and occurs more frequently in female patients (Kaufman et al., 1997).

1. *Reactive Metabolite Involvement*

Felbamate toxicity is presumably caused by the formation of the reactive atropaldehyde metabolite, which is a Michael acceptor that can readily bind to endogenous proteins (Thompson et al., 1996). Atropaldehyde is formed through the hydrolysis of felbamate by esterases to a monocarbamate, which undergoes further oxidation to an aldehyde carbamate that can either be detoxified by aldehyde dehydrogenase or undergo spontaneous elimination of carbon dioxide and ammonia to form atropaldehyde. Additionally, another relatively stable oxazolidine metabolite can reversibly cycle to the aldehyde carbamate, and this may contribute to the delivery of atropaldehyde to distant sites such as the bone marrow.

The identification of atropaldehyde mercapturic acids in the urine of both humans and rats treated with felbamate confirms its formation *in vivo* (Thompson et al., 1997). Glutathione adducts of atropaldehyde are likely protective; however, atropaldehyde irreversibly binds to glutathione transferase M1-1 and inhibits its activity *in vitro* (Dieckhaus et al., 2001). In theory, this could affect the antioxidant status of the cell, but it is less likely to be significant *in vivo*. Atropaldehyde was also found to bind human serum albumin and this interaction is slowly reversible (Roller et al., 2002). This could be a mechanism of detoxification by sequestering the reactive metabolite, but it could also be a mechanism to transport atropaldehyde to distal targets. In mouse bone marrow cells there is evidence that the monocarbamate can induce apoptosis *in vitro* (Husain et al., 2002), which may be related to the development of aplastic anemia. Interestingly, using an antibody against atropaldehyde, covalent adducts were not detected in the liver or bone marrow of rodents treated with felbamate or the monocarbamate metabolite (Popovic et al., 2004). These findings may be due to the lack of sensitivity of the anti-atropaldehyde antibody because it is highly unlikely that covalent adducts were not formed. In contrast, covalent adducts have been observed in the liver of rats treated with radiolabelled felbamate (Leone et al., 2007), which may be a more sensitive method of detection.

2. *Attempts to Develop a Rodent Model*

To date all attempts to develop a rodent model of felbamate-induced IDRs have been unsuccessful (Table II). One issue is that the first step in forming the reactive metabolite, hydrolysis, is a major metabolic pathway in

TABLE II Attempts to Create An Animal Model of Felbamate-Induced IDRs

Species	*Treatment*	*Cotreatments*	*Duration of treatment*	*End point observations*
Popovic et al. (2004)				
Female Sprague Dawley rat	Felbamate 800mg/kg/day in diet	None	1 Week	No changes in complete blood cell counts, or liver enzyme (aspartate transaminase and ALT) levels
Female BN rat	Felbamate 800mg/kg/day in diet	None; poly (I:C); poly (I:C) + ketoprofen	5 Weeks	
Female Lewis rat	Felbamate 800mg/kg/day in diet	None; poly (I:C); poly (I:C) + ketoprofen	2 Weeks	
Female C57BL/6 mice	Felbamate 800mg/kg/day in diet	None; poly (I:C); poly (I:C) + ketoprofen	2 Weeks	
Male BN rat	Felbamate 2.3g/kg/day in methylcellulose by gavage	None; poly (I:C)	1 Week/ 1 month	
Male BALB/c mice	Felbamate 2.3g/kg/day in methylcellulose by gavage	None; poly (I:C)	1 Month	
Female C57BL/6 mice	Monocarbamate felbamate 200mg/kg/day in methylcellulose by interperitoneal injection	None	1 Week	
Female BN rat	Felbamate 2.3g/kg/day in methylcellulose by gavage	Aminobenzotriazole; buthionine sulfoximine; dicoumerol; valproic acid	Up to 4 days	
Dieckhaus et al. (2000)				
Male Sprague Dawley rat	Felbamate 350mg/kg/day by gavage	None; buthionine sulfoximine	4 Weeks	No observable liver toxicity as measured through neutrophil infiltration; no observable bone marrow toxicity as measured by loss of blood cell precursors
Male Sprague Dawley rat	Monocarbamate felbamate 50–300mg/kg/day (incremental increase) by gavage	None; buthionine sulfoximine	9 Weeks	
Male Gunn rat	Felbamate 600–1200mg/kg/day (incremental increase) by gavage	None; buthionine sulfoximine	5 Weeks	
Male Gunn rat	Monocarbamate 300–900mg/kg/day (incremental increase) by gavage	None; buthionine sulfoximine	5 Weeks	

Rats and mice were treated with felbamate and various other interventions including metabolic and immune modulators; however, all attempts to develop an animal model were unsuccessful.

humans but a minor pathway in rodents. To overcome this problem, animals were treated with the hydrolyzed monocarbamate metabolite, but this also did not lead to bone marrow or liver toxicity (Dieckhaus et al., 2000; Popovic et al., 2004). A mild and transient increase in serum ALT has been found in rats and dogs treated chronically with felbamate; however, this did not translate into histopathological findings, and the effects in the dogs may have been due to direct toxicity (McGee et al., 1998). In a gene expression array in rats, felbamate-induced hepatic gene changes indicative of oxidative stress, which could be another mechanism of felbamate toxicity, and such pathways may also be necessary to induce an immune response (Leone et al., 2007). Regardless, there is evidence suggesting immune involvement because the aldehyde carbamate, but not felbamate or the monocarbamate, was able to stimulate an immunogenic response in the popliteal lymph node assay in BALB/c mice (Popovic et al., 2004). This demonstrates the essential nature of forming atropaldehyde in eliciting an immune response even though in most animals and humans this is not sufficient to result in significant injury.

V. Animal Models of Generalized Hypersensitivity Reactions

A. Sulfonamides

Sulfonamide-induced IDRs typically manifest as generalized hypersensitivity reactions including fever, skin rash, blood dyscrasias, systemic organ toxicity, and a lupus-like syndrome (reviewed in Cribb et al., 1996). There is a common misconception that all sulfonamide drugs induce IDRs and cross reactivity exists between these drugs; however, of the sulfonamide drugs that cause these reactions, the toxicity is presumed to be due to the arylamine moiety, which can be metabolized into reactive hydroxylamine and nitroso metabolites independent of the sulfonamide group (Fig. 5; Uetrecht, 2002). These reactive species can bind to biological molecules and induce cell stress/

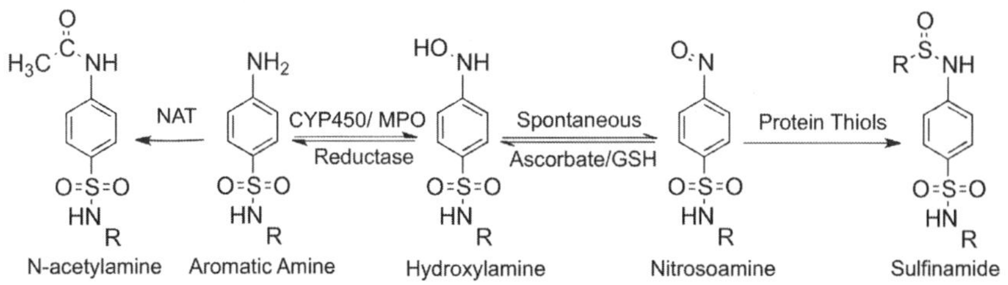

FIGURE 5 Metabolic scheme for the formation of reactive metabolites of arylamine sulfonamides. N-acetylation by N-acetyltransferase (NAT) of the arylamine blocks formation of the hydroxylamine and nitroso metabolites by P450 or myeloperoxidase (MPO). The nitroso metabolite can react with thiol-containing nucleophiles such as endogenous protein thiols to form sulfinamide adducts.

toxicity or form potential antigenic substances. Thus, only the antimicrobial sulfonamides such as sulfamethoxazole, sulfadimethoxine, and sulfadiazine have been implicated in idiosyncratic sulfonamide hypersensitivity (Fig. 6). Extensive studies in rodents found that sulfamethoxazole formed antigenic adducts in antigen presenting cells, and when these cells were adoptively transferred to naïve mice, splenocyte proliferation was induced upon stimulation with nitroso-sulfamethoxazole *ex vivo* (Elsheikh et al., 2010). Although this demonstrates a model of immunogenicity, no rodent model of sulfonamide hypersensitivity currently exists because rodents do not exhibit clinical signs of hypersensitivity to sulfonamides.

1. Dog Model

In contrast, case reports of sulfonamide hypersensitivity in dogs are abundant in the literature (reviewed in Trepanier, 2004). The lack of N-acetylation in the dogs, due to the absence of the N-acetyltransferase gene and protein expression (Trepanier et al., 1997), may increase the susceptibility of dogs to sulfonamide hypersensitivity by down-regulating detoxification pathways and inducing greater bioactivation through oxidative pathways. Cats are also sensitive to sulfonamides, although to a lesser extent than dogs, and an overall incidence of 0.25% has been reported for dermatological and systemic reactions to sulfonamides in dogs and cats (Noli et al., 1995). Despite the fact that dogs provide a

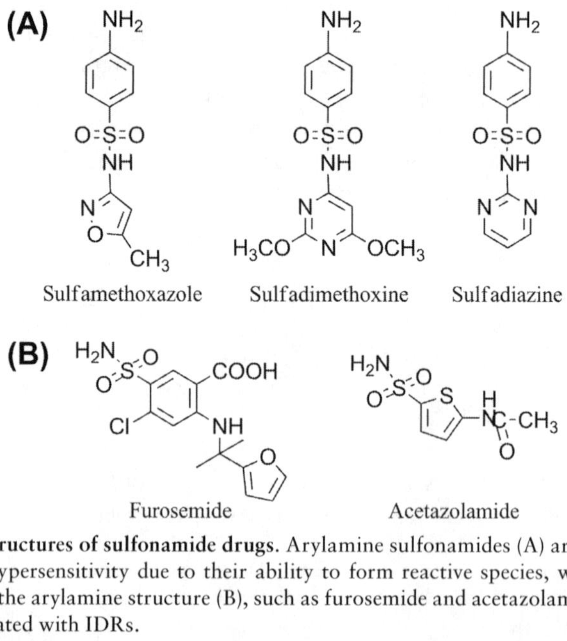

FIGURE 6 Structures of sulfonamide drugs. Arylamine sulfonamides (A) are implicated in sulfonamide hypersensitivity due to their ability to form reactive species, whereas sulfonamide lacking the arylamine structure (B), such as furosemide and acetazolamide, are generally not associated with IDRs.

naturally occurring animal model of sulfonamide hypersensitivity, the ethical and practical issues of using them for experimentation are limiting. Existing studies have mainly been performed on privately owned dogs after the development of sulfonamide hypersensitivity. The time to onset of hypersensitivity in dogs is at least 5 days after sulfonamide initiation and the most common symptoms include fever, thrombocytopenia, hepatopathy, and neutropenia (Trepanier et al., 2003). Female dogs were found to have a greater incidence of hypersensitivity than male dogs, and the reactions were more prevalent in Samoyeds and miniature Schnauzers. Interestingly, sulfonamide-induced polyarthritis occurs almost exclusively in dogs and is more prevalent in larger breeds such as Doberman pinchers (Trepanier, 1999). In addition, dogs with hepatopathy, including hepatic necrosis, cholestasis, and lymphocytic infiltration, had a poorer outcome (Trepanier et al., 2003).

Immune involvement in sulfonamide hypersensitivity has also been investigated in dogs. Fifty percent of the sulfonamide hypersensitive dogs were found to have sulfonamide-serum adducts and anti-drug antibodies, whereas these adducts were not detected in the dogs that were tolerant to sulfonamides (Lavergne et al., 2006). Anti-myeloperoxidase antibodies were also found in the serum of both sulfonamide hypersensitive and tolerant dogs, although they were significantly higher in dogs that did not survive (Lavergne et al., 2007). Several studies have been performed to investigate the involvement of the nitroso metabolite. Similar to the immunogenic rodent model, female beagles were treated for 2 weeks with nitroso-sulfamethoxazole and then rechallenged with sulfamethoxazole after a 1 week recovery. Although sulfamethoxazole adducts were found in the spleen, anti-drug antibodies were not detected and none of the dogs developed hypersensitivity (Lavergne et al., 2005). High doses of the nitroso metabolite would likely cause acute hemolysis and the maximal dose of the administered nitroso metabolite was about 1/5 the usual clinical dose of the drug. The nitroso metabolite is very rapidly reduced back to the hydroxylamine and to a lesser extent the parent drug. Therefore, the lack of response may have been due to the limited exposure, but given the idiosyncratic nature of the hypersensitivity, it is also likely that there are additional factors that determine an animal's susceptibility.

VI. Animal Models of Generalized Autoimmunity

A. Penicillamine

D-Penicillamine has been used in the treatment of rheumatoid arthritis and Wilson's disease. However, its use is limited because of a relative high incidence of a variety of adverse autoimmune reactions (Stein et al., 1980).

1. BN Rat Model

In animals, similar adverse effects have been observed; in BN rats D-penicillamine can induce a disease which is characterized by dermatitis, vasculitis, production of anti-nuclear antibodies, formation of circulating immune complexes, deposits of IgG along the glomerular basement membrane, hepatic necrosis, arthritis, and weight loss (Donker et al., 1984; Tournade et al., 1990). D-penicillamine-induced autoimmunity is idiosyncratic as it occurs only in BN rats, and the incidence is only 50–80% in this highly inbred strain of rat. In addition, there is a delay of about 3 weeks between starting treatment and the onset of the autoimmune syndrome, which is typical of an idiosyncratic reaction. The dose–response curve in the BN rat model is unusual; a dose of 20mg/day is required to induce the syndrome and an increase to 50mg/day does not significantly increase the incidence, but at 10mg/day the incidence is zero, and in fact, this low dose leads to immune tolerance and subsequent treatment with 20mg/day does not lead to autoimmunity. Even though it is an immune-mediated reaction, the time to onset is not shortened on rechallenge.

2. Macrophage Activation

Penicillamine is chemically reactive without metabolism; it can react with protein thiols to form mixed disulfides, and it reacts with aldehydes to form a thiazolidine ring (Howard-Lock et al., 1986). One of the signaling pathways between macrophages and T cells involves reaction of an aldehyde on macrophages with an amine on T cells, forming a reversible imine linkage (Rhodes, 1989). When spleen cells isolated from BN rats were incubated with D-penicillamine, it was found that penicillamine preferentially binds to macrophages (Li et al., 2009). Furthermore, a microarray study showed that after a 6-h incubation with D-penicillamine, several known macrophage activation markers were upregulated (Li & Uetrecht, 2009). All of the above data suggest that the irreversible reaction of penicillamine with the aldehyde groups on macrophages leads to activation of macrophages, and in some cases this can lead to a generalized autoimmune syndrome.

The incidence of D-penicillamine-induced autoimmunity can be influenced by manipulation of the immune system. The incidence and severity of autoimmunity in the BN rat can be increased by a single dose of poly (I:C), which mimics viral RNA and stimulates macrophages through toll-like receptor 3 (Sayeh & Uetrecht, 2001). Lipopolysaccharide, a toll-like receptor 4 agonist, shares a similar but smaller effect than poly (I:C) (Masson & Uetrecht, 2004). As mentioned above, 2 weeks of D-penicillamine low dose treatment (5–10mg/day) prior to a dose of 20mg/day leads to tolerance in 100 percent of BN rats (Masson & Uetrecht, 2004). Adoptive transfer of spleen cells from a tolerant animal led to tolerance in naïve animals, thus indicating that it is immune tolerance. $CD4^+$ T cells appear to be the major cell responsible for this tolerance; when tolerized animals are treated with 20mg/day their $CD4^+$ T cells express increased levels of IL-10 and transforming growth factor beta mRNA (Masson & Uetrecht, 2004). One dose of misoprostol (a prostaglandin E analog) prevents penicillamine-induced autoimmunity. Treatment of tolerized animals with a combination of poly (I:C) and penicillamine partially overcomes tolerance, and it also appears that depletion of macrophages during tolerance induction partially prevents the induction of tolerance.

3. *Involvement of Th17 Cells*

Recently, it was shown that a spike in IL-6 twenty-four hours after the start of penicillamine treatment predicted which animals would develop autoimmunity weeks later. By 7 days, the IL-6 levels had returned to normal, only to increase again when autoimmunity developed. IL-6 is required for the development of Th17 cells, and it was found that IL-17 and interleukin-22 (IL-22), which are characteristic cytokines produced by Th17 cells, were increased in animals that developed autoimmunity. Furthermore, the percentage of IL-17 producing $CD4^+$ T cells was significantly increased in the sick animals. These data strongly suggest that Th17 cells are involved in penicillamine-induced autoimmunity (Zhu et al., 2011). Retinoic acid is reported to inhibit the development of Th17 cells (Mucida et al., 2007) so we expected that it would prevent penicillamine-induced autoimmunity. However, retinoic acid cotreatment had just the opposite effect: it increased the incidence and severity of penicillamine-induced autoimmunity and increased the number of Th17 cells in the circulation (Zhu, X., unpublished observation).

This animal model appears to be a valid representation of the autoimmune reactions induced by penicillamine in humans. The basic mechanism appears to involve direct activation of macrophages with the production of IL-6, but it is not clear in this highly inbred strain of animals why only some of the animals produce an early spike in IL-6, which appears to be essential for the later development of autoimmunity. The activation of macrophages may be an essential step in the initiation of IDRs in general.

B. Propylthiouracil

Propylthiouracil is an antithyroid drug associated with a relatively high incidence of IDRs including agranulocytosis, hepatitis, and a lupus-like syndrome. Drug-dependent antibodies were found in patients with propylthiouracil-induced agranulocytosis (Fibbe et al., 1986), and activated neutrophils have been found to oxidize propylthiouracil to reactive metabolites *in vitro* (Waldhauser & Uetrecht, 1991), which could be implicated in causing this reaction. Anti-nuclear antibodies and anti-neutrophil cytoplasmic antibodies have also been detected in humans with propylthiouracil-induced lupus (Aloush et al., 2006). Given these findings, and the fact that the characteristics of propylthiouracil-induced IDRs such as the delay in onset are typical of other IDRs, it is likely that they are immune-mediated.

1. Cat Model

It was also found that cats treated with propylthiouracil for hyperthyroidism often developed a lupus-like syndrome similar to what is observed in humans (Peterson et al., 1984). Further investigation found that about 50% of healthy cats treated with 150mg/day developed anti-nuclear antibodies and clinical signs of lethargy, lymphadenopathy, and hemolytic anemia 3–4 weeks after the initiation of propylthiouracil treatment (Aucoin et al., 1985). Interestingly, the incidence of lupus-like disease was higher in healthy cats compared to cats with hyperthyroidism, which could be attributed to increased clearance and decreased bioavailability in cats with hyperthyroidism (Peterson et al., 1988). Propylthiouracil rechallenged cats developed clinical symptoms only slightly earlier than the time to onset during the initial clinical episode (Aucoin et al., 1985), which suggests a lack of immune memory even though this is clearly an immune-mediated IDR. Propylthiouracil-treated cats that develop clinical symptoms also have anti-myeloperoxidase antibodies and anti-native DNA autoantibodies (Waldhauser & Uetrecht, 1996; Aucoin et al., 1988). When we tried to continue these studies in cats, we noted that after 1992 none of the animals developed autoimmunity, which could not be explained by differences in experimental procedures or genetic differences (mongrel cats were used for these studies). We suspect that the supplementation of cat chow with taurine, which commenced in 1992 to prevent cardiomyopathy in cats, was the reason for this abrupt change in response to propylthiouracil. Taurine deficiency alters the activity of polymorphonuclear cells in cats and induces dramatic changes to their immune system (Schuller-Levis et al., 1990). Therefore we suspect that a dietary deficiency in taurine could be a risk factor for propylthiouracil-induced autoimmunity, although to our knowledge this hypothesis has not been tested.

C. Procainamide/Hydralazine

Procainamide, an antiarrhythmic, and hydralazine, an antihypertensive, are associated with the highest incidence of drug-induced autoimmunity in humans (Rubin, 2005). The onset of lupus can be delayed for years after initiating drug treatment; however, it is intriguing that the majority of patients on procainamide or hydralazine develop anti-nuclear antibodies regardless of whether or not they develop clinical symptoms of autoimmunity. Procainamide-treated patients that developed a lupus-like syndrome were found to form IgG anti-[(H2A-H2B)-DNA] antibodies that were not detected in asymptomatic patients, which could potentially differentiate between those that develop autoimmune disease and those that do not (Rubin et al., 1995).

The lack of successful animal models that replicate the autoimmunity induced by procainamide and hydralazine could be attributed to an inability to break self-tolerance. An attempt to overcome central T cell tolerance, by injecting the reactive hydroxylamine metabolite of procainamide into the thymus of mice, induced the production of IgG anti-chromatin antibodies but not clinical symptoms of autoimmune disease (Kretz-Rommel et al., 1997). However, intrathymic injection of any cytotoxic agent may interfere with central tolerance and lead to autoimmunity that is not specific to the drug.

Hydralazine reacts irreversibly with aldehyde groups, and by a mechanism similar to that proposed for penicillamine (Howard-Lock et al., 1986), it also appears to activate macrophages and other antigen presenting cells (Li et al., 2009). Procainamide is oxidized to a reactive metabolite by the myeloperoxidase system of macrophages and this may also lead to their activation. As such, the activation of macrophages may play an important role in the ability of these two drugs to induce autoimmune reactions.

1. Inhibition of DNA Methylation

Epigenetic changes in DNA methylation have also been implicated in drug-induced autoimmune diseases (Hewagama & Richardson, 2009). DNA methylation of deoxycytosine in CpG sequences by DNA methyltransferases is an inherent mechanism to silence genes by blocking transcription. Demethylation of DNA enables transcription, and if unregulated, it could lead to gene overexpression. Inhibition of DNA methylation could be involved in the pathogenesis of autoimmunity because T cells from lupus patients have been reported to have decreased levels of methylated deoxycytosine (Richardson et al., 1990). Both procainamide and hydralazine were found to inhibit T cell DNA methylation *in vitro*, and these cells proliferated in the presence of autologous macrophages without antigen stimulation (Cornacchia et al., 1988). Similar findings were observed when mouse $CD4^+$ T cells were treated with procainamide, and when adoptively transferred, syngeneic mice developed anti-DNA and anti-histone antibodies, in addition to multi-organ effects such as glomerulonephritis, resembling chronic graft-versus-host disease. When untreated cells were adoptively transferred, these effects were not observed (Quddus et al., 1993; Yung et al., 1995). The effects appear to be specific to the amine and hydrazine moieties because both the N-acetylated metabolites and the analog that lacks the hydrazine group do not lead to autoreactivity in T cells or in mice after adoptive transfer (Yung et al., 1997).

Further investigation found that procainamide competitively inhibits DNA methyltransferase activity, whereas hydralazine acts on the ERK signaling pathway to decrease expression of DNA methyltransferase, which could explain the delay in the ability of hydrazine to induce hypomethylation compared to procainamide (Deng et al., 2003). Inhibition of DNA methylation leading to the overexpression of genes in T cells may be involved in self-reactivity. Overexpression of lymphocyte function-associated antigen has been observed in the procainamide-treated $CD4^+$ T cells that are autoreactive, and adoptive transfer of lymphocyte function-associated antigen overexpressing T cells induces lupus-like symptoms in syngeneic mice (Yung et al., 1996). Human T cells from lupus patients also have higher levels of this antigen (Richardson et al., 1992). Overexpression of lymphocyte function-associated antigen has been proposed to stabilize the affinity of the T cell receptor to MHC molecules to become autoreactive. Although treatment of animals with procainamide or hydralazine does not lead directly to clinically evident autoimmunity, this mechanism is likely involved in the induction of autoimmunity by some drugs.

D. Mercury

Exposure to mercury can result in the development of an autoimmune syndrome, which shares much of the same pathology as D-penicillamine-induced autoimmunity. Some characteristic manifestations include lymphocyte proliferation, and the production of autoantibodies, such as anti-nuclear, anti-chromatin, anti-histone and anti-DNA antibodies and circulation of immune complexes (Fournie et al., 2002). It has been shown that several strains of rodents, especially BN rats, can develop an autoimmune syndrome following treatment with mercuric chloride. In BN rats, autoimmunity reached its peak 10 days after the continuous administration of mercuric chloride and declined after 20 days (Aten et al., 1988). Lewis rats are protected from the autoimmune syndrome, possibly through the development of a Th1 response (Bagenstose et al., 1999). In A.SW mice (MHC-H2s haplotype), anti-nuclear and anti-nucleolar autoantibodies were elicited by repeated injections of mercuric chloride (Mirtcheva et al., 1989). This appears to be a Th2 response supported by the production of interleukin-4 (IL-4) and IL-10 by $CD4^+$ T cells, as well as IgG1 and immunoglobulin E (IgE) secretion during the first week of treatment (Hultman & Hansson-Georgiadis, 1999). It was also reported that 10-week mercuric chloride treatment induced autoimmunity in female SJL/N mice (Hultman & Enestrom, 1992). The similarity in the characteristics of this model when compared to the penicillamine model suggests that the mechanism is also similar, but studies have not been performed to determine if mercuric chloride can activate macrophages.

VII. Conclusion

Most attempts to develop valid animal models of IDRs have ended in failure, and negative results are often not published (some the data in this review will never be published anywhere else). Probably the two best models are NVP-induced skin rash in rats and penicillamine-induced autoimmunity in BN rats because they are easily reproducible and have very similar characteristics to the IDR that occurs in humans. Sulfamethoxazole-induced hypersensitivity reactions in dogs and propylthiouracil-induced autoimmunity in cats also appear to be very similar to the IDR that occurs in humans, but they are not very practical for detailed studies because of the species involved and the low incidence. These animal models clearly involve an adaptive immune response, and although it is still a matter for debate, it is likely that the vast majority of what we would call IDRs are mediated by the adaptive immune system. This would explain their idiosyncratic nature; it is well accepted that some people are allergic to things such as peanuts, but most people are not. As discussed earlier, many models such as the inflammagen model have characteristics so different from the IDRs that occur in humans that it is very unlikely that they provide any mechanistic insights.

If IDRs are mediated by the adaptive immune system then it might be possible to produce animal models by a combination of drug and something to stimulate an immune response. However, in general, this strategy has failed. One issue is that most agents such as toll-like receptor agonists that stimulate the immune system also inhibit P450 synthesis and thereby lead to decreased reactive metabolite formation. A more basic issue is that a specific MHC and T cell receptor may be required in order to mount a significant immune response (Uetrecht, 2009). This is consistent with the finding that in the case of some IDRs, if a patient does not have a specific MHC they will not have an IDR to a specific drug. But even if they do have the appropriate MHC, it is still unlikely that they will have an IDR to the drug; this is likely due, at least in part, to their T cell receptor repertoire. This is in contrast to an immune response to a pathogen in which most patients will have an immune response. The basis for this difference is presumably because the pathogen expresses many antigens and so there are more chances that at least one antigen will fit some combination of MHC and T cell receptor of an individual. In addition, pathogens stimulate toll-like receptors, but do not require P450-mediated bioactivation; therefore, the fact that they inhibit P450 synthesis is not an issue. Furthermore, the major immunogen produced by a drug is likely to be a drug-modified protein, the major portion of which is a self protein, and T cells with receptors that have a strong affinity for these proteins would have been deleted in the thymus during development. Therefore, the major response to most drug-modified proteins is likely to be immune tolerance, and this is consistent with the fact that drugs that can cause severe IDRs usually cause a much higher incidence of a mild IDR that resolves despite continued treatment with the drug. If the IDR is immune-mediated then this resolution despite continued treatment presumably involves immune tolerance.

If these hypotheses are correct, then in order to be successful in producing an IDR animal model it would require the right combination of MHC and T cell receptors, as well as overcoming immune tolerance to an immunogen that is mostly self protein. This problem is analogous to the problem of treating cancer by stimulation of an immune response against tumor antigens that are not present on normal cells. Some anti-tumor responses have been achieved, but ultimately the result is immune tolerance. This raises the question of why it was so easy to develop an animal model of NVP-induced skin rash. It is clearly immune-mediated, but it does not require a specific MHC/T cell receptor combination as demonstrated by the fact that we were able to get a rash in all strains of rats that we tested as long as we controlled the formation of the reactive metabolite. Conversely, we have not been able to induce a skin rash in mice with NVP.

The NVP model has been very useful in testing mechanistic hypotheses as detailed above. We were able to clearly show that it is immune-mediated because sensitivity could be transferred to naïve animals with spleen cells from a sensitized animal. We were able to clearly define the metabolic pathway involved and that would be virtually impossible to do in humans, especially in the case of NVP, because there are several potential reactive metabolites. We also found that even though a specific metabolic pathway was required to induce the immune response and rash, ultimately the T cells from the affected animals also responded to the parent drug; this demonstrates that what T cells from patients with an IDR respond to cannot be used to infer what chemical species induced the immune response. This assumption was the basis for the pharmacological interaction hypothesis, but it would be impossible to test this assumption in humans. The NVP model is currently being used to determine the sequence of events leading up to the skin rash, again virtually impossible to do in humans. Without understanding how reactive metabolites initiate an immune response it will be impossible to interpret covalent binding data because not all covalent bindings are associated with the same risk of IDRs.

However, the NVP model is only one model, and it would be dangerous to assume that it represents the mechanism of all IDRs. It is reasonable to assume that a finding such as the fact that what chemical species T cells from a patient responds to cannot be used to infer what species initiated the immune response can be generalized. In contrast, it is unlikely that the mechanism by which different drugs initiate an immune response is exactly the same for different drugs, and it even appears that not all IDRs are caused by reactive metabolites. In addition to acting as a hapten, possible ways in which different drugs or their reactive metabolites could initiate an immune response include: causing cell damage/induction of a danger signal, especially through mitochondrial damage or endoplasmic reticulum stress; inhibition of DNA methylation; and direct activation of antigen presenting cells. These hypotheses require further testing.

Many of the characteristics of the two animal models that we have studied most extensively are quite different and this likely reflects mechanistic differences. Specifically, the penicillamine model is both strain- and individual-specific, i.e. not all animals develop autoimmunity, while the NVP model is not strain dependent and we can achieve an incidence of 100%. Penicillamine-induced autoimmunity is made worse with poly (I:C), but it has no effect in the NVP model. Low dose pretreatment for 2 weeks prevents the IDR in both models, but this represents immune tolerance that can be transferred to a naïve animal in the penicillamine model, while in the NVP model, the principal mechanism involves induction of P450, and this tolerance can be overcome with a P450 inhibitor. Retinoic acid made penicillamine autoimmunity worse but appeared to be partially protective in the NVP model. This highlights the importance of developing more valid IDR animal models in order to get a sense of the range of mechanisms by which a drug can induce an IDR. To reiterate, valid animal models are essential to rigorously test mechanistic hypotheses, and a better understanding of how drugs cause IDRs would likely provide better ways to prevent them, including better methods to screen drug candidates for IDR risk.

Acknowledgments

This work was supported by grants from the Canadian Institutes for Health Research.

Conflict of Interest: The authors have no conflict of interest to declare. J.U. is the Canada Research Chair in Adverse Drug Reactions.

Abbreviations

12-OH-NVP	12-hydroxy-nevirapine
ALT	alanine transaminase
BN	Brown Norway
DILI	drug-induced liver injury
HLA	human leukocyte antigen
IDR	idiosyncratic drug reaction
IgG	immunoglobulin G
IL-6	interleukin-6
IL-10	interleukin-10
IL-17	interleukin-17
INF-γ	interferon-gamma
INH	isoniazid
MHC	major histocompatibility complex

NK	natural killer
NKT	natural killer T
NVP	nevirapine
P450	cytochrome P450
Poly (I:C)	polyinosine-polycytidylic acid
S-100	supernatant of syngeneic liver homogenate after 100,000*g* centrifugation
SOD2	superoxide dismutase-2
Th17	T helper 17

References

Adams, D. H., Ju, C., Ramaiah, S. K., Uetrecht, J., & Jaeschke, H. (2010). Mechanisms of immune-mediated liver injury. *Toxicological Sciences*, *115*, 307–321.

Ali, H., Khalaf, L., Nicholls, P. J., & Poole, A. (1990). Comparison of in vitro and in vivo haemotoxic effects of aminoglutethimide and glutethimide. *Toxicology In Vitro*, *4*, 381–383.

Aloush, V., Litinsky, I., Caspi, D., & Elkayam, O. (2006). Propylthiouracil-induced autoimmune syndromes: two distinct clinical presentations with different course and management. *Seminars in Arthritis and Rheumatism*, *36*, 4–9.

Antunes, A. M., Duarte, M. P., Santos, P. P., da Costa, G. G., Heinze, T. M., Beland, F. A., et al. (2008). Synthesis and characterization of DNA adducts from the HIV reverse transcriptase inhibitor nevirapine. *Chemical Research in Toxicology*, *21*, 1443–1456.

Antunes, A. M., Godinho, A. L., Martins, I. L., Justino, G. C., Beland, F. A., & Marques, M. M. (2010a). Amino acid adduct formation by the nevirapine metabolite, 12-hydroxynevirapine–a possible factor in nevirapine toxicity. *Chemical Research in Toxicology*, *23*, 888–899.

Antunes, A. M., Godinho, A. L., Martins, I. L., Oliveira, M. C., Gomes, R. A., Coelho, A. V., et al. (2010b). Protein adducts as prospective biomarkers of nevirapine toxicity. *Chemical Research in Toxicology*, *23*, 1714–1725.

Aten, J., Bosman, C. B., Rozing, J., Stijnen, T., Hoedemaeker, P. J., & Weening, J. J. (1988). Mercuric chloride-induced autoimmunity in the brown Norway rat. Cellular kinetics and major histocompatibility complex antigen expression. *American Journal of Pathology*, *133*, 127–138.

Aucoin, D. P., Peterson, M. E., Hurvitz, A. I., Drayer, D. E., Lahita, R. G., Quimby, F. W., et al. (1985). Propylthiouracil-induced immune-mediated disease in the cat. *Journal of Pharmacology and Experimental Therapeutics*, *234*, 13–18.

Aucoin, D. P., Rubin, R. L., Peterson, M. E., Reidenberg, M. M., Drayer, D. E., Hurvitz, A. I., et al. (1988). Dose dependent induction of anti-native DNA antibodies in cats by propylthiouracil. *Arthritis & Rheumatism*, *31*, 688–692.

Bagenstose, L. M., Salgame, P., & Monestier, M. (1999). Cytokine regulation of a rodent model of mercuric chloride-induced autoimmunity. *Environmental Health Perspectives*, *107*(Suppl. 5), 807–810.

Bersoff-Matcha, S. J., Miller, W. C., Aberg, J. A., van Der Horst, C., Hamrick, H. J., Jr., Powderly, W. G., et al. (2001). Sex differences in nevirapine rash. *Clinical Infectious Diseases*, *32*, 124–129.

Boelsterli, U. A., & Hsiao, C. J. J. (2008). The heterozygous Sod2+/– mouse: modeling the mitochondrial role in drug toxicity. *Drug Discovery Today*, *13*, 982–988.

Bourdi, M., Amouzadeh, H. R., Rushmore, T. H., Martin, J. L., & Pohl, L. R. (2001). Halothane-induced liver injury in outbred guinea pigs: role of trifluoroacetylated protein adducts in animal susceptibility. *Chemical Research in Toxicology*, *14*, 362–370.

Bourdi, M., Masubuchi, Y., Reilly, T. P., Amouzadeh, H. R., Martin, J. L., George, J. W., et al. (2002). Protection against acetaminophen-induced liver injury and lethality by interleukin 10: role of inducible nitric oxide synthase. *Hepatology*, *35*, 289–298.

Cai, P., Nakagawa, T., & Uetrecht, J. (2011). Development of an animal model of amodiaquine-induced liver injury. *The Toxicologist*, *120*, 90.

Cai, P., & Uetrecht, J. (2009). Amodiaquine-induced liver toxicity in the rat. *The Toxicologist*, *108*, 238.

Chen, J., Mannargudi, B. M., Xu, L., & Uetrecht, J. (2008). Demonstration of the metabolic pathway responsible for nevirapine-induced skin rash. *Chemical Research in Toxicology*, *21*, 1862–1870.

Chen, M., & Gandolfi, J. (1997). Characterization of the humoral immune response and hepatotoxicity after multiple halothane exposures in guinea pigs. *Drug Metabolism Reviews*, *29*, 103–122.

Chen, X., Tharmanathan, T., Mannargudi, B., Gou, H., & Uetrecht, J. P. (2009). A study of the specificity of lymphocytes in nevirapine-induced skin rash. *Journal of Pharmacology and Experimental Therapeutics*, *331*, 836–841.

Chen, Y., & Sun, R. (2011). Toll-like receptors in acute liver injury and regeneration. *International Immunopharmacology*10.1016/j.intimp.2011.1004.1023.

Cheng, L., You, Q., Yin, H., Holt, M. P., & Ju, C. (2010). Involvement of natural killer T cells in halothane-induced liver injury in mice. *Biochemical Pharmacology*, *80*, 255–261.

Christie, G., Breckenridge, A. M., & Park, B. K. (1989). Drug-protein conjugates–XVIII. Detection of antibodies towards the antimalarial amodiaquine and its quinone imine metabolite in man and the rat. *Biochemical Pharmacology*, *38*, 1451–1458.

Chu, K. M., Boulle, A. M., Ford, N., Goemaere, E., Asselman, V., & Van Cutsem, G. (2010). Nevirapine-associated early hepatotoxicity: incidence, risk factors, and associated mortality in a primary care ART programme in South Africa. *PLoS One*, *5*, e9183.

Clarke, J. B., Maggs, J. L., Kitteringham, N. R., & Park, B. K. (1990). Immunogenicity of amodiaquine in the rat. *International Archives of Allergy & Applied Immunology*, *91*, 335–342.

Clarke, J. B., Neftel, K., Kitteringham, N. R., & Park, B. K. (1991). Detection of antidrug IgG antibodies in patients with adverse drug reactions to amodiaquine. *International Archives of Allergy & Applied Immunology*, *95*, 369–375.

Clay, K. D., Hanson, J. S., Pope, S. D., Rissmiller, R. W., Purdum, P. P., & Banks, P. M. (2006). Brief communication: severe hepatotoxicity of telithromycin: three case reports and literature review. *Annals of Internal Medicine*, *144*, 415–420.

Cocconi, G. (1994). First generation aromatase inhibitors–aminoglutethimide and testololactone. *Breast Cancer Research and Treatment*, *30*, 57–80.

Coleman, M. D., Khalaf, L. F., & Nicholls, P. J. (2003). Aminoglutethimide-induced leucopenia in a mouse model: effects of metabolic and structural determinates. *Environmental Toxicology and Pharmacology*, *15*, 27–32.

Connolly, M. K., Ayo, D., Malhotra, A., Hackman, M., Bedrosian, A. S., Ibrahim, J., et al. (2011). Dendritic cell depletion exacerbates acetaminophen hepatotoxicity. *Hepatology* In Press, doi:10.1002/hep.24429.

Cornacchia, E., Golbus, J., Maybaum, J., Strahler, J., Hanash, S., & Richardson, B. (1988). Hydralazine and procainamide inhibit T cell DNA methylation and induce autroreactivity. *Journal of Immunology*, *140*, 2197–2200.

Cribb, A. E., Lee, B. L., Trepanier, L. A., & Spielberg, S. P. (1996). Adverse reactions to sulphonamide and sulphonamide-trimethoprim antimicrobials: clinical syndromes and pathogenesis. *Adverse Drug Reactions and Toxicological Reviews*, *15*, 9–50.

Dahlin, D. C., Miwa, G. T., Lu, A. Y., & Nelson, S. D. (1984). N-acetyl-*p*-benzoquinone imine: a cytochrome P-450-mediated oxidation product of acetaminophen. *The Proceedings of the National Academy of Sciences USA*, *81*, 1327–1331.

Degoul, F., Sutton, A., Mansouri, A., Cepanec, C., Degott, C., Fromenty, B., et al. (2001). Homozygosity for alanine in the mitochondrial targeting sequence of superoxide dismutase and risk for severe alcoholic liver disease. *Gastroenterology*, *120*, 1468–1474.

Deng, C., Lu, Q., Zhang, Z., Rao, T., Attwood, J., Yung, R., et al. (2003). Hydralazine may induce autoimmunity by inhibiting extracellular signal-regulated kinase pathway signaling. *Arthritis & Rheumatism*, *48*, 746–756.

Deng, X., Luyendyk, J. P., Ganey, P. E., & Roth, R. A. (2009). Inflammatory stress and idiosyncratic hepatotoxicity: hints from animal models. *Pharmacological Reviews*, *61*, 262–282.

Deng, X., Stachlewitz, R. F., Liguori, M. J., Blomme, E. A. G., Waring, J. F., Luyendyk, J. P., et al. (2006). Modest inflammation enhances diclofenac hepatotoxicity in rats: role of neutrophils and bacterial translocation. *Journal of Pharmacology and Experimental Therapeutics*, *319*, 1191–1199.

Diao, H., Kon, S., Iwabuchi, K., Kimura, C., Morimoto, J., Ito, D., et al. (2004). Osteopontin as a mediator of NKT cell function in T cell-mediated liver diseases. *Immunity*, *21*, 539–550.

Dieckhaus, C. M., Miller, T. A., Sofia, R. D., & Macdonald, T. L. (2000). A mechanistic approach to understanding species differences in felbamate bioactivation: relevance to drug-induced idiosyncratic reactions. *Drug Metabolism and Disposition*, *28*, 814–822.

Dieckhaus, C. M., Roller, S. G., Santos, W. L., Sofia, R. D., & Macdonald, T. L. (2001). Role of gluathione-S-transferases A1-1, M1-1, P1-1 in the detoxificaiton of 2-phenylpropenal, a reactive felbamate metabolite. *Chemical Research in Toxicology*, *2001*, 511–516.

Dieterich, D. T., Robinson, P. A., Love, J., & Stern, J. O. (2004). Drug-induced liver injury associated with the use of nonnucleoside reverse-transcriptase inhibitors. *Clinical Infectious Diseases*, *38*(Suppl. 2), 80–89.

Donker, A. J., Venuto, R. C., Vladutiu, A. O., Brentjens, J. R., & Andres, G. A. (1984). Effects of prolonged administration of D-penicillamine or captopril in various strains of rats. Brown Norway rats treated with D-penicillamine develop autoantibodies, circulating immune complexes, and disseminated intravascular coagulation. *Clinical Immunology and Immunopathology*, *30*, 142–155.

Egger, H., Bartlett, F., Itterly, W., Rodebaugh, R., & Shimanskas, C. (1982). Metabolism of aminoglutethimide in the rat. *Drug Metabolism and Disposition*, *10*, 405–412.

Eghtesadi-Araghi, P. (2008). Halothane hepatitis in Iran: a review of 59 cases. *World Journal of Gastroenterology*, *14*, 5322.

Elsheikh, A., Lavergne, S. N., Castrejon, J. L., Farrell, J., Wang, H., Sathish, J., et al. (2010). Drug antigenicity, immunogenicity, and costimulatory signaling: evidence for formation of a functional antigen through immune cell metabolism. *Journal of Immunology*, *185*, 6448–6460.

Fan, H., & Cook, J. A. (2004). Molecular mechanisms of endotoxin tolerance. *Journal of Endotoxin Research*, *10*, 71–84.

Ferguson, N. M., & Novak, A. F. (1966). Attempts at induced agranulocytosis in rats using dipyrone. *The Journal of Pharmaceutical Sciences*, *55*, 1306–1308.

Fibbe, W. E., Claas, F. H. J., Van der Star-Dijlstra, W., Schaafsma, M. R., Meyboom, R. H. B., & Falkenburg, J. H. F. (1986). Agranulocytosis induced by propylthiouracil: evidence of a drug dependent antibody reacting with granulocytes, monocytes and haematopoietic progenitor cells. *British Journal of Haematology*, *64*, 363–373.

Fishel, B., Tishler, M., Caspi, D., & Yaron, M. (1989). Fatal aplastic anaemia and liver toxicity caused by D-penicillamine treatment of rheumatoid arthritis. *Annals of Rheumatic Diseases*, *48*, 609–610.

Fournie, G. J., Saoudi, A., Druet, P., & Pelletier, L. (2002). Th2-type immunopathological manifestations induced by mercury chloride or gold salts in the rat: signal transduction pathways, cellular mechanisms and genetic control. *Autoimmunity Reviews*, *1*, 205–212.

Fujimoto, K., Kumagai, K., Ito, K., Arakawa, S., Ando, Y., Oda, S. I, et al. (2009). Sensitivity of liver injury in heterozygous Sod2 knockout mice treated with troglitazone or acetaminophen. *Toxicologic Pathology*, *37*, 193–200.

Furst, S. M., Luedke, D., Gaw, H. H., Reich, R., & Gandolfi, A. J. (1997). Demonstration of a cellular immune response in halothane-exposed guinea pigs. *Toxicology and Applied Pharmacology*, *143*, 245–255.

Gardner, I., Leeder, J. S., Chin, T., Zahid, N., & Uetrecht, J. P. (1998). A comparison of the covalent binding of clozapine and olanzapine to human neutrophils in vitro and in vivo. *Molecular Pharmacology*, *53*, 999–1008.

Gatanaga, H., Yazaki, H., Tanuma, J., Honda, M., Genka, I., Teruya, K., et al. (2007). HLA-Cw8 primarily associated with hypersensitivity to nevirapine. *AIDS*, *21*, 264–265.

Gong, Y., Klingenberg, S. L., & Gluud, C. (2006). Systematic review and meta-analysis: D-Penicillamine vs. placebo/no intervention in patients with primary biliary cirrhosis–Cochrane Hepato-Biliary Group. *Alimentary Pharmacology & Therapeutics*, *24*, 1535–1544.

Goss, P. E., Jarman, M., & Griggs, L. J. (1985). Metabolism of aminoglutethimide in humans: quantification and clinical relevance of induced metabolism. *British Journal of Cancer*, *51*, 259–262.

Grant, S. M., Langtry, H. D., & Brogden, R. N. (1989). Ranitidine. An updated review of its pharmacodynamic and pharmacokinetic properties and therapeutic use in peptic ulcer disease and other allied diseases. *Drugs*, *37*, 801–870.

Guest, I., Sokoluk, B., MacCrimmon, J., & Uetrecht, J. (1998). Examination of possible toxic and immune mechanisms of clozapine-induced agranulocytosis. *Toxicology*, *131*, 53–65.

Harris, A. L., Hughes, G., Barrett, A. J., Abusrewil, S., Dowsett, M., & Smith, I. E. (1986). Agranulocytosis associated with aminoglutethimide: pharmacological and marrow studies. *British Journal of Cancer*, *54*, 119–122.

Harrison, A. C., Kitteringham, N. R., Clarke, J. B., & Park, B. K. (1992). The mechanism of bioactivation and antigen formation of amodiaquine in the rat. *Biochemical Pharmacology*, *43*, 1421–1430.

Hastings, K. L., Thomas, C., Brown, A. P., & Gandolfi, A. J. (1995). Trifluoroacetylation potentiates the humoral immune response to halothane in the guinea pig. *Immunopharmacology and Immunotoxicology*, *17*, 201–213.

Hewagama, A., & Richardson, B. (2009). The genetics and epigenetics of autoimmune diseases. *Journal of Autoimmunity*, *33*, 3–11.

Hoffman, A. M., Butt, E. M., & Hickey, N. G. (1934). Neutropenia following amidopyrine. *JAMA*, *102*, 1213–1214.

Horn, D. M., Neeb, L. A., Colacino, J. M., & Richardson, F. C. (1997). Fialuridine is phosphorylated and inhibits DNA synthesis in isolated rat hepatic mitochondria. *Antiviral Research*, *34*, 71–74.

Howard-Lock, H. E., Lock, C. J., Mewa, A., & Kean, W. F. (1986). D-penicillamine: chemistry and clinical use in rheumatic disease. *Seminars in Arthritis and Rheumatism*, *15*, 261–281.

Hughes, S. W. M., & Burley, D. M. (1970). Aminoglutethimide: a 'side-effect' turned therapeutic advantage. *Postgraduate Medical Journal*, *46*, 409–416.

Hultman, P., & Enestrom, S. (1992). Dose-response studies in murine mercury-induced autoimmunity and immune-complex disease. *Toxicology and Applied Pharmacology*, *113*, 199–208.

Hultman, P., & Hansson-Georgiadis, H. (1999). Methyl mercury-induced autoimmunity in mice. *Toxicology and Applied Pharmacology*, *154*, 203–211.

Husain, Z., Pinto, C., Sofia, R. D., & Yunis, E. J. (2002). Felbamate-induced apoptosis of hematopoietic cells is mediated by redox-sensitive and redox-independent pathways. *Epilepsy Research*, *48*, 57–69.

Iorio, R., D'Ambrosi, M., Marcellini, M., Barbera, C., Maggiore, G., Zancan, L., et al. (2004). Serum transaminases in children with Wilsons disease. *Journal of Pediatric Gastroenterology and Nutrition*, *39*, 331–336.

Ip, J., & Uetrecht, J. (2006). In vitro and animal models of drug-induced blood dyscrasias. *Environmental Toxicology and Pharmacology*, *21*, 135–140.

Ip, J., & Uetrecht, J. P. (2008). Testing the hypothesis that selenium deficiency is a risk factor for clozapine-induced agranulocytosis in rats. *Chemical Research in Toxicology*, *21*, 874–878.

Ip, J., Wilson, J. X., & Uetrecht, J. P. (2008). Testing the hypothesis that vitamin C deficiency is a risk factor for clozapine-induced agranulocytosis using guinea pigs and ODS rats. *Chemical Research in Toxicology*, *21*, 869–873.

Ip, J. R. T. (2009). *Investigation of The Mechanisms of Drug-induced Agranulocytosis*. (Doctoral dissertation), Toronto, ON: University of Toronto.

Iverson, S., Kautiainen, A., Ip, J., & Uetrecht, J. P. (2010). Effect of clozapine on neutrophil kinetics in rabbits. *Chemical Research in Toxicology*, *23*, 1184–1191.

Jaeschke, H. (2007). Troglitazone hepatotoxicity: are we getting closer to understanding idiosyncratic liver injury? *Toxicological Sciences*, *97*, 1–3.

Jaeschke, H., Williams, C. D., Ramachandran, A., & Bajt, M. L. (2011). Acetaminophen hepatotoxicity and repair: the role of sterile inflammation and innate immunity. *Liver International* In Press, doi:10.1111/j.1478-3231.2011.02501.x.

Jollow, D. J., Mitchell, J. R., Potter, W. Z., Davis, D. C., Gillette, J. R., & Brodie, B. B. (1973). Acetaminophen-induced hepatic necrosis. II. Role of covalent binding in vivo. *Journal of Pharmacology and Experimental Therapeutics*, *187*, 195–202.

Ju, C., Reilly, T. P., Bourdi, M., Radonovich, M. F., Brady, J. N., George, J. W., et al. (2002). Protective role of Kupffer cells in acetaminophen-induced hepatic injury in mice. *Chemical Research in Toxicology*, *15*, 1504–1513.

Kashimshetty, R., Desai, V. G., Kale, V. M., Lee, T., Moland, C. L., Branham, W. S., et al. (2009). Underlying mitochondrial dysfunction triggers flutamide-induced oxidative liver injury in a mouse model of idiosyncratic drug toxicity. *Toxicology and Applied Pharmacology*, *238*, 150–159.

Kass, G. E. (2006). Mitochondrial involvement in drug-induced hepatic injury. *Chemico-Biological Interactions*, *163*, 145–159.

Kaufman, D. W., Kelly, J. P., Anderson, K. T., Harmon, D. C., & Shapiro, S. (1997). Evaluation of case reports of aplastic anemia among patients treated with felbamate. *Epilepsia*, *38*, 1265–1269.

Keane, N. M., Nolan, D., Phillips, E. J., Lucas, A. D., Almeida, C. A., Martin, A. M., et al. (2007). Use of the ELISpot assay to detect abacavir- and nevirapine-induced IFN-responses in PBMC from HIV-infected patients with abacavir or nevirpine hypersensitivity reactions. Paper presented at the the 4th International AIDS Society Meeting, Sydney, Australia.

Kharasch, E. D. (2008). Adverse drug reactions with halogenated anesthetics. *Clinical Pharmacology & Therapeutics*, *84*, 158–162.

Kobayashi, E., Kobayashi, M., Tsuneyama, K., Fukami, T., Nakajima, M., & Yokoi, T. (2009). Halothane-induced liver injury is mediated by interleukin-17 in mice. *Toxicological Sciences*, *111*, 302–310.

Kokoszka, J. E., Coskun, P., Espositio, L. A., & Wallace, D. C. (2001). Increased mitochondrial oxidative stress in the Sod2 (+/–) mouse results in the age-related decline of mitochondrial function culminating in increased apoptosis. *Proceedings of the Academy of Natural Sciences*, *98*, 2278–2283.

Kretz-Rommel, A., Duncan, S. R., & Rubin, R. L. (1997). Autoimmunity caused by disruption of central T cell tolerance: a murine model of drug-induced lupus. *Journal of Clinical Investigations*, *99*, 1888–1896.

Kumar, A., Bhat, A., Gupta, D. K., Goel, A., & Malaviya, A. N. (1985). D-Penicillamine-induced acute hypersensitivity pneumonitis and cholestatic hepatitis in a patient with rheumatoid arthritis. *Clinical and Experimental Rheumatology*, *3*, 337–339.

Langier, S., Sade, K., & Kivity, S. (2010). Regulatory T cells: the suppressor arm of the immune system. *Autoimmunity Reviews*, *10*, 112–115.

Lavergne, S. N., Danhof, R. S., Volkman, E. M., & Trepanier, L. A. (2006). Association of drug-serum protein adducts and anti-drug antibodies in dogs with sulphonamide hypersensitivity: a naturally occurring model of idiosyncratic drug toxicity. *Clinical & Experimental Allergy*, *36*, 907–915.

Lavergne, S. N., Drescher, N. J., & Trepanier, L. A. (2007). Anti-myeloperoxidase and anti-cathepsin G antibodies in sulphonamide hypersensitivity. *Clinical & Experimental Allergy*, *38*, 199–207.

Lavergne, S. N., Volkman, E. M., Maki, J. E., Yoder, A. R., & Trepanier, L. A. (2005). Evaluation of the clinical, immunologic, and biochemical effects of nitroso sulfamethoxazole administration to dogs: a pilot study. *Toxicology*, *208*, 63–72.

Lebovitz, R. M., Zhang, H., Vogel, H., Cartwright, J., Jr., Dionne, L., Lu, N., et al. (1996). Neurodegeneration myocardial injury and perinatal death in mitochondrial superoxidase dismutase deficient mice. *Proceedings of the Academy of Natural Sciences*, *93*, 9782–9787.

Lee, Y. H., Chung, M. C.M., Lin, Q., & Boelsterli, U. A. (2008). Troglitazone-induced hepatic mitochondrial proteome expression dynamics in heterozygous Sod2+/– mice: two-stage oxidative injury. *Toxicology and Applied Pharmacology*, *231*, 43–51.

Leone, A. M., Kao, L. M., McMillian, M. K., Nie, A. Y., Parker, J. B., Kelley, M. F., et al. (2007). Evaluation of felbamate and other antiepileptic drug toxicity potential based on hepatic protein covalent binding and gene expression. *Chemical Research in Toxicology*, *20*, 600–608.

Li, J., Kourteva, G., Hilton, H., Cai, P., Workman, H., Haggerty, H., et al. (2011a). Changes in hepatic gene expression induced by amodiaquine in rats. *The Toxicologist*, *120*, 323.

Li, J., Mannargudi, B., & Uetrecht, J. P. (2009). Covalent binding of penicillamine to macrophages: implications for penicillamine-induced autoimmunity. *Chemical Research in Toxicology*, *22*, 1277–1284.

Li, J., & Uetrecht, J. (2010). The danger hypothesis as applied to idiosyncratic drug reactions. *Handbook of Experimental Pharmacology*, *196*, 493–509.

Li, J., & Uetrecht, J. P. (2009). D-Penicillamine-induced autoimmunity: relationship to macrophage activation. *Chemical Research in Toxicology*, *22*, 1526–1533.

Li, J., Workman, H., Cai, P., Kourteva, G., Hilton, H., Haggerty, H., et al. (2011b). Immunological aspects of an animal model of amodiaquine-induced liver toxicity. *The Toxicologist*, *120*, 323.

Liu, F., Cai, P., Li, J., & Uetrecht, J. (2011). Study of liver lymphocytes in amodiaquine-induced hepatotoxicity in Brown Norway rats. *The Toxicologist*, *120*, 93.

Liu, Z. C., & Uetrecht, J. P. (1995). Clozapine is oxidized by activated human neutrophils to a reactive nitrinium ion that irreversibly binds to the cells. *Journal of Pharmacology and Experimental Therapeutics*, *275*, 1476–1483.

Lohse, A. W., Manns, M., Dienes, H. P., Meyer zum Buschenfelde, K. H., & Cohen, I. R. (1990). Experimental autoimmune hepatitis: disease induction, time course and T-cell reactivity. *Hepatology*, *11*, 24–30.

Luyendyk, J. P., Maddox, J. F., Cosma, G. N., Ganey, P. E., Cockrell, G. L., & Roth, R. A. (2003). Ranitidine treatment during a modest inflammatory response precipitates idiosyncrasy-like liver injury in rats. *Journal of Pharmacology and Experimental Therapeutics*, *307*, 9–16.

MacGregor, T. R., & Hall, D. B. (2007). Case-control exploration of relationships between early rash or liver toxicity and plasma concentrations of nevirapine and primary metabolites. *HIV Clinical Trials*, *8*, 391–399.

Maddrey, W. C., & Boitnott, J. K. (1973). Isoniazid hepatitis. *Annals of Internal Medicine*, *79*, 1–12.

Martin, A. M., Nolan, D., Gaudieri, S., Almeida, C. A., Nolan, R., James, I., et al. (2004). Predisposition to abacavir hypersensitivity conferred by HLA-B*5701 and a haplotypic Hsp70-Hom variant. *Proceedings of the National Academy of Sciences*, *101*, 4180–4185.

Martin, A. M., Nolan, D., James, I., Cameron, P., Keller, J., Moore, C., et al. (2005). Predisposition to nevirapine hypersensitivity associated with HLA-DRB1*0101 and abrogated by low CD4 T-cell counts. *AIDS*, *19*, 97–99.

Masson, M. J., & Uetrecht, J. P. (2004). Tolerance induced by low dose D-penicillamine in the Brown Norway rat model of drug-induced autoimmunity is immune-mediated. *Chemical Research in Toxicology*, *17*, 82–94.

Masubuchi, Y., Bourdi, M., Reilly, T. P., Graf, M. L., George, J. W., & Pohl, L. R. (2003). Role of interleukin-6 in hepatic heat shock protein expression and protection against acetaminophen-induced liver disease. *Biochemical and Biophysical Research Communications*, *304*, 207–212.

Masubuchi, Y., Kano, S., & Horie, T. (2006). Mitochondrial permeability transition as a potential determinant of hepatotoxicity of antidiabetic thiazolidinediones. *Toxicology*, *222*, 233–239.

Masubuchi, Y., Suda, C., & Horie, T. (2005). Involvement of mitochondrial permeability transition in acetaminophen-induced liver injury in mice. *Journal of Hepatology*, *42*, 110–116.

McGee, J. H., Erikson, D. J., Galbreath, C., Willigan, D. A., & Sofia, R. D. (1998). Acute, subchronic, and chronic toxicity studies with felbamate, 2-phenyl-1,3-propanediol dicarbamate. *Toxicological Sciences*, *45*, 225–232.

Metushi, I. G., Cai, P., Zhu, X., Nakagawa, T., & Uetrecht, J. P. (2011). A fresh look at the mechanism of isoniazid-induced hepatotoxicity. *Clinical Pharmacology & Therapeutics*, *89*, 911–914.

Mirtcheva, J., Pfeiffer, C., De Bruijn, J. A., Jacquesmart, F., & Gleichmann, E. (1989). Immunological alterations inducible by mercury compounds. III. H-2A acts as an immune response and H-2E as an immune "suppression" locus for HgCl2-induced antinucleolar autoantibodies. *Europen Journal of Immunology*, *19*, 2257–2261.

Mitchell, J. R., Jollow, D. J., Potter, W. Z., Davis, D. C., Gillette, J. R., & Brodie, B. B. (1973). Acetaminophen-induced hepatic necrosis. I. Role of drug metabolism. *Journal of Pharmacology and Experimental Therapeutics*, *187*, 185–194.

Mitchell, J. R., Zimmerman, H. J., Ishak, K. G., Thorgeirsson, U. P., Timbrell, J. A., Snodgrass, W. R., et al. (1976). Isoniazid liver injury: clinical spectrum, pathology, and probable pathogenesis. *Annals of Internal Medicine*, *84*, 181–192.

Moeschlin, S., & Wagner, K. (1952). Agranulocytosis due to the occurrence of leukocyte-agglutinins. *Acta Haematologica*, *8*, 29–41.

Morgan, E. T. (2001). Regulation of cytochrome P450 by inflammatory mediators: why and how. *Drug Metabolism and Disposition*, *29*, 207–212.

Mucida, D., Park, Y., Kim, G., Turovskaya, O., Scott, I., Kronenberg, M., et al. (2007). Reciprocal TH17 and regulatory T cell differentiation mediated by retinoic acid. *Science*, *317*, 256–260.

Myers, T. G., Dietz, E. C., Anderson, N. L., Khairallah, E. A., Cohen, S. D., & Nelson, S. D. (1995). A comparative study of mouse liver proteins arylated by reactive metabolites of acetaminophen and its nonhepatotoxic regioisomer, 3'-hydroxyacetanilide. *Chemical Research in Toxicology*, *8*, 403–413.

Naisbitt, D. J., Ruscoe, J. E., Williams, D., O'Neill, P. M., Pirmohamed, M., & Park, B. K. (1997). Disposition of amodiaquine and related antimalarial agents in human neutrophils: implications for drug design. *Journal of Pharmacology and Experimental Therapeutics*, *280*, 884–893.

Neftel, K. A., Woodtly, W., Schmid, M., Frick, P. G., & Fehr, J. (1986). Amodiaquine induced agranulocytosis and liver damage. *British Medical Journal*, *292*, 721–723.

Nelson, S. D., Mitchell, J. R., Timbrell, J. A., Snodgrass, W. R., & Corcoran, G. B. (1976). Isoniazid and iproniazid: activation of metabolites to toxic intermediates in man and rat. *Science*, *193*, 901–903.

Noli, C., Koeman, J. P., & Willemse, T. (1995). A retrospective evaluation of adverse reactions to trimethoprim-sulphonamide combinations in dogs and cats. *Veterinary Quarterly*, *17*, 123–128.

O'Brien, P. J., Slaughter, M. R., Polley, S. R., & Kramer, K. (2002). Advantages of glutamate dehydrogenase as a blood biomarker of acute hepatic injury in rats. *Laboratory Animals*, *36*, 313–321.

Obach, R. S., Kalgutkar, A. S., Soglia, J. R., & Zhao, S. X. (2008). Can in vitro metabolism-dependent covalent binding data in liver microsomes distinguish hepatotoxic from non-hepatotoxic drugs? An analysis of 18 drugs with consideration of intrinsic clearance and daily dose. *Chemical Research in Toxicology*, *21*, 1814–1822.

Ong, M. M. K., Latchoumycandane, C., & Boelsterli, U. A. (2007). Troglitazone-induced hepatic necrosis in an animal model of silent genetic mitochondrial abnormalities. *Toxicological Sciences*, *97*, 205–213.

Ong, M. M. K., Wang, A. S., Leow, K. Y., Khoo, Y. M., & Boelsterli, U. A. (2006). Nimesulide-induced hepatic mitochondrial injury in heterozygous Sod2+/– mice. *Free Radical Biology & Medicine*, *40*, 420–429.

Padma, P., & Setty, O. H. (1999). Protective effect of *Phyllanthus Fraternus* against carbon tetrachloride-induced mitochondrial dysfunction. *Life Sciences*, *64*, 2411–2417.

Patel, S. M., Johnson, S., Belknap, S. M., Chan, J., Sha, B. E., & Bennett, C. (2004). Serious adverse cutaneous and hepatic toxicities associated with nevirapine use by non-HIV-infected individuals. *Journal of Acquired Immune Deficiency Syndromes*, *35*, 120–125.

Peterson, M. E., Aucoin, D. P., Davis, C. A., & Graves, T. K. (1988). Altered disposition of propylthiouracil in cats with hyperthyroidism. *Research in Veterinary Science*, *45*, 1–3.

Peterson, M. E., Hurvitz, A. I., Leib, M. S., Cavanagh, P. G., & Dutton, R. E. (1984). Propylthiouracil-associated hemolytic anemia, thrombocytopenia, and antinuclear antibodies in cats with hyperthyroidism. *Journal of the American Veterinary Medical Association*, *184*, 806–808.

Pirmohamed, M. (2010). Pharmacogenetics of idiosyncratic adverse drug reactions. *Handbook of Experimental Pharmacology*, *196*, 477–491.

Pollard, R. B., Robinson, P., & Dransfield, K. (1998). Safety profile of nevirapine, a nonnucleoside reverse transcriptase inhibitor for the treatment of human immunodeficiency virus infection. *Clinical Therapeutics*, *20*, 1071–1092.

Pollmächer, T., Haack, M., Schuld, A., Kraus, T., & Hinze-Selch, D. (2000). Effects of antipsychotic drugs on cytokine networks. *Journal of Psychiatric Research*, *34*, 369–382.

Popovic, M., Caswell, J. L., Mannargudi, B., Shenton, J. M., & Uetrecht, J. P. (2006). Study of the sequence of events involved in nevirapine-induced skin rash in Brown Norway rats. *Chemical Research in Toxicology*, *19*, 1205–1214.

Popovic, M., Nierkens, S., Pieters, R., & Uetrecht, J. (2004). Investigating the role of 2 phenylpropenal in felbamate-induced idiosyncratic drug reactions. *Chemical Research in Toxicology*, *17*.

Quddus, J., Johnson, K. J., Gavalchin, J., Amento, E. P., Chrisp, C. E., Yung, R., et al. (1993). Treating activated CD4+Tcells with either of two distinct DNA methyltransferase inhibitors, 5-azacytidine or procainamide, is sufficient to cause a lupus-like disease in syngeneic mice. *Journal of Clinical Investigations*, *92*, 38–53.

Ramachandran, A., Lebofsky, M., Weinman, S. A., & Jaeschke, H. (2011). The impact of partial manganese superoxide dismutase (SOD2)-deficiency on mitochondrial oxidant stress, DNA fragmentation and liver injury during acetaminophen hepatotoxicity. *Toxicology and Applied Pharmacology*, *251*, 226–233.

Reilly, T. P., Brady, J. N., Marchick, M. R., Bourdi, M., George, J. W., Radonovich, M. F., et al. (2001). A protective role for cyclooxygenase-2 in drug-induced liver injury in mice. *Chemical Research in Toxicology*, *14*, 1620–1628.

Remmen, H. V., Salvador, C., Yang, H., Huang, T. T., Epstein, C. J., & Richardson, A. (1999). Characterization of the antioxidant status of the heterozygous manganese superoxide dismutase knockout mouse. *Archives of Biochemistry and Biophysics*, *363*, 91–97.

Reynolds, E. S., & Moslen, M. T. (1977). Halothane hepatotoxicity: enhancement by polychlorinated biphenyl pretreatment. *Anesthesiology*, *47*, 19–27.

Rhodes, J. (1989). Evidence for an intercellular covalent reaction essential in antigen-specific T cell activation. *Journal of Immunology*, *143*, 1482–1489.

Richardson, B., Scheinbart, L., Strahler, J., Gross, L., Hanash, S., & Johnson, M. (1990). Evidence for impared T cell DNA methylation in systemic lupus erythematosus and rheumatoid arthritis. *Arthritis Rheumatism*, *33*, 1665–1673.

Richardson, B. C., Strahler, J. R., Pivirotto, T. S., Quddus, J., Bayliss, G. E., Gross, L. A., et al. (1992). Phenotypic and functional similarities between 5 azacytidine-treated T cells and a T cell subset in patients with active systemic lupus erythematosus. *Arthritis Rheumatism*, *35*, 647–662.

Roller, S. G., Dieckhaus, C. M., Santos, W. L., Sofia, R. D., & Macdonald, T. L. (2002). Interaction between human serum albumin and the felbamate metabolites 4-hydroxy-5-phenyl-[1,3]oxazinan-2-one and 2-phenylpropenal. *Chemical Research in Toxicology*, *15*, 815–824.

Rubin, R. L. (2005). Drug-induced lupus. *Toxicology*, *209*, 135–147.

Rubin, R. L., Burlingame, R. W., Arnott, J. E., Totoritis, M. C., McNally, E. M., & Johnson, A. D. (1995). IgG but not other classes of anti-[(H2A-H2B)-DNA] is an early sign of procainamide induced lupus. *Journal of Immunology*, *154*, 2483–2493.

Ruddy, M. J., Shen, F., Smith, J. B., Sharma, A., & Gaffen, S. L. (2004). Interleukin-17 regulates expression of the CXC chemokine LIX/CXCL5 in osteoblasts: implications for inflammation and neutrophil recruitment. *Journal of Leukocyte Biology*, *76*, 135–144.

Sakurai, K., Zou, J. -P., Tschetter, J. R., Ward, J. M., & Shearer, G. M. (2002). Effect of indoleamine 2,3-dioxygenase on induction of experimental autoimmune encephalomyelitis. *Journal of Neuroimmunology*, *129*, 186–196.

Sarich, T. C., Adams, S. P., Petricca, G., & Wright, J. M. (1999). Inhibition of isoniazid-induced hepatotoxicity in rabbits by pretreatment with an amidase inhibitor. *Journal of Pharmacology and Experimental Therapeutics*, *289*, 695–702.

Sarich, T. C., Youssefi, M., Zhou, T., Adams, S. P., Wall, R. A., & Wright, J. M. (1996). Role of hydrazine in the mechanism of isoniazid hepatotoxicity in rabbits. *Archives in Toxicology*, *70*, 835–840.

Sayeh, E., & Uetrecht, J. P. (2001). Factors that modify penicillamine-induced autoimmunity in Brown Norway rats: failure of the Th1/Th2 paradigm. *Toxicology*, *163*, 195–211.

Scaffidi, P., Misteli, T., & Bianchi, M. E. (2002). Release of chromatin protein HMGB1 by necrotic cells triggers inflammation. *Nature*, *418*, 191–195.

Schuller-Levis, G., Mehta, P. D., Rudelli, R., & Sturman, J. (1990). Immunologic consequences of taurine deficiency in cats. *Journal of Leukocyte Biology*, *47*, 321–331.

Seago, A., Jarman, M., Foster, A. B., & Baker, M. (1985). Identification of hydroxylaminoglutethimide as induced urinary metabolites of aminoglutethimide in C57BL/6 mice. In J. W. Forrod, & L. A. Damani (Eds.), *Biological Oxidation of Nitrogen in Organic Molecules* (pp. 149–1563). Chichester: Ellis Horwood Ltd.

Sharma, A., & Uetrecht, J. (2011). Covalent binding of nevirapine in vitro and in vivo. *The Toxicologist*, *120*, 323.

Shenton, J. M., Chen, J., & Uetrecht, J. P. (2004). Animal models of idiosyncratic drug reactions. *Chemico-Biological Interactions*, *150*, 53–70.

Shenton, J. M., Popovic, M., Chen, J., Masson, M. J., & Uetrecht, J. P. (2005). Evidence of an immune-mediated mechanism for an idiosyncratic nevirapine-induced reaction in the female Brown Norway rat. *Chemical Research in Toxicology*, *18*, 1799–1813.

Shenton, J. M., Teranishi, M., Abu-Asab, M. S., Yager, J. A., & Uetrecht, J. P. (2003). Characterization of a potential animal model of an idiosyncratic drug reaction: nevirapine-induced skin rash in the rat. *Chemical Research in Toxicology*, *16*, 1078–1089.

Shevach, E. M., McHugh, R. S., Piccirillo, C. A., & Thornton, A. M. (2001). Control of T-cell activation by CD4+ CD25+ suppressor T cells. *Immunological Reviews*, *182*, 58–67.

Shimizu, S., Atsumi, R., Itokawa, K., Iwasaki, M., Aoki, T., Ono, C., et al. (2009). Metabolism-dependent hepatotoxicity of amodiaquine in glutathione-depleted mice. *Archives in Toxicology*, *83*, 701–707.

Sipes, I. G., & Brown, B. R., Jr, (1976). An animal model of hepatotoxicity associated with halothane anesthesia. *Anesthesiology*, *45*, 622–628.

Siraki, A. G., Bonini, M. G., Jiang, J., Ehrenshaft, M., & Mason, R. P. (2007). Aminoglutethimide-induced protein free radical formation on myeloperoxidase: a potential mechanism of agranulocytosis. *Chemical Research in Toxicology*, *20*, 1038–1045.

Smith, M. T. (2003). Mechanisms of troglitazone hepatotoxicity. *Chemical Research in Toxicology*, *16*, 679–687.

Sodhi, C. P., Rana, S. V., Mehta, S. K., Vaiphei, K., Attari, S., & Mehta, S. (1997). Study of oxidative-stress in isoniazid-rifampicin induced hepatic injury in young rats. *Drug and Chemical Toxicology*, *20*, 255–269.

Stein, H. B., Patterson, A. C., Offer, R. C., Atkins, C. J., Teufel, A., & Robinson, H. S. (1980). Adverse effects of D-penicillamine in rheumatoid arthritis. *Annals of Internal Medicine*, *92*, 24–29.

Tasduq, S. A., Kaiser, P., Sharma, S. C., & Johri, R. K. (2007). Potentiation of isoniazid-induced liver toxicity by rifampicin in a combinational therapy of antitubercular drugs (rifampicin, isoniazid and pyrazinamide) in Wistar rats: a toxicity profile study. *Hepatology Research*, *37*, 845–853.

Thompson, C. D., Gulden, P. H., & Macdonald, T. L. (1997). Identification of modified atropaldehyde mercapturic acids in rat and human urine after felbamate administration. *Chemical Research in Toxicology*, *10*, 457–462.

Thompson, C. D., Kinter, M. T., & Macdonald, T. L. (1996). Synthesis and in vitro reactivity of 3-carbamoyl-2-phenylpropionaldehyde and 2-phenylpropenal: putative reactive metabolites of felbamate. *Chemical Research in Toxicology*, *9*, 1225–1229.

Tingle, M. D., Jewell, H., Maggs, J. L., O'Neill, P. M., & Park, B. K. (1995). The bioactivation of amodiaquine by human polymorphonuclear leucocytes in vitro: chemical mechanisms and the effects of fluorine substitution. *Biochemical Pharmacology*, *50*, 1113–1119.

Tournade, H., Pelletier, L., Pasquier, R., Vial, M. C., Mandet, C., & Druet, P. (1990). D-Penicillamine-induced autoimmunity in Brown-Norway rats. Similarities with HgCl2-induced autoimmunity. *Journal of Immunology*, *144*, 2985–2991.

Trepanier, L. A. (1999). Delayed hypersensitivity reactions to sulphonamides: syndromes, pathogenesis and management. *Veterinary Dermatology*, *10*, 241–248.

Trepanier, L. A. (2004). Idiosyncratic toxicity associated with potentiated sulfonamides in the dog. *Journal of Veterinary Pharmacology and Therapeutics*, *27*, 129–138.

Trepanier, L. A., Danhof, R., Toll, J., & Watrous, D. (2003). Clinical findings in 40 dogs with hypersensitivity associated with administration of potentiated sulfonamides. *Journal of Veterinary Internal Medicine*, *17*, 647–652.

Trepanier, L. A., Ray, K., Winand, N. J., Spielberg, S. P., & Cribb, A. E. (1997). Cytosolic arylamine N-acetyltransferase (NAT) deficiency in the dog and other canids due to absence of NAT genes. *Biochemical Pharmacology*, *54*, 73–80.

Uetrecht, J. (1992). The role of leukocyte-generated reactive metabolites in the pathogenesis of idiosyncratic drug reactions. *Drug Metabolism Reviews*, *24*, 299–366.

Uetrecht, J. (2002). N-oxidation of drugs associated with idiosyncratic drug reactions. *Drug Metabolism Reviews*, *34*, 651–665.

Uetrecht, J. (2005). Role of animal models in the study of drug-induced hypersensitivity reactions. *AAPS Journal*, *7*, E914–921.

Uetrecht, J. (2007). Idiosyncratic drug reactions: current understanding. *Annual Review of Pharmacology and Toxicology*, *47*, 513–539.

Uetrecht, J. (2009). Immunoallergic drug-induced liver injury in humans. *Seminars in Liver Disease*, *29*, 383–392.

Uetrecht, J. P., Ma, H. M., MacKnight, E., & McClelland, R. (1995). Oxidation of aminopyrine by hypochlorite to a reactive dication: possible implications for aminopyrine-induced agranulocytosis. *Chemical Research in Toxicology*, *8*, 226–233.

Usui, T., Mise, M., Hashizume, T., Yabuki, M., & Komuro, S. (2009). Evaluation of the potential for drug-induced liver injury based on in vitro covalent binding to human liver proteins. *Drug Metabolism and Disposition*, *37*, 2383–2392.

Vitezica, Z. G., Milpied, B., Lonjou, C., Borot, N., Ledger, T. N., Lefebvre, A., et al. (2008). HLA-DRB1*01 associated with cutaneous hypersensitivity induced by nevirapine and efavirenz. *AIDS*, *22*, 540–541.

Waldhauser, L., & Uetrecht, J. (1991). Oxidation of propylthiouracil to reactive metabolites by activated neutrophils: implications for agranulocytosis. *Drug Metabolism and Disposition*, *19*, 354–359.

Waldhauser, L., & Uetrecht, J. (1996). Antibodies to myeloperoxidase in propylthiouracil-induced autoimmune disease in the cat. *Toxicology*, *114*, 155–162.

Waring, J. F., Liguori, M. J., Luyendyk, J. P., Maddox, J. F., Ganey, P. E., & Stachlewitz, R. F. (2005). Microarray analysis of lipopolysaccharide potentiation of trovafloxacin-induced liver injury in rats suggests a role for proinflammatory chemokines and neutrophils. *Journal of Pharmacology and Experimental Therapeutics*, *316*, 1080–1087.

Warrington, R. J., McPhilips-Feener, S., & Rutherford, W. J. (1982). The predictive value of the lymphocyte transformation test in isoniazid-associated hepatitis. *Clinical Allergy*, *12*, 217–222.

Warrington, R. J., Tse, K. S., Gorski, B. A., Schwenk, R., & Sehon, A. H. (1978). Evaluation of isoniazid-associated hepatitis by immunological tests. *Clinical & Experimental Immunology*, *32*, 97–104.

Williams, D. P., Pirmohamed, M., Naisbitt, D. J., Uetrecht, J. P., & Park, B. K. (2000). Induction of metabolism-dependent and -independent neutrophil apoptosis by clozapine. *Molecular Pharmacology*, *58*, 207–216.

Wong, K. H., Chan, K. C., & Lee, S. S. (2001). Sex differences in nevirapine rash. *Clinical Infectious Diseases*, *33*, 2096–2098.

You, Q., Cheng, L., & Ju, C. (2010). Generation of T cell responses targeting the reactive metabolite of halothane in mice. *Toxicology Letters*, *194*, 79–85.

You, Q., Cheng, L., Reilly, T. P., Wegmann, D., & Ju, C. (2006). Role of neutrophils in a mouse model of halothane-induced liver injury. *Hepatology*, *44*, 1421–1431.

Yuan, J., Guo, S., Hall, D., Cammett, A. M., Jayadev, S., Distel, M., et al. (2011). Toxicogenomics of nevirapine-associated cutaneous and hepatic adverse events among populations of African, Asian, and European descent. *Aids*, *25*, 1271–1280.

Yung, R., Chang, S., Hemati, N., Johnson, K., & Richardson, B. (1997). Mechanisms of drug induced lupus IV: comparison of procainamide and hydralazine with analogs in vitro and in vivo. *Arthritis & Rheumatism*, *40*, 1436–1443.

Yung, R., Powers, D., Johnson, K., Amento, E., Carr, D., Laing, T., et al. (1996). Mechanisms of drug induced lupus II: T cells overexpressing lymphocyte function-associated antigen 1 become autroreactive and cause lupuslike disease in syngeneic mice. *Journal of Clinical Investgations*, *97*, 2866–2871.

Yung, R. L., Quddus, J., Chrisp, C. E., Johnson, K. J., & Richardson, B. C. (1995). Mechanisms of drug induced lupus I: cloned Th2 cells modified with DNA methylation inhibitors in vitro cause autoimmunity in vivo. *Journal of Immunology*, *154*, 3025–3035.

Zhu, X., Li, J., Liu, F., & Uetrecht, J. P. (2011). Involvement of T helper 17 cells in D-penicillamine-induced autoimmune disease in Brown Norway rats. *Toxicological Sciences*, *120*, 331–338.

Zimmerman, H. (1999). In *Hepatotoxicity: The Adverse Effects of Drugs and Other Chemicals on The Liver* (second ed.). Philadelphia: Lippincott Williams and Wilkins.

Ann K. Daly

Institute of Cellular Medicine, Newcastle University Medical School, Framlington Place, Newcastle upon Tyne, United Kingdom

Genetic Polymorphisms Affecting Drug Metabolism: Recent Advances and Clinical Aspects

Abstract

Though current knowledge of pharmacogenetic factors relevant to drug metabolism is fairly comprehensive and this should facilitate translation to the clinic, there are a number of gaps in knowledge. Recent studies using both conventional and novel approaches have added to our knowledge of pharmacogenetics of drug metabolism. Genome-wide association studies have provided new insights into the major contribution of cytochromes P450 to response to therapeutic agents such as coumarin anticoagulants and clopidogrel as well as to caffeine and nicotine. Recent advances in understanding of factors affecting gene expression, both regulation by transcription factors and by microRNA and epigenetic factors, have added to understanding of variation in expression of genes such as CYP3A4 and CYP2E1. The implementation of testing for pharmacogenetic polymorphisms in prescription of selected anticancer drugs and cardiovascular agents is considered in detail, with current controversies and barriers to implementation of pharmacogenetic testing assessed. Though genotyping for thiopurine methyltransferase is now common prior to prescription of thiopurines, genotyping for other pharmacogenetic polymorphisms prior to drug prescription remains uncommon. However, it seems likely that it will become more widespread as both increased evidence that certain pharmacogenetic tests are valuable and cost-effective and more accessible genotyping methods become available.

Advances in Pharmacology, Volume 63
1054-3589/12 $35.00
http://dx.doi.org/10.1016/B978-0-12-398339-8.00004-5

I. Introduction

Pharmacogenetics is often defined as the study of genetic factors affecting drug response. This includes the genetics of drug metabolism which up to the present is the most widely studied aspect of pharmacogenetics. Our understanding of genetic factors that affect metabolism of prescribed drugs is now generally very comprehensive, though some gaps in knowledge and detail on aspects such as the contribution of factors affecting gene expression still exist. This article will consider in particular advances in genetic aspects of drug metabolism that have taken place in the past 5 years as well as the current situation with regard to application of this knowledge to clinical practice.

There are now a number of examples of therapeutically important drugs whose metabolism is affected to a clinically significant extent by genetic polymorphism. Regulatory authorities worldwide have initiated consultation on how to implement existing knowledge on all aspects of pharmacogenetics to enable safer prescribing of drugs and in some cases guidelines have already been issued. There is still considerable potential for further progress in this area and a number of novel associations linking particular metabolic polymorphisms to outcome of treatment have emerged quite recently. Some key examples of this type of association will be considered individually.

II. Recent Advances in the Pharmacogenetics of Cytochromes P450

A. Background

A range of polymorphisms has been described in 50 or more genes encoding human cytochromes P450 (CYP). Many of these are functionally significant and occur at relatively high population frequencies. These high frequencies may be because the nonessential nature of many CYP-mediated reactions and the overlapping substrate specificity of these enzymes mean that absence or low activity of a particular isoform is generally not a serious problem. In the case of four isoforms important in drug metabolism, CYP2D6, CYP2C19, CYP2A6 and CYP3A5, there is complete absence of active enzyme in significant number of individuals (Table I). In addition, polymorphisms resulting in either decreased or increased activity are common in genes encoding most cytochrome P450 isoforms relevant to drug metabolism (see Table I). For at least three different CYP genes, higher than normal activity due to the existence of copy number variants or upstream polymorphisms can also occur. Detailed descriptions of the importance of individual isoforms in drug metabolism and the types of genetic polymorphisms that may affect this metabolism are provided in several recent review articles (Daly, 2010b;

TABLE I Polymorphisms in Cytochromes P450 Relevant to Drug Metabolism and Their Functional Importance

Gene	*Common variant alleles*	*Functional effect*	*Reference*
CYP1A2	*CYP1A2*1F*	High induced activity	Sachse et al. (1999)
CYP2A6	*CYP2A6*2 & *4*	Absence of activity	Fernandez-Salguero et al. (1995); Oscarson et al. (1999)
	*CYP2A6*1X2A & *1X2B*	High activity	Rao et al. (2000); Fukami et al. (2007)
CYP2B6	*CYP2B6*2, *5 & *6*	?Decreased activity	Lang et al. (2001)
CYP2C8	*CYP2C8*2, *3 & *4*	?Decreased activity	Bahadur et al. (2002); Dai et al. (2001)
	*CYP2C8*5*	Absence of activity	Soyama et al. (2002)
CYP2C9	*CYP2C9*2 & *3*	Low activity	Rettie et al. (1994); Sullivan-Close et al. (1996)
	*CYP2C9*6*	No activity	Kidd et al. (2001)
CYP2C19	*CYP2C19*2 & *3*	No activity	de Morais et al. (1994a, b)
	*CYP2C19*17*	High activity	Sim et al. (2006)
CYP2D6	*CYP2D6*3, *4, *5 & *6*	No activity	Gaedigk et al. (1991); Kagimoto et al. (1990); Saxena et al. (1994)
	*CYP2D6*10 & *17*	Low activity	Johansson et al. (1994); Masimirembwa et al. (1996)
	*CYP2D6*1XN & *2XN*	High activity	Johansson et al. (1993)
CYP3A5	*CYP3A5*3*	No expression	Kuehl et al. (2001)

Only selected alleles and CYP isoforms are shown. Full details are available elsewhere (http://www.cypalleles.ki.se/, accessed September 2011).

Ingelman-Sundberg & Sim, 2010; Ingelman-Sundberg et al., 2007; Rodriguez-Antona et al., 2010). There is also a website which provides detailed descriptions of individual variants (http://www.cypalleles.ki.se/, accessed September 2011). However, as summarized in Table I, the effect on enzyme activity of certain variant alleles in CYP2B6 and CYP2C8 is still unclear with disagreement between studies, possibly because some effects could be substrate-dependent, though this has not been demonstrated directly.

B. Impact of Genome-wide Association Studies

Much of the current knowledge on sequence variation and its phenotypic effect in the cytochromes P450 was obtained from detailed investigations of sequences following cloning and localization of the various genes to particular regions of the human genome. This knowledge was mainly available prior to the sequencing of the human genome or the HapMap project (Manolio et al., 2008), though the availability of additional genomic information from these sources has still been informative. Since 2007, genome-wide association (GWA) studies on disease susceptibility and other individual traits ranging from height to coffee consumption have provided additional information on the effects of genetic variability on these traits (Burton et al., 2007). These studies involve genotyping approx. one million single nucleotide polymorphisms (often referred to as SNPs) scattered throughout the human genome and determining statistically whether genotype distribution for each is different between cases and controls or correlates with a particular measurable characteristic. More details of the methods used are provided in recent review articles (Hardy & Singleton, 2009; Hirschhorn, 2009). A number of these GWA studies are concerned with pharmacogenetics (Daly, 2010a) with several adding to our understanding of the role of cytochrome P450 in drug metabolism, as summarized in Table II.

In particular, the GWA studies with findings relevant to cytochrome P450 were concerned with response to coumarin anticoagulants and clopidogrel, with factors affecting smoking intensity and with factors affecting coffee consumption. Four GWA studies on genetic factors affecting various aspects of the coumarin anticoagulants warfarin and acenocoumarol, particularly dose requirement to achieve the required level of anticoagulation, have appeared (Cha et al., 2010; Cooper et al., 2008; Takeuchi et al., 2009; Teichert et al., 2009). They are largely confirmatory of previous candidate gene studies and are discussed in more detail in Section IV.B.1. Response to another agent used in treatment of cardiovascular disease, the antiplatelet drug clopidogrel has also been studied by a GWA study with this study confirming that the most important factor in response is genotype for the main metabolizing enzyme CYP2C19, as discussed in more detail in Section IV.B.2. (Shuldiner et al., 2009).

TABLE II Genome-Wide Association Studies Showing Significant Roles for Cytochrome P450 Genes

Subject of study	*Significant CYP gene*	*References*
Warfarin dose requirement	CYP2C9 and CYP4F2[a]	Cha et al. (2010); Cooper et al. (2008); Takeuchi et al. (2009)
Acenocoumarol dose requirement	CYP2C9 and CYP4F2[a]	Teichert et al. (2009)
Response to clopidogrel	CYP2C19	Shuldiner et al. (2009)
Smoking behavior	CYP2A6[b]	Thorgeirsson et al. (2010)
Caffeine intake	CYP1A2[c]	Cornelis et al. (2011); Sulem et al. (2011)

[a] VKORC1 gene is also genome-wide significant.

[b] CHRNB3–CHRNA6 gene region is also genome-wide significant.

[c] AhR gene is also genome-wide significant.

A GWA study on smoking behavior found a strong association with the main nicotine metabolizing cytochrome P450, CYP2A6 (Thorgeirsson et al., 2010). A polymorphism in linkage disequilibrium with *CYP2A6*2*, an allele which is well established to be associated with absence of CYP2A6 enzyme activity, was associated with reduced smoking quantity. This had been shown previously by studying CYP2A6 directly but the GWA also found some evidence for an additional role for CYP2B6 in smoking behavior and also enabled the relative overall contribution of the CYP2A6 variant (odds ratio 0.39 for cigarettes smoked per day) to this process to be assessed in more detail. As with the GWA study on coumarin anticoagulant response, genes which encode the nicotinic acetylcholine receptor, the target for nicotine, were also important predictors of response in the GWA study on smoking behavior.

Recently, two GWA studies on coffee consumption have provided valuable insights into genetic polymorphism in CYP1A2 (Cornelis et al., 2011; Sulem et al., 2011). These findings are particularly interesting because, though it has been well established that individuals vary in their ability to metabolize caffeine, clear correlations between CYP1A2 genotype and caffeine metabolism have not been made previously. Both recent studies involved very large sample sizes (5000 and 40,000 subjects respectively) and found that polymorphisms close to the CYP1A2 gene and the gene for its transcriptional regulator AhR predict the amount of caffeine consumed per day. There are still limitations; though highly statistically significant associations were found, the overall contribution of the two genes to caffeine consumption is still small (only in the region of 0.2 cups a day per allele for each gene) with other factors also likely to be involved. Also, the underlying mechanisms by which the effects occur is still unclear except that for CYP1A2, there is a relationship between the most statistically significant polymorphism and *CYP1A2*1F* which was previously reported to be associated with higher CYP1A2 activity when induction via AhR had occurred (Sachse et al., 1999). However, it seems likely that the main genetic polymorphisms affecting CYP1A2 activity and hence coffee consumption may lie elsewhere in the gene, possibly further upstream. These findings are also likely to be applicable to prescribed drugs whose main route of metabolism is by CYP1A2. Examples of these include clozapine, theophylline and several fluoroquinolone antimicrobials (Faber et al., 2005).

Using a slightly different approach involving the DMET™ gene chip (http://www.affymetrix.com/browse/products.jsp?productId=131412&categoryId=35657#1_1, accessed September 2011) which enables genotyping for a large number of genetic polymorphisms relevant to drug disposition but does not cover the entire genome, novel data showing that CYP4F2 genotype for a nonsynonymous polymorphism contributes to warfarin dose requirement was obtained (Caldwell et al., 2008). CYP4F2 had been previously demonstrated to contribute to metabolism of fatty acids and vitamin E (Sontag & Parker, 2007; Stec et al., 2007). Following the finding on the apparent relevance to warfarin treatment, it was demonstrated that CYP4F2 also contributes to vitamin K1 oxidation with the nonsynonymous polymorphism resulting in decreased activity *in vitro* (McDonald et al., 2009). CYP4F2 has a limited role in drug metabolism but it contributes to metabolism of fingolimod, a new treatment for relapsing multiple sclerosis (Jin et al., 2011).

Using the DMET™ chip described above or a variety of other contemporary genotyping techniques, a comprehensive genotype profile for all genes relevant to phases I and II metabolism together with transporter genes and transcription factors relevant to drug disposition can be obtained without difficulty. When investigating genotype–phenotype relationships by genotyping samples for many different polymorphisms, care needs to be taken to perform appropriate correction for multiple testing to avoid detecting spurious associations. Finding significant associations may therefore require larger sample sizes than those used normally in, for example, detailed pharmacokinetic studies in phase I clinical trials.

C. Genetic Factors Affecting Cytochrome P450 Expression

The studies described in Section II.B above have added to understanding of genetic factors directly affecting levels or activity of cytochrome P450s. Other likely contributors to interindividual variability in cytochrome P450 activity include variation in transcription factors, regulation by microRNA and epigenetics involving differential gene methylation. The general area of transcription factor regulation of CYP expression is complex and beyond the scope of this article but there are a few examples where either polymorphisms affecting transcription factors or polymorphisms in transcription factor binding sites on CYPs can affect overall expression.

It is clear that all CYPs show considerable interindividual variation in expression. Whether the majority of this variation can be explained by genetic polymorphisms in the coding or regulatory regions of genes varies between CYP isoforms. In the case of CYP2D6, it is possible to predict overall activity and hepatic expression on the basis of genotype. One reason for this is that CYP2D6 is not inducible and regulation of its expression at the transcriptional level seems relatively simple. For other CYPs with well-studied genetic polymorphisms including CYP2C19 and CYP2C9, the situation is less clearcut. The known polymorphisms make an important contribution to overall variation in activity but other factors, potentially both additional genetic factors and environmental factors, are also likely to important determinants of activity. This is also the case for both CYP3A4 and CYP2E1 but for these CYPs, despite extensive genetic studies, it is not currently possible to predict activity by genotyping for known polymorphisms in either coding or non-coding regions of the genes.

There is emerging data on the relevance of polymorphisms in the nuclear receptor gene superfamily to activity for some cytochromes P450. In particular, though nonsynonymous polymorphisms in *NR1I2* which encodes PXR are rare, a number of non-coding polymorphisms have been identified and studied in detail. Evidence that several of these non-coding polymorphisms are functionally significant has been obtained using a variety of *in vitro* and *in vivo* approaches (Zhang et al., 2001; Hustert et al., 2001; Lamba et al., 2008; Sandanaraj et al., 2008; Andrews et al., 2010; Schipani et al., 2010). In the case of the main other nuclear receptor superfamily member that contributes to induction of drug metabolizing cytochromes P450 CAR which is encoded by *NR1I3*, there is less information on polymorphisms and their functional significance. However, as in the case of PXR, a number of coding and non-coding polymorphisms have been detected with non-synonymous polymorphisms rare (Ikeda et al., 2003; Lamba, 2008). A recent report suggests that a synonymous polymorphism which can be used to tag a common CAR haplotype is associated with a higher than normal plasma concentration of the antiretroviral drug efavirenz (Wyen et al., 2011) but other data on functional effects of common CAR polymorphisms is currently very limited.

When P450 induction occurs, genotype for upstream polymorphisms in the induced cytochrome P450 gene together with nuclear receptor genotype may combine to predict overall P450 activity post-induction. For example, rifampicin inducibility of CYP2B6 appears to be affected by genotype for a promoter-region CYP2B6 polymorphism in the *CYP2B6*22* allele (Li et al., 2010). Somewhat similarly, an upstream polymorphism in CYP2C9 within the *CYP2C9*1B* allele was shown previously not to have any effect on warfarin dose requirement (King et al., 2004) but has recently been demonstrated to be relevant to clearance and maintenance dose requirement for phenytoin, another CYP2C9 substrate (Chaudhry et al., 2010). This appears to be due to two separate upstream polymorphisms within *CYP2C9*1B* affecting the level of CAR- and PXR-mediated induction by phenytoin. Other CYP2C9 substrates which also act as autoinducers may show similar genotype-dependent induction patterns.

Since CYP3A4 is the most abundant CYP in most human livers and is also the most important in terms of number of drugs metabolized, understanding the factors that determine variation in levels of expression is of considerable interest. Two recent studies have attempted to do this. The first found that up to 25% of variability could be explained by genetic polymorphisms in the CYP3A4 promoter region together with genotypes for a number of different transcription factors including pregnane X-receptor (PXR), HNF-4α and FoxA2 (Lamba et al., 2010). The second study compared the CYP3A4 upstream regulatory region with that for other CYP3A genes, including CYP3A5 and various non-human CYP3A genes, and concluded that the unique complexity of this region in CYP3A4 which includes binding sites for a number of different nuclear receptors means that it is not possible to predict activity from genotype due to the unusual sensitivity of this gene to endogenous and exogenous nuclear receptor ligands (Qiu et al., 2010).

In addition to polymorphisms affecting transcription factors and transcription factor binding sites, regulation of gene expression by microRNAs (miRNA) should be considered as a possible predictor of CYP gene expression. It is increasingly clear that these small (approx. 22bp) RNA molecules interact with mRNA targets, often in the 3′-noncoding region, to affect mRNA levels which can result in either increased degredation rates or stabilization. Alternatively, binding of an miRNA can affect translation rate. Both the miRNA molecules and their target mRNAs are subject to genetic polymorphism. Data on the possible relevance of such polymorphisms to regulation of CYP levels is still limited. One recent survey suggests that fewer genes concerned with pharmacokinetics are regulated by miRNAs compared with those involved with pharmacodynamics or other functions (Rukov et al., 2011) so this form of regulation may not be of great overall importance for the CYPs. There are two more general pharmacogenetic examples involving non-CYP genes (dihydrofolate reductase and SULT1A1) where polymorphisms in the target gene affect miRNA binding and hence overall enzyme activity (Mishra et al., 2007; Yu et al., 2010). For CYP genes, several different miRNA binding sites have been characterized. In the case of one of these, located at the 3'-end of the CYP2E1 gene, a correlation between levels of the miRNA (miR-378), CYP2E1 mRNA and CYP2E1 protein in human liver has been demonstrated (Mohri et al., 2010).

Epigenetic mechanisms are a further possible determinant level of CYP expression. There is increasing interest in epigenetics as a predictor of disease susceptibility generally as well as its possible contribution to pharmacogenetic variation (epipharmacogenetics) (for review see Ingelman-Sundberg & Gomez (2010)). Epigenetics is concerned with the study of DNA and histone modification by various mechanisms including methylation and acetylation. There is tissue specificity but patterns of modification can be maintained during mitosis. Patterns of DNA methylation of specific genes can be inherited with preferential expression possible of either the maternal or paternal form (imprinting). This form of epigenetic inheritance is important in certain rare diseases but probably only affects a subset of genes. More general DNA or histone modification is of more relevance to variation in CYP expression. However, in this case, the level of modification will be determined primarily by environmental factors (including drug treatment) and will therefore not be predictable by studying germ-line DNA, though it may be measurable by studying DNA or chromatin derived from a specific CYP gene from a tissue of interest. For example, in an epigenetic study on CYP1A2, it was found that the extent of methylation of a CpG island close to the translation start site inversely correlated with hepatic CYP1A2 mRNA levels (Ghotbi et al., 2009). Though the impact of pharmacoepigenetic factors will be important in relation to issues such as drug–drug interactions, applying epigenetic information on drug metabolism by CYPs to individualising drug therapy in the way that has already been done for some pharmacogenetic polymorphisms (see Section IV for specific examples) is difficult because of the likely need to study liver tissue.

Recently, expression quantitative trait locus (eQTL) analysis relating genotype for polymorphisms genome-wide to levels of gene expression determined by expression microarray analysis has been applied to human liver samples in several independent studies (Schadt et al., 2008; Innocenti et al., 2011; Schroder et al., 2011). The eQTL studies have generally not demonstrated strong associations between cytochrome P450 genotype and expression and also there is generally poor overall agreement between findings in the three studies. However, two of the studies report significant correlations between CYP3A5 genotype and expression. The first of the three eQTL studies was recently extended to a systems biology study of genetic and genomic factors affecting individual cytochrome P450 isoform expression and activity with additional data on enzyme activity for common P450 isoforms added. There was not only a good correlation between gene expression and enzyme activity for most isoforms but also correlations between activity measurements for different isoforms were seen. A network underlying P450 transcriptional regulation was described with three non-P450 genes, *EHHADH*, *SLC10A1* and *AKR1D1* appearing to regulate overall P450 expression (Yang et al., 2010). Each of these genes has some indirect biological plausibility for a connection to P450 in that all are responsive to transcription factors which also regulate P450 genes. These findings are interesting and novel but need to be confirmed independently. It seems likely that further bioinformatic-based approaches of this type will enable a more complete integration of the overall effect of genetic and non-genetic factors on cytochrome P450 gene expression.

III. Recent Advances in the Pharmacogenetics of Non-P450 Metabolism

As for the cytochromes P450, the pharmacogenetics of metabolism involving either non-P450 phase I metabolism or phase II conjugation reactions is mostly already well established with only limited advances reported on the fundamental aspects in the last 5 years. There are still gaps in knowledge in some areas, including pharmacogenetics of carboxyesterases (Sanghani et al., 2009) and amino acid conjugation (Knights et al., 2007), but the extent of variation in these metabolic reactions as well as their overall importance appears to be insufficient to stimulate detailed investigations. In terms of overall importance in drug metabolism as well as the extent to which they have been studied, the UGT family ranks second after the CYP superfamily. In particular, pharmacogenetic aspects of glucuronidation have been well studied. In recent reviews (Bock, 2010; Guillemette et al., 2010), detailed information on the individual isoforms including their substrate specificities and the main genetic polymorphisms affecting them is provided. The issue concerning effects on expression by multiple transcription factors and potential for additional effects on activity by epigenetic factors discussed in detail for the CYPs is also relevant for UGTs, especially since a number are subject to regulation by several different nuclear receptors.

Acetyltransferases and methyltransferases do not appear to be inducible and thus direct prediction of individual phenotypes from genetic information is more feasible. This is certainly the case for N-acetyltransferase 2 (NAT2) and thiopurine methyltransferase (TPMT) where genetic polymorphisms associated with absence of enzyme activity are relatively common and there is a clear relationship between genotype and phenotype. TPMT is discussed in more detail in Section IV.A.1 in relation to thiopurine drug therapy.

Pharmacogenetic knowledge of the sulfotransferases is less complete but SULT1A1 is the sulfotransferase isoform investigated in most detail. Two relatively recent findings on SULT1A1 pharmacogenetics are of particular interest. The first involved the finding that additional copies of this gene coding for apparently active enzyme are not uncommon, especially in African Americans and also that some individuals have a deletion of *SULT1A1* (Hebbring et al., 2007). Further studies on this gene have investigated polymorphisms in the 3'-untranslated region with three common polymorphisms in strong linkage disequilibrium detected (Yu et al., 2010). Genotype for these polymorphisms, when combined with copy number variation information, was a strong predictor of SULT1A1 activity in individuals of European ethnic origin. One 3'-untranslated region polymorphism was demonstrated to interact with the miRNA miR-631 with stronger binding to the variant sequence predicting decreased stability, providing an interesting explanation for the function significance of the polymorphism. As discussed in Section II.C, miRNA regulation of gene expression is likely to be an important general regulatory mechanism and the *SULT1A1* polymorphism is currently the best example of this applied to drug metabolism. Though SULT1A1 is likely to contribute to the metabolism of a relatively large number of drugs, the overall importance of polymorphism in this gene in terms of drug response or toxicity is still unclear.

There is also a large amount of pharmacogenetic data on the glutathione *S*-transferases (GSTs), another gene superfamily that encodes enzymes that contribute to conjugation (for review see Board (2011)). The best-studied polymorphisms are the large deletions in *GSTM1* and *GSTT1* which are each associated with absence of enzyme activity. However, there are up to 10 different GST families, all subject to polymorphisms to some extent. In general, the overall importance of genetic polymorphism in GST to drug metabolism is unimportant with some important exceptions. Because of their chemical properties, a range of anticancer drugs undergo metabolism by GST so GST polymorphisms may be particularly important in this therapeutic area (for review see Bosch et al. (2006)). In addition, for adverse drug reactions involving reactive metabolite formation such as those seen in drug-induced liver injury, there is some evidence that the GSTM1 and T1 deletions may be associated with increased susceptibility to toxicity (Andrade et al., 2009). Otherwise, the main importance of GST polymorphisms is likely to be in relation to diseases linked to xenobiotic exposure or variation in metabolism of endogenous compounds.

IV. Clinical Relevance of Polymorphic Metabolism – Some Contemporary Examples

A. Anticancer Drugs

Polymorphic metabolism affecting anticancer drugs is of particular interest for a number of reasons including the narrow therapeutic window for these drugs and the fact that the specialist nature of cancer chemotherapy may make implementation of pharmacogenetic testing easier than in more general medicine. One of the earliest and most successful examples of use of a pharmacogenetic test, that of TPMT in relation to thiopurine use, falls within the area of cancer chemotherapy. This example is discussed in detail together with newer examples of UGT1A1 and irinotecan, CYP2D6 and tamoxifen, CYP2B6 and cyclophosphamide and dihydropyrimidine dehydrogenase (DPD) and 5-fluorouracil. Pharmacogenetic tests on tumor material are also important in cancer chemotherapy but as they do not relate to drug metabolism are outside the scope of this article.

1. Thiopurines and TPMT

Thiopurine methyltransferase (TPMT) metabolizes the cytotoxic drug 6-mercaptopurine which is widely used in treatment of childhood acute lymphoblastic leukemia (ALL). This enzyme also metabolizes thioguanine, another anti-cancer drug, and azathioprine, a 6-mercaptopurine precursor which is used as an immunosuppressant. Approximately 0.3% of various European populations lack detectable TPMT activity and 11% have intermediate levels (Weinshilboum & Sladek, 1980). The molecular basis of the polymorphism is now very well understood and it is well established that in individuals with undetectable activity, the toxic effects of treatment with standard doses of thioguanines are life-threatening due to high concentrations of thioguanine nucleotides being formed (for reviews see Evans (2004) and Marsh & Van Booven (2009)). TPMT status can be determined either by genotyping or by phenotyping, which involves measurement of enzyme levels in erythrocytes. Recent surveys suggest that TPMT testing prior to initiation of treatment with either 6-mercaptopurine or azathioprine is now common in a number of countries worldwide (Ford & Berg, 2010; Gardiner & Begg, 2005; Relling et al., 2011; van den Akker-van Marle et al., 2006). International recommendations giving guidance on testing and interpretation of results are now available (Relling et al., 2011; Swen et al., 2011). Most of the data showing the value and cost-effectiveness for TPMT testing relates to the use of azathioprine in inflammatory diseases in adults rather than 6-mercaptopurine in childhood leukemia, mainly because azathioprine is used widely in these common conditions and childhood leukemia requiring 6-mercaptopurine treatment is rarer (Meggitt et al., 2006; Newman et al., 2011; Teml et al., 2007). However, data from studies on azathioprine can also be extrapolated to 6-mercaptopurine use. An important difference is that in leukemia patients with TPMT deficiency the recommended starting dose for 6-mercaptopurine is a 10-fold lower than normal dose, whereas for inflammatory conditions for which azathioprine treatment in an option, use of an alternative drug in TPMT-deficient patients would be more usual (Relling et al., 2011).

2. *Irinotecan and UGT1A1*

Irinotecan is a camptothecin analog which, following metabolism by carboxyesterase to an active metabolite (SN38), acts as a topoisomerase I inhibitor. The overall metabolic pathway for irinotecan is complex but glucuronidation by UGT1A1 is an important detoxicating step for SN38 (Nagar & Blanchard, 2006). UGT1A1 is also the main enzyme responsible for the glucuronidation of bilirubin and is subject to a well-characterized polymorphism which results in a raised serum bilirubin and a condition called Gilbert's syndrome. The most common polymorphism giving rise to Gilbert's syndrome is a 2bp insertion in the promoter region (*UGT1A1*28* allele) but certain SNPs which result in amino acid substitutions can also give rise to the condition (Burchell et al., 2000). Individuals homozygous or heterozygous for polymorphisms associated with Gilbert's syndrome appear to be at increased risk of toxicity with irinotecan (Nagar & Blanchard, 2006). The US Food and Drug Administration (FDA)-approved drug label recommends that *UGT1A1*28* genotyping should be performed prior to administration of this drug due to the increased risk of neutropenia in patients homozygous for this allele (http://www.pfizer.com/files/products/uspi_camptosar.pdf, accessed September 2011). The FDA has also licensed a genotyping test for *UGT1A1*28* (http://twt.com/clinical/ivd/ugt1a1.html, accessed September 2011). However, there are still some issues that need to be addressed in relation to the value of UGT1A1 genotyping in patients receiving irinotecan. In a detailed review of published studies linking *UGT1A1* genotype and either irinotecan pharmacokinetics or irinotecan-associated toxicity (Nagar & Blanchard, 2006), it was stated that the majority of published pharmacokinetic studies reported that possession of either *UGT1A1*28* or another "Gilbert's" allele was associated with a lower SN38-glucuronide over SN38 ratio as expected due to lower rates of glucuronide formation. However, when clinical studies examining UGT1A1 genotype in relation to toxicity were considered, there was less agreement. The various studies disagreed on whether *UGT1A1*28* was a risk factor for either severe diarrhea or neutropenia though there was some indication that *UGT1A1*28* might be associated with an increased risk of neutropenia but with a decreased risk of diarrhea. In addition to UGT1A1, other members of the UGT1A family can also glucuronidate SN38. Apparent associations between toxicity and other UGT1A genes including UGT1A6, UGT1A7 and UGT1A9 have also been reported (Carlini et al., 2005; Girard et al., 2006). Interpretation of these studies is complicated by the strong linkage disequilibrium within the UGT1A locus but it is possible that genotyping for additional polymorphisms may provide a better prediction of susceptibility to toxicity. The frequency of *UGT1A1*28* is lower in non-European populations but a number of other polymorphisms which give rise to the same phenotype are more common in other ethnic groups (Hall et al., 1999). The relationship between *UGT1A1*28* and neutropenia also appears to be dose dependent. For example, though possession of at least one *UGT1A1*28* allele is a significant risk factor for neutropenia at moderate to high irinotecan doses (Hoskins et al., 2007), this does not hold at lower doses (Schulz et al., 2009). Further assessment suggests that use of lower doses may not be effective in most patients and, if *UGT1A1*28* homozygotes can be excluded from treatment, those with other genotypes may benefit from relatively high doses (Toffoli et al., 2010).

Some recent studies have considered additional pharmacogenetic factors to *UGT1A1*28* genotype in susceptibility to irinotecan toxicity. There is now evidence that additional UGT1A1 polymorphisms such as −3156G>A also contribute (Innocenti et al., 2009; McLeod et al., 2010). ABC transporter genotype, particularly that for ABCC2, may be an additional toxicity predictor (Innocenti et al., 2009).

In general, though there is now considerable data to suggest that *UGT1A1*28* genotype is an important predictor of neutropenia related to irinotecan, additional genetic factors may need to be considered to provide a comprehensive individual risk prediction. For another important irinotecan toxicity, diarrhea, recent studies suggest that inhibition of bacterial intestinal glucuronidase activity toward SN38 glucuronide by use of specific glucuronidase inhibitors may be more effective than defining an "at risk" genotype group for this toxicity (Wallace et al., 2010).

3. *Tamoxifen and CYP2D6*

Tamoxifen is a very successful and widely used treatment for estrogen receptor-positive breast cancer. Its metabolism is complex but relatively recently it was recognized that CYP2D6 produces a 4-hydroxy-N-desmethyltamoxifen metabolite (endoxifen) (Desta et al., 2004; Jin et al., 2005). Endoxifen is found at high plasma levels in many patients and binds strongly to estrogen receptors suggesting it is particularly important in the biological response to tamoxifen (Lim et al., 2006; Murdter et al., 2011). Other metabolites, particularly 4-hydroxytamoxifen, also bind to the estrogen receptor though not as strongly as endoxifen (Murdter et al., 2011). A number of studies suggest that patients positive for one or two CYP2D6 poor metabolizer alleles show an increased incidence of breast cancer relapse though a number of studies also report no CYP2D6 influence (reviewed by Hoskins et al. (2009)). Studies relating plasma endoxifen levels to CYP2D6 genotype show a strong positive correlation with the presence of poor metabolizer alleles associated with the lowest levels of this metabolite (Jin et al., 2005; Lim et al., 2006; Murdter et al., 2011). It is possible that CYP2D6 ultrarapid metabolizers may show a different outcome to other genotype groups when treated with tamoxifen but this aspect has not been widely studied except for one study demonstrating that those patients positive for ultrarapid alleles showed highest clinical benefit (Schroth et al., 2010). Tamoxifen is also a substrate for CYP3A4/5 and CYP2C9 and it may therefore be necessary to consider the effect of additional polymorphisms on tamoxifen metabolism (Murdter et al., 2011). A role for *CYP2C19* genotype in determining outcome of treatment has also been suggested (Schroth et al., 2007; van Schaik et al., 2011).

The lack of overall agreement between studies on the relationship between CYP2D6 and outcome of treatment may reflect the overall complexity of tamoxifen metabolism together with issues such as tumor behavior over time and the fact that most studies up to the present have been retrospective (Brauch et al., 2011; Singh et al., 2011). One recent prospective study used CYP2D6 genotype-guided dosing with intermediate or poor metabolizers given double the normal tamoxifen dose. This resulted in the intermediate metabolizers showing similar plasma endoxifen levels to the extensive metabolizers though the levels reached in poor metabolizers were still lower (Irvin et al., 2011). The study indicates that dose adjustment on the basis of genotype is certainly feasible though may not be effective for all CYP2D6 genotypes. However, as stated recently, only when ongoing prospective studies are completed is the issue of relevance of CYP2D6 to tamoxifen treatment likely to be finally resolved (Brauch et al., 2011).

In view of the availability of other effective treatments such as aromatase inhibitors which are suitable for many, though not all, patients, CYP2D6 genotyping may be of value in determining the most appropriate treatment for estrogen receptor-positive breast cancer. However, routine testing is not recommended currently for a number of reasons as discussed by Higgins & Stearns (2011).

4. *Cyclophosphamide*

The oxazaphosphorine cyclophosphamide is one of the most widely used drugs in cancer chemotherapy. It is also used as an immunosuppressive at lower doses. As with the other anticancer drugs discussed in previous sessions, it is a prodrug. In this case, the first activation step involves hydroxylation by cytochromes P450 but there is also a competing CYP-mediated detoxication reaction (for review see Pinto et al. (2009)). A number of different CYP isoforms contribute to these reactions but in general CYP2B6, CYP2C19, CYP2C9 and CYP3A4/5 appear to be the main contributors to the activation step. Each of these is subject to well-studied polymorphisms, though the functional effects of the CYP2B6 variants are less well understood than those of the other isoforms (see Table I). A number of studies have assessed the effect of genotype on response to cyclophosphamide in patients undergoing treatment for a range of diseases. Most studies have determined effects of genotype on relapse and overall survival following treatment. Several report significant effects for CYP2B6 and CYP2C19 genotypes. *CYP2C19*2* homozygosity appears to be associated with a poorer response to treatment (Bray et al., 2010; Melanson et al., 2010; Takada et al., 2004). The relative rarity of this genotype means larger studies are needed to confirm these findings but they are consistent with a recent study using both human liver samples and pharmacokinetic studies on a small number of patients which indicated that carriage of at least one *CYP2C19*2* allele was associated with lower levels of cyclophosphamide activation (Helsby et al., 2010). The situation concerning CYP2B6 as a determinant of cyclophosphamide response is more complicated, mainly because phenotype–genotype relationships for various alleles remain somewhat unclear. However, in a recent study possession of *CYP2B6*6* appeared to be associated with poorer survival in breast cancer patients who had been treated with cyclophosphamide (Bray et al., 2010) and an analogous result was seen in patients who received hematopoietic stem cell grafts following cyclophosphamide conditioning with poorer progression-free survival seen in *CYP2B6*6* homozygotes (Melanson et al., 2010). *CYP2B6*2* and *CYP2B6*5* have also been suggested to be associated with poorer treatment outcomes (Bray et al., 2010; Takada et al., 2004). The precise effects of the *CYP2B6*2*, **5* and **6* alleles on cyclophosphamide activation remain controversial (Helsby & Tingle, 2011) so interpretation of the various *in vivo* findings is difficult and it is not possible to offer any current pharmacogenetic guidelines in relation to cyclophosphamide treatment. As other enzymes including GST isoforms and aldehyde dehydrogenases also contribute to cyclophosphamide activation and metabolism, it has been suggested that GWA studies may provide clearer data on genetic factors affecting response and toxicity (Pinto et al., 2009).

5. *Fluoropyrimidines and DPD*

DPD has a biochemical role in the catabolism of uracil and thymine and is not primarily a drug metabolizing enzyme. However, this enzyme is also responsible for the phase I metabolism of the fluoropyrimidine anticancer drugs 5-fluorouracil and capecitabine. Interindividual variation in the metabolism of 5-fluorouracil has been correlated with levels of DPD in peripheral blood mononuclear cells (Van Kuilenburg et al., 1999). Complete deficiency of DPD has been linked to various physiological abnormalities. It is estimated that up to 3% of the population may be heterozygous for the deficiency and, although they do not suffer physiological abnormalities, these individuals are at increased risk of serious toxic effects if given 5-fluorouracil or capecitabine. The US pack insert for capecitabine (www.accessdata.fda.gov/drugsatfda_docs/label/2000/20896lbl.pdf, accessed September 2011) states that "rarely, unexpected, severe toxicity (e.g., stomatitis, diarrhea, neutropenia and neurotoxicity) associated with 5-fluorouracil has been attributed to a deficiency of DPD activity. A link between decreased levels of DPD and increased, potentially fatal toxic effects of 5-fluorouracil therefore cannot be excluded" but there is no specific requirement currently for genetic testing. A number of common polymorphisms that give rise to DPD deficiency have been identified but these do not appear to explain all cases of low DPD activity, indicating the complex nature of genetics of this enzyme (Collie-Duguid et al., 2000; Van Kuilenburg et al., 2000). In particular, there is recent evidence that polymorphisms in non-coding regions of the gene and large gene deletions may be associated with absence of enzyme activity in some individuals (Amstutz et al., 2009; Van Kuilenburg et al., 2010). Measurement of DPD levels in peripheral blood mononuclear cells is the most sensitive method currently available to predict drug response but the method is relatively cumbersome (Yen & McLeod, 2007). In view of the widespread use of fluoropyrimidines in cancer treatment, it is important that reliable and sensitive methods be available to identify those at risk of serious toxicity due to low or absent DPD activity. Possibly sequencing the entire gene prior to treatment may be feasible in the near future.

B. Cardiovascular Agents

1. *Warfarin and Other Coumarin Anticoagulants*

There is an extensive literature showing that CYP2C9 plays a major role in the metabolism of warfarin and other coumarin anticoagulants (reviewed recently by Jonas & McLeod (2009)). The *CYP2C9*2* and *CYP2C9*3* alleles were originally shown to be significant predictors of low warfarin dose requirement (Steward et al., 1997; Aithal et al., 1999) and have been subsequently demonstrated to affect coumarin anticoagulant dose requirement in a large number of studies (Jonas & McLeod, 2009). Most of these studies suggest that 10–15% of interindividual variation in anticoagulant dose requirement relates to CYP2C9 polymorphisms. The relatively recent cloning of the gene encoding the coumarin anticoagulant target VKORC1 (Li et al., 2004; Rost et al., 2004) led to further population studies that showed that genotype for this gene contributed in the region of 25% to variability in dose requirement (Jonas & McLeod, 2009). More recently, as discussed in Section II.B above, a small contribution by CYP4F2 to dose requirement due to its role in vitamin K metabolism has been demonstrated. Non-genetic factors such as age and body size are also predictors of dose requirement. A number of recent GWA studies have confirmed the relative contributions of both CYP2C9 and VKORC1 and, to a small extent, CYP4F2 to dose requirement (Cha et al., 2010; Cooper et al., 2008; Takeuchi et al., 2009; Teichert et al., 2009). Though the overall contribution of VKORC1 genotype to coumarin anticoagulant dose requirement is clearly greater than that from CYP2C9, the main determinant of pharmacokinetic variability, CYP2C9 alleles, especially *CYP2C9*3*, may be particularly important as determinants of overcoagulation in the period soon after the initiation of treatment with anticoagulant (Higashi et al., 2002; Meckley et al., 2008; Wadelius et al., 2009).

Several studies have examined the value of using genotype and other patient-related factors to set initial warfarin dose (Anderson et al., 2007; Burmester et al., 2011; Caraco et al., 2008; Epstein et al., 2010; Gong et al., 2011; McMillin et al., 2010; Millican et al., 2007). Most of these small studies report no advantage for a genotype-determined dose but they may not have had adequate power to detect all genetic effects. One of these studies focused on CYP2C9 genotypes only and did find improved time to stable INR and a higher percentage of time within therapeutic range in the group with the genotype-guided dose compared with controls receiving standard care (Caraco et al., 2008). Another obtained data showing that provision of information on genotype for both CYP2C9 and VKORC1 to the treating physician resulted in better outcomes for warfarin treatment (Epstein et al., 2010). Larger randomized controlled trials to determine whether dose adjustment on the basis of genotype including CYP2C9 genotype leads to better outcomes during early treatment with warfarin and other anticoagulants compared with standard care are in progress (van Schie et al., 2009; French et al., 2010).

2. *Clopidogrel*

A number of independent studies indicate that the antiplatelet agent clopidogrel is less effective in individuals with at least one variant CYP2C19 allele because of a major role for CYP2C19 in activation of this prodrug (Brandt et al., 2007; Collet et al., 2009; Giusti et al., 2007; Hulot et al., 2006;

Kim et al., 2008; Mega et al., 2009; Simon et al., 2009). Though clopidogrel was developed quite recently and was first licensed in the US and Europe in the 1990s, the important contribution of CYP2C19 to its activation was not appreciated until studies on response by measurement of platelet aggregation rate in volunteers of known genotype were performed (Hulot et al., 2006). A subsequent *in vitro* metabolism study showed that though a number of different CYPs contribute to clopidogrel activation, CYP2C19 makes an important contribution to both the steps involved (Kazui et al., 2010). Despite the large number of studies showing an apparent association between CYP2C19 genotype, especially the *CYP2C19*2* allele, and susceptibility to adverse cardiovascular events in patients treated with clopidogrel, the relationship is still not completely clear. A recent meta analysis on the risk of further cardiovascular events in patients treated with clopidogrel following percutaneous coronary intervention confirmed a significant association for carriage of at least one *CYP2C19*2* allele (Mega et al., 2010). However, a subsequent meta analysis and systematic review of a larger number of studies found that a small increase in risk for *CYP2C19*2* carriage was abolished when correction was made for various biases such as small study numbers (Bauer et al., 2011). Response to clopidogrel has also been investigated by a GWA study (Shuldiner et al., 2009). The main study concerned response to the drug in a healthy volunteer group by measuring platelet aggregation. The most significant polymorphism is in strong linkage disequilibrium with a polymorphism in the cytochrome P450 *CYP2C19*2* allele. No polymorphisms outside the *CYP2C* locus showed genome-wide significance, providing no evidence for a strong effect by other genetic factors on clopidoprel response. In 2010, the FDA added a boxed warning to the clopidogrel label stating that CYP2C19 poor metabolizers may not benefit from treatment with this drug and that a genetic test to determine CYP2C19 status is available (http://www.fda.gov/Drugs/DrugSafety/PostmarketDrugSafetyInformationforPatientsandProviders/ucm203888.htm, accessed September 2011).

It was recently suggested that genotype for the *PON1* gene which encodes the esterase paraoxonase 1 was an important predictor for clopidogrel response (Bouman et al., 2011). However, three subsequent independent studies failed to confirm this finding, finding instead that CYP2C19 poor metabolizer alleles were important predictors of treatment outcome (Lewis et al., 2011; Sibbing et al., 2011; Trenk et al., 2011). At present, therefore, though a role for *PON1* genotype in predicting response to clopidogrel cannot be ruled out, the evidence for an effect is limited.

Some guidelines for clopidogrel therapy in patients with acute coronary syndrome or undergoing percutaneous coronary intervention have been formulated recently by the Clinical Pharmacogenetics Implementation Consortium (CPIC) (Scott et al., 2011). These provide a strong recommendation for use of prasugrel or another alternative to clopidogrel in CYP2C19 poor metabolizers and a moderate recommendation for this in those heterozygous for *CYP2C19*2*. As mentioned in the guidelines, data on other CYP2C19 "poor metabolizer" alleles is too limited to allow clear guidelines to be provided. The possibility that higher doses of clopidogrel might be a useful alternative to use of another platelet inhibitor, especially in those heterozygous for *CYP2C19*2* has also been considered. In one study where genotyping was not performed, use of a higher than normal concentration did not result in a lower rate of serious cardiovascular events in patients treated by percutaneous coronary intervention compared with a group treated at the standard dose (Price et al., 2011). However, in a relatively small healthy volunteer study, an improved antiplatelet response and higher levels of active metabolite were seen in a group of 10 CYP2C19 poor metabolizers given a high dose regimen over a 4 day period (Simon et al., 2011).

A further complicating factor in clopidogrel therapy is that another CYP2C19 variant allele, *CYP2C19*17*, includes an upstream polymorphism which apparently increases transcription levels and is associated with higher levels of gene expression (Sim et al., 2006). There is some data suggesting that patients homozygous for *CYP2C19*17* who are treated with clopidogrel are more likely to develop a bleeding complication (Sibbing et al., 2010) but this still requires independent confirmation. At present, the CPIC prescribing guidelines suggest use of standard dosing with clopidogrel for those homozygous or heterozygous for *CYP2C19*17* (Scott et al., 2011).

In spite of an extensive recent literature, not all aspects of genetic factors predicting clopidogrel response are completely clear. As recommended by the FDA (http://www.fda.gov/Drugs/DrugSafety/PostmarketDrugSafetyInformationforPatientsandProviders/ucm203888.htm, accessed September 2011), further prospective randomized clinical trials based on genotype-guided dosing are needed to understand fully the relationship between CYP2C19 genotype and response to clopidogrel before routine genotyping prior to treatment is recommended.

C. Other Drugs

1. *Codeine*

The very widely used analgesic drug codeine is an important CYP2D6 substrate. It is activated to morphine exclusively by CYP2D6 with morphine generally accepted to be the main contributor to analgesia, though there may be some analgesic effect also from codeine-6-glucuronide which is formed independently of CYP2D6 (Lotsch et al., 2006). The failure of CYP2D6 poor metabolizers to respond effectively to codeine treatment was established in several independent studies in the 1980s and early 1990s (Sindrup & Brosen, 1995). Similar reports continue to appear. For example, in a recent study on 45 mothers prescribed codeine for analgesia after delivery by Caesarian section, the two CYP2D6 poor metabolizers reported no analgesia from this drug (VanderVaart et al., 2011).

A number of case-reports concerning excessive activation of codeine in ultrarapid metabolizers with one additional copy of CYP2D6 have appeared relatively recently. In the first, a patient prescribed a cough medicine containing codeine suffered life-threatening opioid intoxication (Gasche et al., 2004). This individual had at least three copies of CYP2D6 on genotyping. The second concerned the death of a breast-fed baby 13 days after birth (Koren et al., 2006). His mother had been prescribed codeine for pain post-delivery. Post-mortem examination of stored breast milk samples showed a morphine level at least four times higher than expected and the mother was found to have a CYP2D6 gene duplication with the infant an extensive metabolizer. In a case–control study on mothers and babies who had suffered CNS depression following codeine prescription, two mothers whose babies exhibited severe toxicity not only had CYP2D6 gene duplications but also had the *UGT2B7*2/*2* genotype which may be associated with a decreased glucuronidation rate of morphine (Madadi et al., 2009). There is a suggestion that high levels of morphine described in some case reports on codeine toxicity could result from concurrent intake of codeine and heroin rather than a problem CYP2D6 genotype (He et al., 2008) but no evidence is available to confirm this directly. A study involving codeine administration to healthy volunteers of known CYP2D6 genotype showed that ultrarapid metabolizers were significantly more likely than extensive metabolizers to suffer sedation (Kirchheiner et al., 2006), though there was overlap between the two phenotypes. Whether all ultrarapid metabolizers with one or more additional copies of CYP2D6 are at risk of toxicity with codeine remains unclear. Ideally larger studies to investigate this are needed but performing these may be challenging because CYP2D6 ultrarapid metabolizers are relatively rare, especially in Northern European populations.

V. Conclusion

Despite over 50 years of pharmacogenetics studies, implementation of genotyping relating to metabolic polymorphisms in the clinic remains low. There is a single example, that of TPMT, of very successful clinical translation though there are also some examples of pharmacogenetic polymorphisms unrelated to metabolism where genotyping is normally performed including *HLA-B*5701* in relation to abacavir and *HLA-B*1502* in Asians prescribed certain antiepileptic drugs. There is now considerable potential for introducing additional pharmacogenetic tests in the cases of the coumarin anticoagulants and clopidogrel together with tamoxifen, especially if prospective data showing benefit and cost-effectiveness can be obtained. Up to recently, access to pharmacogenetic tests was a limitation for many prescribers with most testing only available in specialist laboratories and results taking days or weeks to become available. However, there is an increasing range of simple tests available (Aomori et al., 2009; Howard et al., 2011; Litos et al., 2011). These involve a range of different technologies but all are simple to use and can be performed in hours either in a local laboratory or directly at the point of care.

In therapeutic areas such as psychiatry where CYP2D6 contributes to metabolism of a range of drugs, progress on clinical translation has been disappointing. This may reflect not only the nature of psychiatric disease, especially the complex phenotypes, but also the failure up to now to consider additional genetic factors so that both drug metabolism and the drug target are covered. The increasing possibilities for genome-wide studies, involving both genotyping for polymorphisms and genome-wide sequencing, means that it will be feasible to evaluate a number of different genetic factors in an open manner without preselection of genes (Daly, 2010a). This may lead to the development of new tests and an improved ability to interpret data from existing tests.

Conflict of Interest: The author has no conflicts of interest to declare.

Abbreviations

CYP	cytochrome P450
GST	glutathione S-transferase
TPMT	thiopurine methyltransferase
UGT	UDP-glucuronosyltransferase
SULT	sulfotransferase
DPD	dihydropyrimidine dehydrogenase
FDA	US Food and Drug Administration
SNP	single nucleotide polymorphism
GWA	genome-wide association
miRNA	microRNA
AhR	Aromatic hydrocarbon receptor
PXR	pregnane X-receptor

References

Aithal, G. P., Day, C. P., Kesteven, P. J. L., & Daly, A. K. (1999). Association of polymorphisms in the cytochrome P450 CYP2C9 with warfarin dose requirement and risk of bleeding complications. *Lancet*, *353*, 717–719.

Amstutz, U., Farese, S., Aebi, S., & Largiader, C. R. (2009). Dihydropyrimidine dehydrogenase gene variation and severe 5-fluorouracil toxicity: a haplotype assessment. *Pharmacogenomics*, *10*, 931–944.

Anderson, J. L., Horne, B. D., Stevens, S. M., Grove, A. S., Barton, S., Nicholas, Z. P., et al. (2007). Randomized trial of genotype-guided versus standard warfarin dosing in patients initiating oral anticoagulation. *Circulation*, *116*, 2563–2570.

Andrade, R. J., Agundez, J. A., Lucena, M. I., Martinez, C., Cueto, R., & Garcia-Martin, E. (2009). Pharmacogenomics in drug induced liver injury. *Current Drug Metabolism*, *10*, 956–970.

Andrews, E., Armstrong, M., Tugwood, J., Swan, D., Glaves, P., Pirmohamed, M., et al. (2010). A role for the pregnane X receptor in flucloxacillin-induced liver injury. *Hepatology*, *51*, 1656–1664.

Aomori, T., Yamamoto, K., Oguchi-Katayama, A., Kawai, Y., Ishidao, T., Mitani, Y., et al. (2009). Rapid single-nucleotide polymorphism detection of cytochrome P450 (CYP2C9) and vitamin K epoxide reductase (VKORC1) genes for the warfarin dose adjustment by the SMart-amplification process version 2. *Clinical Chemistry*, *55*, 804–812.

Bahadur, N., Leathart, J. B. S., Mutch, E., Steimel-Crespi, D., Dunn, S. A., Gilissen, R., et al. (2002). CYP2C8 polymorphisms in Caucasians and their relationship with paclitaxel 6alpha-hydroxylase activity in human liver microsomes. *Biochemical Pharmacology*, *64*, 1579–1589.

Bauer, T., Bouman, H. J., van Werkum, J. W., Ford, N. F., Berg, Ten, et al. (2011). Impact of CYP2C19 variant genotypes on clinical efficacy of antiplatelet treatment with clopidogrel: systematic review and meta-analysis. *British Medical Journal*, *343*, d4588.

Board, P. (2011). Glutathione transferases. Preface. *Drug Metabolism Reviews*, *43*, 91.

Bock, K. W. (2010). Functions and transcriptional regulation of adult human hepatic UDP-glucuronosyl-transferases (UGTs): mechanisms responsible for interindividual variation of UGT levels. *Biochemical Pharmacology*, *80*, 771–777.

Bosch, T. M., Meijerman, I., Beijnen, J. H., & Schellens, J. H. (2006). Genetic polymorphisms of drug-metabolising enzymes and drug transporters in the chemotherapeutic treatment of cancer. *Clinical Pharmacokinetics*, *45*, 253–285.

Bouman, H. J., Schomig, E., van Werkum, J. W., Velder, J., Hackeng, C. M., Hirschhauser, C., et al. (2011). Paraoxonase-1 is a major determinant of clopidogrel efficacy. *Nature Medicine*, *17*, 110–116.

Brandt, J. T., Close, S. L., Iturria, S. J., Payne, C. D., Farid, N. A., Ernest, C. S., II, et al. (2007). Common polymorphisms of CYP2C19 and CYP2C9 affect the pharmacokinetic and pharmacodynamic response to clopidogrel but not prasugrel. *Journal of Thrombosis and Haemostasis*, *5*, 2429–2436.

Brauch, H. B., Schroth, W., Ingle, J. N., & Goetz, M. P. (2011). CYP2D6 and tamoxifen: awaiting the denouement. *Journal of Clinical Oncology*, *29*, 4589–4590.

Bray, J., Sludden, J., Griffin, M. J., Cole, M., Verrill, M., Jamieson, D., et al. (2010). Influence of pharmacogenetics on response and toxicity in breast cancer patients treated with doxorubicin and cyclophosphamide. *British Journal of Cancer*, *102*, 1003–1009.

Burchell, B., Soars, M., Monaghan, G., Cassidy, A., Smith, D., & Ethell, B. (2000). Drug-mediated toxicity caused by genetic deficiency of UDP-glucuronosyltransferases. *Toxicology Letters*, *112–113*, 333–340.

Burmester, J. K., Berg, R. L., Yale, S. H., Rottscheit, C. M., Glurich, I. E., Schmelzer, J. R., et al. (2011). A randomized controlled trial of genotype-based Coumadin initiation. *Genetics in Medicine*, *13*, 509–518.

Burton, P. R., Clayton, D. G., Cardon, L. R., Craddock, N., Deloukas, P., Duncanson, A., et al. (2007). Genome-wide association study of 14,000 cases of seven common diseases and 3,000 shared controls. *Nature*, *447*, 661–678.

Caldwell, M. D., Awad, T., Johnson, J. A., Gage, B. F., Falkowski, M., Gardina, P., et al. (2008). CYP4F2 genetic variant alters required warfarin dose. *Blood*, *111*, 4106–4112.

Caraco, Y., Blotnick, S., & Muszkat, M. (2008). CYP2C9 genotype-guided warfarin prescribing enhances the efficacy and safety of anticoagulation: a prospective randomized controlled study. *Clinical Pharmacology & Therapeutics*, *83*, 460–470.

Carlini, L. E., Meropol, N. J., Bever, J., Andria, M. L., Hill, T., Gold, P., et al. (2005). UGT1A7 and UGT1A9 polymorphisms predict response and toxicity in colorectal cancer patients treated with capecitabine/irinotecan. *Clinical Cancer Research*, *11*, 1226–1236.

Cha, P. C., Mushiroda, T., Takahashi, A., Kubo, M., Minami, S., Kamatani, N., et al. (2010). Genome-wide association study identifies genetic determinants of warfarin responsiveness for Japanese. *Human Molecular Genetics*, *19*, 4735–4744.

Chaudhry, A. S., Urban, T. J., Lamba, J. K., Birnbaum, A. K., Remmel, R. P., Subramanian, M., et al. (2010). CYP2C9*1B promoter polymorphisms, in linkage with CYP2C19*2, affect phenytoin autoinduction of clearance and maintenance dose. *Journal of Pharmacology and Experimental Therapeutics*, *332*, 599–611.

Collet, J. P., Hulot, J. S., Pena, A., Villard, E., Esteve, J. B., Silvain, J., et al. (2009). Cytochrome P450 2C19 polymorphism in young patients treated with clopidogrel after myocardial infarction: a cohort study. *Lancet*, *373*, 309–317.

Collie-Duguid, E. S., Etienne, M. C., Milano, G., & McLeod, H. L. (2000). Known variant DPYD alleles do not explain DPD deficiency in cancer patients. *Pharmacogenetics*, *10*, 217–223.

Cooper, G. M., Johnson, J. A., Langaee, T. Y., Feng, H., Stanaway, I. B., Schwarz, U. I., et al. (2008). A genome-wide scan for common genetic variants with a large influence on warfarin maintenance dose. *Blood*, *112*, 1022–1027.

Cornelis, M. C., Monda, K. L., Yu, K., Paynter, N., Azzato, E. M., Bennett, S. N., et al. (2011). Genome-wide meta-analysis identifies regions on 7p21 (AHR) and 15q24 (CYP1A2) as determinants of habitual caffeine consumption. *PLoS Genetics*, *7*, e1002033.

Dai, D., Zeldin, D. C., Blaisdell, J. A., Chanas, B., Coulter, S. J., Ghanayem, B. I., et al. (2001). Polymorphisms in human CYP2C8 decrease metabolism of the anticancer drug paclitaxel and arachidonic acid. *Pharmacogenetics*, *11*, 597–607.

Daly, A. K. (2010a). Genome-wide association studies in pharmacogenomics. *Nature Reviews Genetics*, *11*, 241–246.

Daly, A. K. (2010b). Pharmacogenetics and human genetic polymorphisms. *Biochemical Journal*, *429*, 435–449.

de Morais, S. M. F., Wilkinson, G. R., Blaisdell, J., Meyer, U. A., Nakamura, K., & Goldstein, J. A. (1994a). Identification of a new genetic defect responsible for the polymorphism of *(S)*-mephenytoin metabolism in Japanese. *Molecular Pharmacology*, *46*, 594–598.

de Morais, S. M. F., Wilkinson, G. R., Blaisdell, J., Nakamura, K., Meyer, U. A., & Goldstein, J. A. (1994b). The major genetic defect responsible for the polymorphism of *S*-mephenytoin metabolism in humans. *The Journal of Biological Chemistry*, *269*, 15,419–15,422.

Desta, Z., Ward, B. A., Soukhova, N. V., & Flockhart, D. A. (2004). Comprehensive evaluation of tamoxifen sequential biotransformation by the human cytochrome P450 system *in vitro*: prominent roles for CYP3A and CYP2D6. *Journal of Pharmacology and Experimental Therapeutics*, *310*, 1062–1075.

Epstein, R. S., Moyer, T. P., Aubert, R. E., O'Kane, D. J., Xia, F., Verbrugge, R. R., et al. (2010). Warfarin genotyping reduces hospitalization rates results from the MM-WES (Medco-Mayo Warfarin Effectiveness study). *Journal of the American College of Cardiology*, *55*, 2804–2812.

Evans, W. E. (2004). Pharmacogenetics of thiopurine S-methyltransferase and thiopurine therapy. *Therapeutic Drug Monitoring*, *26*, 186–191.

Faber, M. S., Jetter, A., & Fuhr, U. (2005). Assessment of CYP1A2 activity in clinical practice: why, how, and when? *Basic & Clinical Pharmacology & Toxicology*, *97*, 125–134.

Fernandez-Salguero, P., Hoffman, S. M. G., Cholerton, S., Mohrenweiser, H., Raunio, H., Pelkonen, O., et al. (1995). A genetic polymorphism in coumarin 7-hydroxylation: sequence of the human *CYP2A* genes and identification of variant *CYP2A6* alleles. *The American Journal of Human Genetics*, *57*, 651–660.

Ford, L. T., & Berg, J. D. (2010). Thiopurine S-methyltransferase (TPMT) assessment prior to starting thiopurine drug treatment; a pharmacogenomic test whose time has come. *Journal of Clinical Pathology*, *63*, 288–295.

French, B., Joo, J., Geller, N. L., Kimmel, S. E., Rosenberg, Y., Anderson, J. L., et al. (2010). Statistical design of personalized medicine interventions: the Clarification of Optimal Anticoagulation through Genetics (COAG) trial. *Trials*, *11*, 108.

Fukami, T., Nakajima, M., Yamanaka, H., Fukushima, Y., McLeod, H. L., & Yokoi, T. (2007). A novel duplication type of CYP2A6 gene in African–American population. *Drug Metabolism and Disposition*, *35*, 515–520.

Gaedigk, A., Blum, M., Gaedigk, R., Eichelbaum, M., & Meyer, U. A. (1991). Deletion of the entire cytochrome P450 gene as a cause of impaired drug metabolism in poor metabolizers of the debrisoquine/sparteine polymorphism. *The American Journal of Human Genetics*, *48*, 943–950.

Gardiner, S. J., & Begg, E. J. (2005). Pharmacogenetic testing for drug metabolizing enzymes: is it happening in practice? *Pharmacogenetics and Genomics*, *15*, 365–369.

Gasche, Y., Daali, Y., Fathi, M., Chiappe, A., Cottini, S., Dayer, P., et al. (2004). Codeine intoxication associated with ultrarapid CYP2D6 metabolism. *New England Journal of Medicine*, *351*, 2827–2831.

Ghotbi, R., Gomez, A., Milani, L., Tybring, G., Syvanen, A. C., Bertilsson, L., et al. (2009). Allele-specific expression and gene methylation in the control of CYP1A2 mRNA level in human livers. *Pharmacogenomics Journal*, *9*, 208–217.

Girard, H., Villeneuve, L., Court, M. H., Fortier, L. C., Caron, P., Hao, Q., et al. (2006). The novel UGT1A9 intronic I399 polymorphism appears as a predictor of 7-ethyl-10-hydroxycamptothecin glucuronidation levels in the liver. *Drug Metabolism and Disposition*, *34*, 1220–1228.

Giusti, B., Gori, A. M., Marcucci, R., Saracini, C., Sestini, I., Paniccia, R., et al. (2007). Cytochrome P450 2C19 loss-of-function polymorphism, but not CYP3A4 IVS10 + 12G/A and P2Y12 T744C polymorphisms, is associated with response variability to dual antiplatelet treatment in high-risk vascular patients. *Pharmacogenetics and Genomics*, *17*, 1057–1064.

Gong, I. Y., Tirona, R. G., Schwarz, U. I., Crown, N., Dresser, G. K., Larue, S., et al. (2011). Prospective evaluation of a pharmacogenetics-guided warfarin loading and maintenance dose regimen for initiation of therapy. *Blood*.

Guillemette, C., Levesque, E., Harvey, M., Bellemare, J., & Menard, V. (2010). UGT genomic diversity: beyond gene duplication. *Drug Metabolism Reviews*, *42*, 24–44.

Hall, D., Ybazeta, G., Destro-Bisol, G., Petzl-Erler, M. L., & Di Rienzo, A. (1999). Variability at the uridine diphosphate glucuronosyltransferase 1A1 promoter in human populations and primates. *Pharmacogenetics*, *9*, 591–599.

Hardy, J., & Singleton, A. (2009). Genomewide association studies and human disease. *New England Journal of Medicine*, *360*, 1759–1768.

He, Y. J., Brockmoller, J., Schmidt, H., Roots, I., & Kirchheiner, J. (2008). Short communication: CYP2D6 ultrarapid metabolism and morphine/codeine ratios in blood: was it codeine or heroin? *Journal of Analytical Toxicology*, *32*, 178–182.

Hebbring, S. J., Adjei, A. A., Baer, J. L., Jenkins, G. D., Zhang, J., Cunningham, J. M., et al. (2007). Human SULT1A1 gene: copy number differences and functional implications. *Human Molecular Genetics*, *16*, 463–470.

Helsby, N., & Tingle, M. (2011). The importance of correct assignment of CYP2B6 genetic variants with respect to cyclophosphamide metabolizer status. *American Journal of Hematology*, *86*, 383–384. author reply 384.

Helsby, N. A., Hui, C. Y., Goldthorpe, M. A., Coller, J. K., Soh, M. C., Gow, P. J., et al. (2010). The combined impact of CYP2C19 and CYP2B6 pharmacogenetics on cyclophosphamide bioactivation. *British Journal of Clinical Pharmacology*, *70*, 844–853.

Higashi, M. K., Veenstra, D. L., Kondo, L. M. L., Wittkowsky, A. K., Srinouanprachanh, S. L., Farin, F. M., et al. (2002). Association between CYP2C9 genetic variants and anticoagulation-related outcomes during warfarin therapy. *Journal of American Medical Association*, *287*, 1690–1698.

Higgins, M. J., & Stearns, V. (2011). Pharmacogenetics of endocrine therapy for breast cancer. *Annual Review of Medicine*, *62*, 281–293.

Hirschhorn, J. N. (2009). Genomewide association studies–illuminating biologic pathways. *New England Journal of Medicine*, *360*, 1699–1701.

Hoskins, J. M., Carey, L. A., & McLeod, H. L. (2009). CYP2D6 and tamoxifen: DNA matters in breast cancer. *Nature Reviews Cancer*, *9*, 576–586.

Hoskins, J. M., Goldberg, R. M., Qu, P., Ibrahim, J. G., & McLeod, H. L. (2007). UGT1A1*28 genotype and irinotecan-induced neutropenia: dose matters. *Journal of the National Cancer Institute*, *99*, 1290–1295.

Howard, R., Leathart, J. B., French, D. J., Krishan, E., Kohnke, H., Wadelius, M., et al. (2011). Genotyping for CYP2C9 and VKORC1 alleles by a novel point of care assay with HyBeacon(R) probes. *Clinica Chimica Acta*, *412*, 2063–2069.

Hulot, J. S., Bura, A., Villard, E., Azizi, M., Remones, V., Goyenvalle, C., et al. (2006). Cytochrome P450 2C19 loss-of-function polymorphism is a major determinant of clopidogrel responsiveness in healthy subjects. *Blood*, *108*, 2244–2247.

Hustert, E., Zibat, A., Presecan-Siedel, E., Eiselt, R., Mueller, R., Fuss, C., et al. (2001). Natural protein variants of pregnane X receptor with altered transactivation activity toward CYP3A4. *Drug Metabolism and Disposition*, *29*, 1454–1459.

Ikeda, S., Kurose, K., Ozawa, S., Sai, K., Hasegawa, R., Komamura, K., et al. (2003). Twenty-six novel single nucleotide polymorphisms and their frequencies of the NR1I3 (CAR) gene in a Japanese population. *Drug Metabolism and Pharmacokinetics*, *18*, 413–418.

Ingelman-Sundberg, M., & Gomez, A. (2010). The past, present and future of pharmacoepigenomics. *Pharmacogenomics*, *11*, 625–627.

Ingelman-Sundberg, M., & Sim, S. C. (2010). Pharmacogenetic biomarkers as tools for improved drug therapy; emphasis on the cytochrome P450 system. *Biochemical and Biophysical Research Communications*, *396*, 90–94.

Ingelman-Sundberg, M., Sim, S. C., Gomez, A., & Rodriguez-Antona, C. (2007). Influence of cytochrome P450 polymorphisms on drug therapies: pharmacogenetic, pharmacoepigenetic and clinical aspects. *Pharmacology & Therapeutics*, *116*, 496–526.

Innocenti, F., Cooper, G. M., Stanaway, I. B., Gamazon, E. R., Smith, J. D., Mirkov, S., et al. (2011). Identification, replication, and functional fine-mapping of expression quantitative trait loci in primary human liver tissue. *PLoS Genetics*, *7*, e1002078.

Innocenti, F., Kroetz, D. L., Schuetz, E., Dolan, M. E., Ramirez, J., Relling, M., et al. (2009). Comprehensive pharmacogenetic analysis of irinotecan neutropenia and pharmacokinetics. *Journal of Clinical Oncology*, *27*, 2604–2614.

Irvin, W. J., Jr., Walko, C. M., Weck, K. E., Ibrahim, J. G., Chiu, W. K., Dees, E. C., et al. (2011). Genotype-guided tamoxifen dosing increases active metabolite exposure in women with reduced CYP2D6 metabolism: a multicenter study. *Journal of Clinical Oncology*, *29*, 3232–3239.

Jin, Y., Desta, Z., Stearns, V., Ward, B., Ho, H., Lee, K. H., et al. (2005). CYP2D6 genotype, antidepressant use, and tamoxifen metabolism during adjuvant breast cancer treatment. *Journal of National Cancer Institute*, *97*, 30–39.

Jin, Y., Zollinger, M., Borell, H., Zimmerlin, A., & Patten, C. J. (2011). CYP4F enzymes are responsible for the elimination of fingolimod (FTY720), a novel treatment of relapsing multiple sclerosis. *Drug Metabolism and Disposition*, *39*, 191–198.

Johansson, I., Lundqvist, E., Bertilsson, L., Dahl, M. -L., Sjoqvist, F., & Ingelman-Sundberg, M. (1993). Inherited amplification of an active gene in the cytochrome P450 *CYP2D* locus as a cause of ultrarapid metabolism of debrisoquine. *Proceedings of the National Academy of Sciences of the United States of America*, *90*, 11,825–11,829.

Johansson, I., Oscarson, M., Yue, Q. -Y., Bertilsson, L., Sjoqvist, F., & Ingelman-Sundberg, M. (1994). Genetic analysis of the Chinese cytochrome P4502D locus: characterization of variant *CYP2D6* genes present in subjects with diminished capacity for debrisoquine hydroxylation. *Molecular Pharmacology*, *46*, 452–459.

Jonas, D. E., & McLeod, H. L. (2009). Genetic and clinical factors relating to warfarin dosing. *Trends in Pharmacological Sciences*, *30*, 375–386.

Kagimoto, M., Heim, M., Kagimoto, K., Zeugin, T., & Meyer, U. A. (1990). Multiple mutations of the human cytochrome P450IID6 gene (CYP2D6) in poor metabolisers of debrisoquine. *Journal of Biological Chemistry*, *265*, 17,209–17,214.

Kazui, M., Nishiya, Y., Ishizuka, T., Hagihara, K., Farid, N. A., Okazaki, O., et al. (2010). Identification of the human cytochrome P450 enzymes involved in the two oxidative steps in the bioactivation of clopidogrel to its pharmacologically active metabolite. *Drug Metabolism and Disposition*, *38*, 92–99.

Kidd, R. S., Curry, T. B., Gallagher, S., Edeki, T., Blaisdell, J., & Goldstein, J. A. (2001). Identification of a null allele of CYP2C9 in an African-American exhibiting toxicity to phenytoin. *Pharmacogenetics*, *11*, 803–808.

Kim, K., Park, P., Hong, S., & Park, J. Y. (2008). The effect of CYP2C19 polymorphism on the pharmacokinetics and pharmacodynamics of clopidogrel: a possible mechanism for clopidogrel resistance. *Clinical Pharmacology & Therapeutics*, *84*, 236–242.

King, B. P., Khan, T. I., Aithal, G. P., Kamali, F., & Daly, A. K. (2004). Upstream and coding region CYP2C9 polymorphisms: correlation with warfarin dose and metabolism. *Pharmacogenetics*, *14*, 813–822.

Kirchheiner, J., Schmidt, H., Tzvetkov, M., Keulen, J. T., Lotsch, J., Roots, I., et al. (2006). Pharmacokinetics of codeine and its metabolite morphine in ultra-rapid metabolizers due to CYP2D6 duplication. *Pharmacogenomics Journal*, *7*, 257–265.

Knights, K. M., Sykes, M. J., & Miners, J. O. (2007). Amino acid conjugation: contribution to the metabolism and toxicity of xenobiotic carboxylic acids. *Expert Opinion on Drug Metabolism and Toxicology*, *3*, 159–168.

Koren, G., Cairns, J., Chitayat, D., Gaedigk, A., & Leeder, S. J. (2006). Pharmacogenetics of morphine poisoning in a breastfed neonate of a codeine-prescribed mother. *Lancet*, *368*, 704.

Kuehl, P., Zhang, J., Lin, Y., Lamba, J., Assem, M., Schuetz, J., et al. (2001). Sequence diversity in CYP3A promoters and characterization of the genetic basis of polymorphic CYP3A5 expression. *Nature Genetics*, *27*, 383–391.

Lamba, J., Lamba, V., Strom, S., Venkataramanan, R., & Schuetz, E. (2008). Novel single nucleotide polymorphisms in the promoter and intron 1 of human pregnane X receptor/NR1I2 and their association with CYP3A4 expression. *Drug Metabolism and Disposition*, *36*, 169–181.

Lamba, J. K. (2008). Pharmacogenetics of the constitutive androstane receptor. *Pharmacogenomics*, *9*, 71–83.

Lamba, V., Panetta, J. C., Strom, S., & Schuetz, E. G. (2010). Genetic predictors of interindividual variability in hepatic CYP3A4 expression. *Journal of Pharmacology and Experimental Therapeutics*, *332*, 1088–1099.

Lang, T., Klein, K., Fischer, J., Nussler, A. K., Neuhaus, P., Hofmann, U., et al. (2001). Extensive genetic polymorphism in the human CYP2B6 gene with impact on expression and function in human liver. *Pharmacogenetics*, *11*, 399–415.

Lewis, J. P., Fisch, A. S., Ryan, K., O'Connell, J. R., Gibson, Q., Mitchell, B. D., et al. (2011). Paraoxonase 1 (PON1) gene variants are not associated with clopidogrel response. *Clinical Pharmacology & Therapeutics* *90*, 568–574.

Li, H., Ferguson, S. S., & Wang, H. (2010). Synergistically enhanced CYP2B6 inducibility between a polymorphic mutation in CYP2B6 promoter and pregnane X receptor activation. *Molecular Pharmacology*, *78*, 704–713.

Li, T., Chang, C. Y., Jin, D. Y., Lin, P. J., Khvorova, A., & Stafford, D. W. (2004). Identification of the gene for vitamin K epoxide reductase. *Nature*, *427*, 541–544.

Lim, Y. C., Li, L., Desta, Z., Zhao, Q., Rae, J. M., Flockhart, D. A., et al. (2006). Endoxifen, a secondary metabolite of tamoxifen, and 4-OH-tamoxifen induce similar changes in global gene expression patterns in MCF-7 breast cancer cells. *Journal of Pharmacology and Experimental Therapeutics*, *318*, 503–512.

Litos, I. K., Ioannou, P. C., Christopoulos, T. K., Tzetis, M., Kanavakis, E., & Traeger-Synodinos, J. (2011). Quadruple-allele dipstick test for simultaneous visual genotyping of A896G (Asp299Gly) and C1196T (Thr399Ile) polymorphisms in the toll-like receptor-4 gene. *Clinica Chimica Acta*, *412*, 1968–1972.

Lotsch, J., Skarke, C., Schmidt, H., Rohrbacher, M., Hofmann, U., Schwab, M., et al. (2006). Evidence for morphine-independent central nervous opioid effects after administration of codeine: contribution of other codeine metabolites. *Clinical Pharmacology & Therapeutics*, *79*, 35–48.

Madadi, P., Ross, C. J., Hayden, M. R., Carleton, B. C., Gaedigk, A., Leeder, J. S., et al. (2009). Pharmacogenetics of neonatal opioid toxicity following maternal use of codeine during breastfeeding: a case-control study. *Clinical Pharmacology & Therapeutics*, *85*, 31–35.

Manolio, T. A., Brooks, L. D., & Collins, F. S. (2008). A HapMap harvest of insights into the genetics of common disease. *Journal of Clinical Investigations*, *118*, 1590–1605.

Marsh, S., & Van Booven, D. J. (2009). The increasing complexity of mercaptopurine pharmacogenomics. *Clinical Pharmacology & Therapeutics*, *85*, 139–141.

Masimirembwa, C., Persson, I., Bertilsson, L., Hasler, J., & Ingelman-Sundberg, M. (1996). A novel mutant variant of the *CYP2D6* gene (*CYP2D6*17*) common in a black African population: association with diminished debrisoquine hydroxylase activity. *British Journal of Clinical Pharmacology*, *42*, 713–719.

McDonald, M. G., Rieder, M. J., Nakano, M., Hsia, C. K., & Rettie, A. E. (2009). CYP4F2 is a vitamin K1 oxidase: an explanation for altered warfarin dose in carriers of the V433M variant. *Molecular Pharmacology*, *75*, 1337–1346.

McLeod, H. L., Sargent, D. J., Marsh, S., Green, E. M., King, C. R., Fuchs, C. S., et al. (2010). Pharmacogenetic predictors of adverse events and response to chemotherapy in metastatic colorectal cancer: results from North American Gastrointestinal Intergroup Trial N9741. *Journal of Clinical Oncology*, *28*, 3227–3233.

McMillin, G. A., Melis, R., Wilson, A., Strong, M. B., Wanner, N. A., Vinik, R. G., et al. (2010). Gene-based warfarin dosing compared with standard of care practices in an orthopedic surgery population: a prospective, parallel cohort study. *Therapeutic Drug Monitoring*, *32*, 338–345.

Meckley, L. M., Wittkowsky, A. K., Rieder, M. J., Rettie, A. E., & Veenstra, D. L. (2008). An analysis of the relative effects of VKORC1 and CYP2C9 variants on anticoagulation related outcomes in warfarin-treated patients. *Thrombosis and Haemostasis*, *100*, 229–239.

Mega, J. L., Close, S. L., Wiviott, S. D., Shen, L., Hockett, R. D., Brandt, J. T., et al. (2009). Cytochrome p-450 polymorphisms and response to clopidogrel. *New England Journal of Medicine*, *360*, 354–362.

Mega, J. L., Simon, T., Collet, J. P., Anderson, J. L., Antman, E. M., Bliden, K., et al. (2010). Reduced-function CYP2C19 genotype and risk of adverse clinical outcomes among patients treated with clopidogrel predominantly for PCI: a meta-analysis. *JAMA*, *304*, 1821–1830.

Meggitt, S. J., Gray, J. C., & Reynolds, N. J. (2006). Azathioprine dosed by thiopurine methyltransferase activity for moderate-to-severe atopic eczema: a double-blind, randomised controlled trial. *Lancet*, *367*, 839–846.

Melanson, S. E., Stevenson, K., Kim, H., Antin, J. H., Court, M. H., Ho, V. T., et al. (2010). Allelic variations in CYP2B6 and CYP2C19 and survival of patients receiving cyclophosphamide prior to myeloablative hematopoietic stem cell transplantation. *American Journal of Hematology*, *85*, 967–971.

Millican, E. A., Lenzini, P. A., Milligan, P. E., Grosso, L., Eby, C., Deych, E., et al. (2007). Genetic-based dosing in orthopedic patients beginning warfarin therapy. *Blood*, *110*, 1511–1515.

Mishra, P. J., Humeniuk, R., Mishra, P. J., Longo-Sorbello, G. S., Banerjee, D., & Bertino, J. R. (2007). A miR-24 microRNA binding-site polymorphism in dihydrofolate reductase gene leads to methotrexate resistance. *Proceedings of the National Academy of Sciences of the United States of America*, *104*, 13,513–13,518.

Mohri, T., Nakajima, M., Fukami, T., Takamiya, M., Aoki, Y., & Yokoi, T. (2010). Human CYP2E1 is regulated by miR-378. *Biochemical Pharmacology*, *79*, 1045–1052.

Murdter, T. E., Schroth, W., Bacchus-Gerybadze, L., Winter, S., Heinkele, G., Simon, W., et al. (2011). Activity levels of tamoxifen metabolites at the estrogen receptor and the impact of genetic polymorphisms of phase I and II enzymes on their concentration levels in plasma. *Clinical Pharmacology & Therapeutics*, *89*, 708–717.

Nagar, S., & Blanchard, R. L. (2006). Pharmacogenetics of uridine diphosphoglucuronosyltransferase (UGT) 1A family members and its role in patient response to irinotecan. *Drug Metabolism Reviews*, *38*, 393–409.

Newman, W. G., Payne, K., Tricker, K., Roberts, S. A., Fargher, E., Pushpakom, S., et al. (2011). A pragmatic randomized controlled trial of thiopurine methyltransferase genotyping prior to azathioprine treatment: the TARGET study. *Pharmacogenomics*, *12*, 815–826.

Oscarson, M., McLellan, R. A., Gullsten, H., Yue, Q. Y., Lang, M. A., Bernal, M. L., et al. (1999). Characterisation and PCR-based detection of a CYP2A6 gene deletion found at a high frequency in a Chinese population. *FEBS Letters*, *448*, 105–110.

Pinto, N., Ludeman, S. M., & Dolan, M. E. (2009). Drug focus: pharmacogenetic studies related to cyclophosphamide-based therapy. *Pharmacogenomics*, *10*, 1897–1903.

Price, M. J., Berger, P. B., Teirstein, P. S., Tanguay, J. F., Angiolillo, D. J., Spriggs, D., et al. (2011). Standard- vs high-dose clopidogrel based on platelet function testing after percutaneous coronary intervention: the GRAVITAS randomized trial. *JAMA*, *305*, 1097–1105.

Qiu, H., Mathas, M., Nestler, S., Bengel, C., Nem, D., Godtel-Armbrust, U., et al. (2010). The unique complexity of the CYP3A4 upstream region suggests a nongenetic explanation of its expression variability. *Pharmacogenetics and Genomics*, *20*, 167–178.

Rao, Y., Hoffmann, E., Zia, M., Bodin, L., Zeman, M., Sellers, E. M., et al. (2000). Duplications and defects in the CYP2A6 gene: identification, genotyping, and *in vivo* effects on smoking. *Molecular Pharmacology*, *58*, 747–755.

Relling, M. V., Gardner, E. E., Sandborn, W. J., Schmiegelow, K., Pui, C. H., Yee, S. W., et al. (2011). Clinical Pharmacogenetics Implementation Consortium guidelines for thiopurine methyltransferase genotype and thiopurine dosing. *Clinical Pharmacology & Therapeutics*, *89*, 387–391.

Rettie, A. E., Wienkers, L. C., Gonzalez, F. J., Trager, W. F., & Korzekwa, K. R. (1994). Impaired *(S)*-warfarin metabolism catalysed by the R144C allelic variant of CYP2C9. *Pharmacogenetics*, *4*, 39–42.

Rodriguez-Antona, C., Gomez, A., Karlgren, M., Sim, S. C., & Ingelman-Sundberg, M. (2010). Molecular genetics and epigenetics of the cytochrome P450 gene family and its relevance for cancer risk and treatment. *Human Genetics*, *127*, 1–17.

Rost, S., Fregin, A., Ivaskevicius, V., Conzelmann, E., Hortnagel, K., Pelz, H. J., et al. (2004). Mutations in VKORC1 cause warfarin resistance and multiple coagulation factor deficiency type 2. *Nature*, *427*, 537–541.

Rukov, J. L., Vinther, J., & Shomron, N. (2011). Pharmacogenomics genes show varying perceptibility to microRNA regulation. *Pharmacogenetics and Genomics*, *21*, 251–262.

Sachse, C., Brockmoller, J., Bauer, S., & Roots, I. (1999). Functional significance of a C→A polymorphism in intron 1 of the cytochrome P450 CYP1A2 gene tested with caffeine. *British Journal of Clinical Pharmacology*, *47*, 445–449.

Sandanaraj, E., Lal, S., Selvarajan, V., Ooi, L. L., Wong, Z. W., Wong, N. S., et al. (2008). PXR pharmacogenetics: association of haplotypes with hepatic CYP3A4 and ABCB1 messenger RNA expression and doxorubicin clearance in Asian breast cancer patients. *Clinical Cancer Research*, *14*, 7116–7126.

Sanghani, S. P., Sanghani, P. C., Schiel, M. A., & Bosron, W. F. (2009). Human carboxylesterases: an update on CES1, CES2 and CES3. *Protein & Peptide Letters*, *16*, 1207–1214.

Saxena, R., Shaw, G. L., Relling, M. V., Frame, J. N., Moir, D. T., Evans, W. E., et al. (1994). Identification of a new variant CYP2D6 single base pair deletion in exon 3 and its association with the poor metabolizer phenotype. *Human Molecular Genetics*, *3*, 923–926.

Schadt, E. E., Molony, C., Chudin, E., Hao, K., Yang, X., Lum, P. Y., et al. (2008). Mapping the genetic architecture of gene expression in human liver. *PLoS Biology*, *6*, e107.

Schipani, A., Siccardi, M., D'Avolio, A., Baietto, L., Simiele, M., Bonora, S., et al. (2010). Population pharmacokinetic modeling of the association between 63396C->T pregnane X receptor polymorphism and unboosted atazanavir clearance. *Antimicrobial Agents and Chemotheraphy*, *54*, 5242–5250.

Schroder, A., Klein, K., Winter, S., Schwab, M., Bonin, M., Zell, A., et al. (2011). Genomics of ADME gene expression: mapping expression quantitative trait loci relevant for absorption, distribution, metabolism and excretion of drugs in human liver. *Pharmacogenomics Journal*, Oct 18, doi: 10.1038/tpj.2011.44. [Epub ahead of print].

Schroth, W., Antoniadou, L., Fritz, P., Schwab, M., Muerdter, T., Zanger, U. M., et al. (2007). Breast cancer treatment outcome with adjuvant tamoxifen relative to patient CYP2D6 and CYP2C19 genotypes. *Journal of Clinical Oncology*, *25*, 5187–5193.

Schroth, W., Hamann, U., Fasching, P. A., Dauser, S., Winter, S., Eichelbaum, M., et al. (2010). CYP2D6 polymorphisms as predictors of outcome in breast cancer patients treated with tamoxifen: expanded polymorphism coverage improves risk stratification. *Clinical Cancer Research*, *16*, 4468–4477.

Schulz, C., Heinemann, V., Schalhorn, A., Moosmann, N., Zwingers, T., Boeck, S., et al. (2009). UGT1A1 gene polymorphism: impact on toxicity and efficacy of irinotecan-based regimens in metastatic colorectal cancer. *World Journal of Gastroenterology*, *15*, 5058–5066.

Scott, S. A., Sangkuhl, K., Gardner, E. E., Stein, C. M., Hulot, J. S., Johnson, J. A., et al. (2011). Clinical Pharmacogenetics Implementation Consortium guidelines for cytochrome P450-2C19 (CYP2C19) genotype and clopidogrel therapy. *Clinical Pharmacology & Therapeutics*, *90*, 328–332.

Shuldiner, A. R., O'Connell, J. R., Bliden, K. P., Gandhi, A., Ryan, K., Horenstein, R. B., et al. (2009). Association of cytochrome P450 2C19 genotype with the antiplatelet effect and clinical efficacy of clopidogrel therapy. *JAMA*, *302*, 849–857.

Sibbing, D., Koch, W., Gebhard, D., Schuster, T., Braun, S., Stegherr, J., et al. (2010). Cytochrome 2C19*17 allelic variant, platelet aggregation, bleeding events, and stent thrombosis in clopidogrel-treated patients with coronary stent placement. *Circulation*, *121*, 512–518.

Sibbing, D., Koch, W., Massberg, S., Byrne, R. A., Mehilli, J., Schulz, S., et al. (2011). No association of paraoxonase-1 Q192R genotypes with platelet response to clopidogrel and risk of stent thrombosis after coronary stenting. *European Heart Journal*, *32*, 1605–1613.

Sim, S. C., Risinger, C., Dahl, M. L., Aklillu, E., Christensen, M., Bertilsson, L., et al. (2006). A common novel CYP2C19 gene variant causes ultrarapid drug metabolism relevant for the drug response to proton pump inhibitors and antidepressants. *Clinical Pharmacology & Therapeutics*, *79*, 103–113.

Simon, T., Bhatt, D. L., Bergougnan, L., Farenc, C., Pearson, K., Perrin, L., et al. (2011). Genetic polymorphisms and the impact of a higher clopidogrel dose regimen on active metabolite exposure and antiplatelet response in healthy subjects. *Clinical Pharmacology & Therapeutics*, *90*, 287–295.

Simon, T., Verstuyft, C., Mary-Krause, M., Quteineh, L., Drouet, E., Meneveau, N., et al. (2009). Genetic determinants of response to clopidogrel and cardiovascular events. *New England Journal of Medicine*, *360*, 363–375.

Sindrup, S. H., & Brosen, K. (1995). The pharmacogenetics of codeine hypoalgesia. *Pharmacogenetics*, *5*, 335–346.

Singh, M. S., Francis, P. A., & Michael, M. (2011). Tamoxifen, cytochrome P450 genes and breast cancer clinical outcomes. *Breast*, *20*, 111–118.

Sontag, T. J., & Parker, R. S. (2007). Influence of major structural features of tocopherols and tocotrienols on their omega-oxidation by tocopherol-omega-hydroxylase. *The Journal of Lipid Research*, *48*, 1090–1098.

Soyama, A., Saito, Y., Komamura, K., Ueno, K., Kamakura, S., Ozawa, S., et al. (2002). Five novel single nucleotide polymorphisms in the CYP2C8 gene, one of which induces a frame-shift. *Drug Metabolism and Pharmacokinetics*, *17*, 374.

Stec, D. E., Roman, R. J., Flasch, A., & Rieder, M. J. (2007). Functional polymorphism in human CYP4F2 decreases 20-HETE production. *Physiological Genomics*, *30*, 74–81.

Steward, D. J., Haining, R. L., Henne, K. R., Davis, G., Rushmore, T. H., Trager, W. F., et al. (1997). Genetic association between sensitivity to warfarin and expression of CYP2C9*3. *Pharmacogenetics*, *7*, 361–367.

Sulem, P., Gudbjartsson, D. F., Geller, F., Prokopenko, I., Feenstra, B., Aben, K. K., et al. (2011). Sequence variants at CYP1A1–CYP1A2 and AHR associate with coffee consumption. *Human Molecular Genetics*, *20*, 2071–2077.

Sullivan-Close, T. H., Ghanayem, B. I., Bell, D. A., Zhang, Z. -Y., Kaminsky, L. S., Shenfield, G. M., et al. (1996). The role of the *CYP2C9*-Leu359 allelic variant in the tolbutamide polymorphism. *Pharmacogenetics*, *6*, 341–349.

Swen, J. J., Nijenhuis, M., de Boer, A., Grandia, L., Maitland-van der Zee, A. H., Mulder, H., et al. (2011). Pharmacogenetics: from bench to byte – an update of guidelines. *Clinical Pharmacology & Therapeutics*, *89*, 662–673.

Takada, K., Arefayene, M., Desta, Z., Yarboro, C. H., Boumpas, D. T., Balow, J. E., et al. (2004). Cytochrome P450 pharmacogenetics as a predictor of toxicity and clinical response to pulse cyclophosphamide in lupus nephritis. *Arthritis & Rheumatism*, *50*, 2202–2210.

Takeuchi, F., McGinnis, R., Bourgeois, S., Barnes, C., Eriksson, N., Soranzo, N., et al. (2009). A genome-wide association study confirms VKORC1, CYP2C9, and CYP4F2 as principal genetic determinants of warfarin dose. *PLoS Genetics*, *5*, e1000433.

Teichert, M., Eijgelsheim, M., Rivadeneira, F., Uitterlinden, A. G., van Schaik, R. H., et al. (2009). A genome-wide association study of acenocoumarol maintenance dosage. *Human Molecular Genetics*, *18*, 3758–3768.

Teml, A., Schaeffeler, E., Herrlinger, K. R., Klotz, U., & Schwab, M. (2007). Thiopurine treatment in inflammatory bowel disease: clinical pharmacology and implication of pharmacogenetically guided dosing. *Clinical Pharmacokinetics*, *46*, 187–208.

Thorgeirsson, T. E., Gudbjartsson, D. F., Surakka, I., Vink, J. M., Amin, N., Geller, F., et al. (2010). Sequence variants at CHRNB3-CHRNA6 and CYP2A6 affect smoking behavior. *Nature Genetics*, *42*, 448–453.

Toffoli, G., Cecchin, E., Gasparini, G., D'Andrea, M., Azzarello, G., Basso, U., et al. (2010). Genotype-driven phase I study of irinotecan administered in combination with fluorouracil/leucovorin in patients with metastatic colorectal cancer. *Journal of Clinical Oncology*, *28*, 866–871.

Trenk, D., Hochholzer, W., Fromm, M. F., Zolk, O., Valina, C. M., Stratz, C., et al. (2011). Paraoxonase-1 Q192R polymorphism and antiplatelet effects of clopidogrel in patients undergoing elective coronary stent placement. *Circulation: Cardiovascular Genetics*, *4*, 429–436.

van den Akker-van Marle, M. E., Gurwitz, D., Detmar, S. B., Enzing, C. M., Hopkins, M. M., Gutierrez de Mesa, E., et al. (2006). Cost-effectiveness of pharmacogenomics in clinical practice: a case study of thiopurine methyltransferase genotyping in acute lymphoblastic leukemia in Europe. *Pharmacogenomics*, *7*, 783–792.

Van Kuilenburg, A. B., Haasjes, J., Richel, D. J., Zoetekouw, L., Van Lenthe, H., De Abreu, R. A., et al. (2000). Clinical implications of dihydropyrimidine dehydrogenase (DPD) deficiency in patients with severe 5-fluorouracil-associated toxicity: identification of new mutations in the DPD gene. *Clinical Cancer Research*, *6*, 4705–4712.

Van Kuilenburg, A. B., Meijer, J., Mul, A. N., Meinsma, R., Schmid, V., Dobritzsch, D., et al. (2010). Intragenic deletions and a deep intronic mutation affecting pre-mRNA splicing in the dihydropyrimidine dehydrogenase gene as novel mechanisms causing 5-fluorouracil toxicity. *Human Genetics*, *128*, 529–538.

Van Kuilenburg, A. B., Vreken, P., Abeling, N. G., Bakker, H. D., Meinsma, R., Van Lenthe, H., et al. (1999). Genotype and phenotype in patients with dihydropyrimidine dehydrogenase deficiency. *Human Genetics*, *104*, 1–9.

van Schaik, R. H., Kok, M., Sweep, F. C., van Vliet, M., van Fessem, M., Meijer-van Gelder, M. E., et al. (2011). The CYP2C19*2 genotype predicts tamoxifen treatment outcome in advanced breast cancer patients. *Pharmacogenomics*, *12*, 1137–1146.

van Schie, R. M., Wadelius, M. I., Kamali, F., Daly, A. K., Manolopoulos, V. G., de Boer, A., et al. (2009). Genotype-guided dosing of coumarin derivatives: the European pharmacogenetics of anticoagulant therapy (EU-PACT) trial design. *Pharmacogenomics*, *10*, 1687–1695.

VanderVaart, S., Berger, H., Sistonen, J., Madadi, P., Matok, I., Gijsen, V. M., et al. (2011). CYP2D6 polymorphisms and codeine analgesia in postpartum pain management: a pilot study. *Therapeutic Drug Monitoring*, *33*, 425–432.

Wadelius, M., Chen, L. Y., Lindh, J. D., Eriksson, N., Ghori, M. J., Bumpstead, S., et al. (2009). The largest prospective warfarin-treated cohort supports genetic forecasting. *Blood*, *113*, 784–792.

Wallace, B. D., Wang, H., Lane, K. T., Scott, J. E., Orans, J., Koo, J. S., et al. (2010). Alleviating cancer drug toxicity by inhibiting a bacterial enzyme. *Science*, *330*, 831–835.

Weinshilboum, R., & Sladek, S. L. (1980). Mercaptopurine pharmacogenetics: monogenic inheritance of erythrocyte thiopurine methyltransferase activity. *American Journal of Human Genetics*, *32*, 651–662.

Wyen, C., Hendra, H., Siccardi, M., Platten, M., Jaeger, H., Harrer, T., et al. (2011). Cytochrome P450 2B6 (CYP2B6) and constitutive androstane receptor (CAR) polymorphisms are associated with early discontinuation of efavirenz-containing regimens. *Journal of Antimicrobial Chemotherapy*, *66*, 2092–2098.

Yang, X., Zhang, B., Molony, C., Chudin, E., Hao, K., Zhu, J., et al. (2010). Systematic genetic and genomic analysis of cytochrome P450 enzyme activities in human liver. *Genome Research*, *20*, 1020–1036.

Yen, J. L., & McLeod, H. L. (2007). Should DPD analysis be required prior to prescribing fluoropyrimidines? *European Journal of Cancer*, *43*, 1011–1016.

Yu, X., Dhakal, I. B., Beggs, M., Edavana, V. K., Williams, S., Zhang, X., et al. (2010). Functional genetic variants in the 3′-untranslated region of sulfotransferase isoform 1A1 (SULT1A1) and their effect on enzymatic activity. *Toxicological Sciences*, *118*, 391–403.

Zhang, J., Kuehl, P., Green, E. D., Touchman, J. W., Watkins, P. B., Daly, A., et al. (2001). The human pregnane X receptor: genomic structure and identification and functional characterization of natural allelic variants. *Pharmacogenetics*, *11*, 555–572.

Edith Sim[1,2], Giannoulis Fakis[3], Nicola Laurieri[1] and Sotiria Boukouvala[3]

[1]Department of Pharmacology, University of Oxford, Mansfield Road, Oxford, United Kingdom
[2]Faculty of Science, Engineering and Computing, Kingston University, Kingston, United Kingdom
[3]Department of Molecular Biology and Genetics, Democritus University of Thrace, Alexandroupolis, Greece

Arylamine *N*-Acetyltransferases – from Drug Metabolism and Pharmacogenetics to Identification of Novel Targets for Pharmacological Intervention

Dedicated to Patrick Hanna who retires from the University of Minnesota in June 2012, an Olympic year. Pat, Medicinal Chemist and friend who has made a true Olympic contribution to the NAT field.

Abstract

Arylamine *N*-acetyltransferases (NATs) are defined as xenobiotic metabolizing enzymes, adding an acetyl group from acetyl coenzyme A (CoA) to arylamines and arylhydrazines. NATs are found in organisms from bacteria and fungi to vertebrates. Several isoenzymes, often polymorphic, may be present in one organism. There are two functional polymorphic NATs in humans and polymorphisms in *NAT2* underpinned pharmacogenetics as a discipline. NAT enzymes have had a role in important metabolic concepts: the identification of acetyl-CoA and endogenous metabolic roles in bacteria and in eukaryotic folate metabolism. In fungi, NAT is linked to formation of unique metabolites.

A broad and exciting canvas of investigations has emerged over the past five years from fundamental studies on NAT enzymes. The role of human NAT1 in breast cancer where it is a biomarker and possible therapeutic target may also underlie NAT's early appearance during mammalian fetal development. Studies of NAT in *Mycobacterium tuberculosis* have identified potential therapeutic targets for tuberculosis whilst the role of NATs in fungi opens up potential toxicological intervention in agriculture.

Advances in Pharmacology, Volume 63 1054-3589/12 $35.00

http://dx.doi.org/10.1016/B978-0-12-398339-8.00005-7

These developments are possible through the combination of genomics, enzymology and structural data. Strong binding of CoA to *Bacillis anthracis* NAT may point to divergent roles of NATs amongst organisms as does differential control of mammalian *NAT* gene expression. The powerful combination of phenotypic investigation following genetic manipulation of *NAT* genes from mice to mycobacteria has been coupled with generation of isoenzyme-specific inhibitors. This battery of molecular and systems biology approaches heralds a new era for NAT research in pharmacology and toxicology.

I. Introduction

Arylamine *N*-acetyltransferases (NATs) constitute a unique family of drug-metabolizing enzymes, which have been important in understanding endogenous metabolism, as well as biotransformation of drugs and other environmental chemicals. This article provides an overview of the important role NATs have had, and are continuing to have, in establishing many important concepts in cellular metabolism and xenobiotic conversion, also reviewing their relevance to pharmacogenetics and carcinogenesis, as well as microbial metabolism in bacteria and fungi.

In humans, mice and rats there are three *NAT* loci, although in humans one of these is a pseudogene. Identifying the human equivalent gene products in mammals has been very important in developing appropriate models, including transgenic mice, for the human NAT enzymes. There is a high degree of homology in all of the mammalian isoenzymes (over 80% identity at the amino acid level). Both human NAT enzymes are polymorphic, as are all three mouse enzymes, and understanding the fast and slow acetylator phenotypes has been established at the molecular level. As with many other functional single nucleotide polymorphisms (SNPs), incorrect folding of the enzymes appears to be the major cause of the slow acetylator type (reviewed by Boukouvala & Fakis, 2005; Sim et al., 2008b). The characterization of polymorphisms in the human *NAT* genes has provided an important resource for pharmacogenetics and personalized medicine, also allowing their use as tools in population genetics and molecular anthropology.

A major area of study has focused on the endogenous role of one of the human isoenzymes, human NAT1. These studies have involved the use of a wide range of approaches, including transgenic mice as models. A further area of investigation has been the control of expression of mammalian genes for NAT, including the beginnings of the important arena of epigenetics (Minchin et al., 2007; Butcher et al., 2008; Wakefield et al., 2010).

There has been a major effort also in studying the bioinformatics of NATs in a wide range of organisms. Structural and functional studies on microbial NATs have recently been described (Sim et al., 2008a, b for review). These homologs are likely to be of importance in agriculture (Glenn & Bacon, 2009), bioremediation (Martins et al., 2009) and pathogenesis (Bhakta et al., 2004), and also as models for deciphering the role of NATs in fundamental cellular metabolism – a role which the NAT enzymes have played repeatedly, and with increasing complexity, since the essential metabolic cofactor acetyl coenzyme A (CoA) was identified (Lipmann, 1945).

Data on the NAT genes and polymorphisms is curated through consensus, by scientists representing the main teams in the field. There have been a series of workshops at approximately 36-month intervals (Table I), and these workshops have been extremely important in forging collaborations which have advanced the studies on these enzymes. There has been a clutch of reviews on the NATs since 2007, following advances in structural studies (Sinclair et al., 2000; Wu et al., 2007; Minchin et al., 2007; Sim et al., 2008b) and also updates on NATs from a genomic perspective (Vagena et al., 2008; Glenn et al., 2010). For those new to the world of NATs, this article review will provide an overview of the field and will then focus on the major findings in the last four years.

II. NAT Enzyme Mechanism

NATs were first identified as transferring an acetyl group from acetyl-CoA to the amino group of an arylhydrazine (e.g. isoniazid and hydralazine) or of an arylamine such as *p*-aminosalicylate (Fig. 1). Early studies used *p*-nitrophenyl acetate (pNPA) as acetyl donor (Riddle & Jencks, 1971), and this has been a useful reagent in more recent studies with purified recombinant enzyme, e.g. from hamster and humans (Liu et al., 2006; Wang et al., 2005a). It has become clear that other alkyl-CoAs can also act as acyl donors and this has been linked with studies establishing the wide range of organisms in which the NAT enzymes are found. Recent studies have demonstrated that propionyl-CoA can be used by a NAT enzyme from

TABLE I International NAT Workshops

Year	*Location*	*Organizer(s)*	*Workshop report*
1998	Kuranda, Queensland, Australia	Rodney F. Minchin	Ilett et al., 1999
2001	Eynsham, Oxfordshire, U.K.	Edith Sim	Rodrigues-Lima et al., 2002
2004	Vancouver, BC, Canada	Charlene A. McQueen	McQueen, 2004
2007	Alexandroupolis, Greece	Giannoulis Fakis Sotiria Boukouvala	Boukouvala et al., 2008
2010	Paris, France	Jean-Marie Dupret Fernando Rodrigues-Lima	Rodrigues-Lima et al., 2011

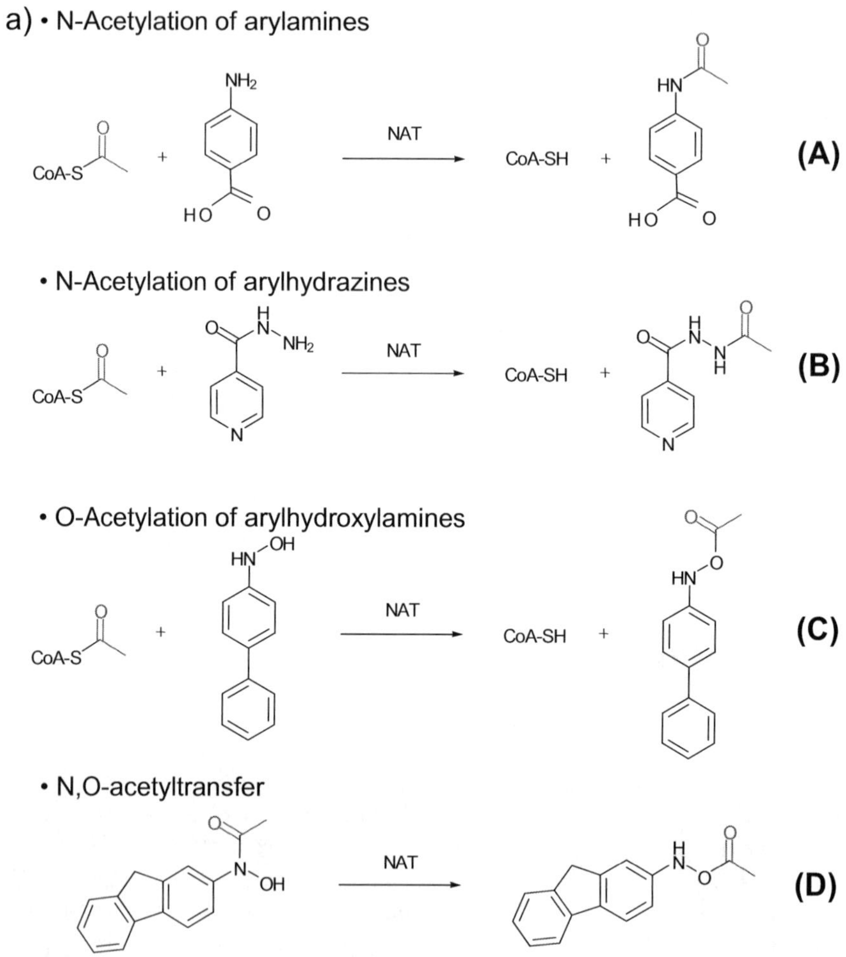

FIGURE 1 Reactions catalyzed by NAT. (a) Reactions illustrated as A–C are acyl-CoA dependent reactions. Reactions C and D are activation reactions which also require an oxidation step of the xenobiotic (the carcinogen 2-aminofluorene is shown in D).

Mycobacterium marinum (Lack et al., 2009) and in the fungus *Fusarium verticllioides*, malonyl-CoA is a very effective acyl donor (Glenn et al., 2003; Glenn & Bacon, 2009).

Identification of the reactions catalyzed by the NAT family of enzymes has established that there is a range of reactions catalyzed and these are summarized along with the activation via cytochrome P450 in Fig. 1.

Once hydroxamic acids are formed through the oxidation of arylamines, the *N*-acetylation and also the *O*-acetylation of arylhydroxylamine have been identified and these reactions are activation reactions. Acetyl-CoA or pNPA can act as the acetyl donor, but a further reaction which is

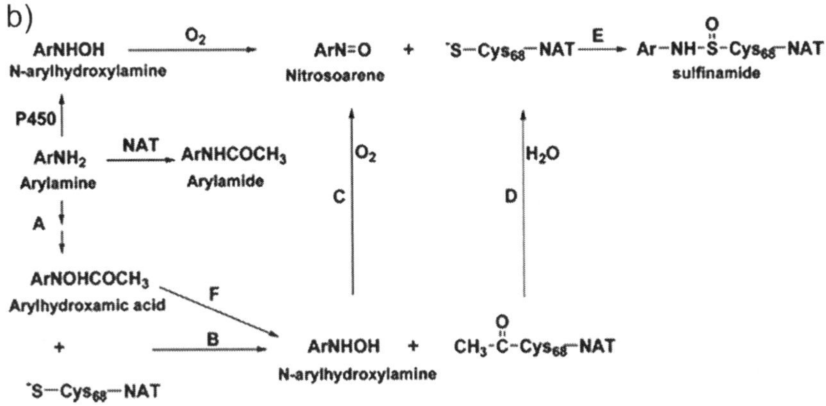

FIGURE 1—cont'd (b) Isoform selective inactivation of human NAT by reactive metabolites (after Liu et al., 2009), in which the reactive oxidized and acetylated metabolite is demonstrated to form an adduct with the active site cysteine rendering the enzyme inactive.

acetyl-CoA independent has been recognized: the transfer of an acetyl group from *N*-acetylhyroxamic acid to the O group to form an *N*-acetoxyester and this is considered to result in the formation of the ultimate carcinogen (Fig. 1) (Liu et al., 2009).

Initial enzyme kinetic studies, using tissue extracts and homogenates, established the nature of the reaction catalyzed by the NATs as a ping-pong-bi-bi mechanism (Riddle & Jencks, 1971). These studies played a major part in establishing that there was an active site cysteine as a result of early inhibition studies with cysteine reactive inhibitors, such as iodoacetamide, which was demonstrated to inhibit mammalian (Andres et al., 1988; Watson et al., 1990) and bird NAT enzymic activity (Jencks et al., 1972; Andres et al., 1983). Studies on pure rabbit enzyme showed specific labeling of cysteine with ^{14}C-iodoacetamide (Andres et al., 1988). Recent studies demonstrating inhibition by mercuric compounds (Ragunathan et al., 2010) and antabuse (Malka et al., 2009) have developed this theme. Other studies have demonstrated suicide inhibition of NAT1 in humans and its hamster equivalent by nitrosoarenes (Liu et al., 2009). The elegant studies demonstrated the formation of a sulphonamide adduct of the recombinant pure enzymes and studies with cytosolic extracts of cultured cells demonstrated the same phenomenon.

Further studies showing oxidation of the active site cysteine as a potential toxicological mechanism have also been demonstrated in bronchial extracts (Dairou et al., 2009) and in lens (Dairou et al., 2005).

The work of Watanabe et al. (1992), through functional and sequencing studies of the NAT homolog from *Salmonella typhimurium*, was instrumental in identifying which cysteine in the eukaryotic NATs was likely to be involved in the active site. These studies were supported by site-directed mutagenesis of the human NAT2 in which cysteine 68 was replaced by alanine with a loss of activity (Dupret & Grant, 1992).

Structural studies identified cysteine, histidine and aspartate at the active site of the NAT enzyme from *S. typhimurium* and showed that the proposed active site cysteine could be labeled by a bromacetanilide (Sinclair et al., 2000) (Figs. 2 and 3). These X-ray structures laid the foundation for a clutch of subsequent NAT structures (Sandy et al., 2002; Westwood et al., 2005; Holton et al., 2005; Wu et al., 2007; Fullam et al., 2008; Pluvinage et al., 2011) and also allowed identification of the key conserved residues in all NATs which had been shown to be active in arylamine acetylation (Sandy et al., 2005). Several of those residues are conserved in a recently identified homolog (NAT1 or FDB2) from filamentous fungi which uses malonyl-CoA rather than acetyl-CoA (Glenn & Bacon, 2009).

Hamster NAT2 has been demonstrated to be able to utilize propionyl and butyryl-CoA as acyl donors (Kawamura et al., 2005), albeit less effectively than acetyl-CoA. Interestingly, malonyl-CoA was not an acyl donor with hamster NAT2. Succinyl-CoA is a potent inhibitor of acetylation with hamster NAT2.

The ping-pong-bi-bi mechanism appears universal for all active NATs, and real kinetic constants for NATs from hamster (Wang et al., 2004) and *Pseudomonas aeruginosa* (Westwood & Sim, 2007) confirm this mechanism. It has been demonstrated, for the NATs which have been investigated, including NAT enzymes from hamster (Wang et al., 2004, 2005a, b), pigeon (Riddle & Jencks, 1971), *P. aeruginosa* (Westwood & Sim, 2007) and *S. typhimurium* (Mushtaq et al., 2002), that pNPA will also act as an acetyl donor.

Whilst the reaction mechanism proposed is widely applicable, there are questions which have emerged – isoniazid will bind to the enzyme from *S. typhimurium* in the absence of acetyl-CoA (Delgoda et al., 2003) and recent studies show that CoA will bind extremely strongly to NAT from *Bacillus anthracis* such that, in the crystal structure of the recombinant *B. anthracis*, CoA was found in a cleft despite the protein having been prepared from an *Escherichia coli* cell lysate (Pluvinage et al., 2011). The cleft in which the CoA is bound differs from that of both the human enzyme (Wu et al., 2007) and also the NAT from *M. marinum* (Fullam et al., 2008) (Fig. 2). In the latter cases, CoA had been added following purification. Each of these three enzymes shows a distinct CoA binding cleft – hence it is unlikely that it is the endogenous source of CoA in *B. anthracis* that is the reason for the difference in modes of binding.

One of the questions which emerge repeatedly is whether the NAT enzymes can hydrolyze acetyl-CoA or other alkyl-CoA derivatives in the absence of an acceptor substrate. The studies by Pluvinage et al. (2011), showing the binding of endogenous CoA to *B. anthracis* NAT strongly suggests that this enzyme can hydrolyze acyl-CoA without an arylamine substrate being present.

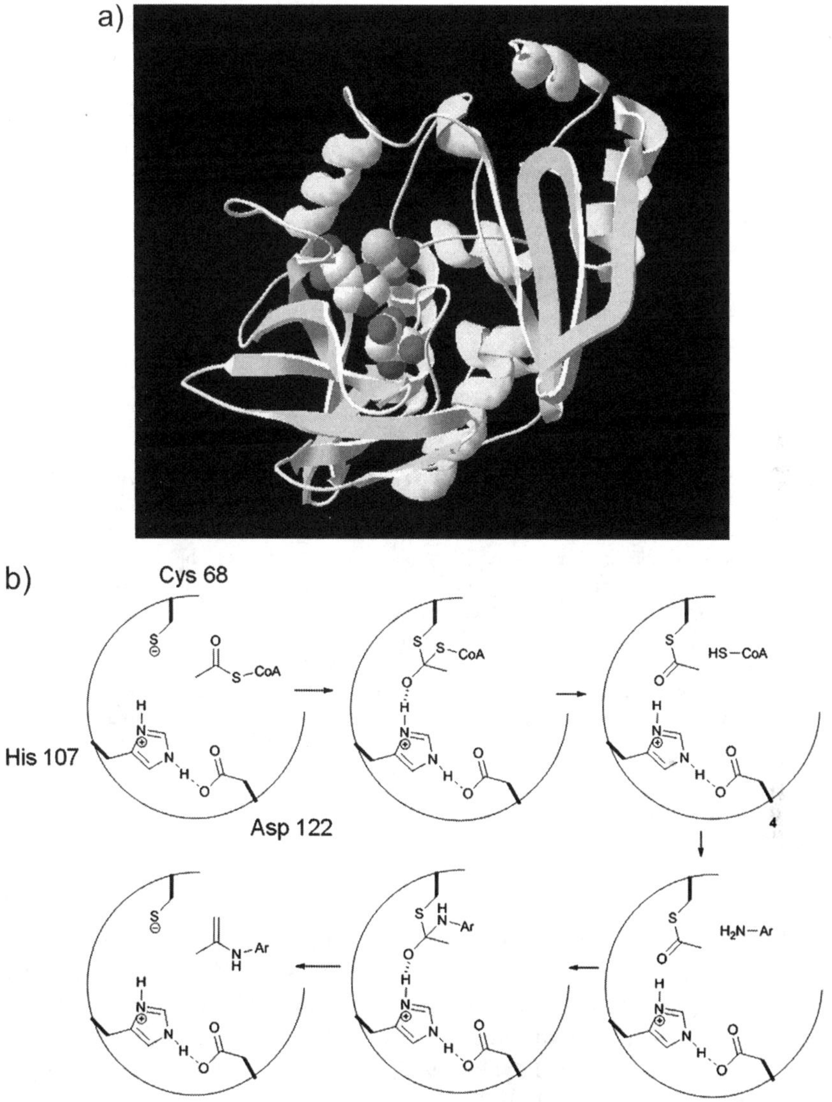

FIGURE 2 **Reaction mechanism of arylamine N-acetyltransferase (a).** Ribbon diagram of structure of NAT from *M. smegmatis* (Sandy et al., 2002; PDB 1W6F) showing the backbone secondary structural elements. The active site residues Cys 70, His110 and Asp 127 are shown space filled to emphasize their proximity. The numbering of the active site residues varies slightly amongst individual members of the family (e.g. Sandy et al., 2005) but all NAT structures show the same juxtaposition of active site residues. (**b**) The proposed mechanism is shown with acetyl-CoA as acyl donor. The residue numbering refers to the human NAT1 amino acid sequence. The formation of the acetyl-enzyme intermediate requires the stabilization of charge across a Cys-His-Asp triad. The acetyl transfer occurs following nucleophilic attack of the acetylated intermediate by the arylamine substrate. The lifetime of an acetylated NAT intermediate differs among NAT species (Wang et al., 2005a, b). The diagram is modified from (Westwood et al., 2006).

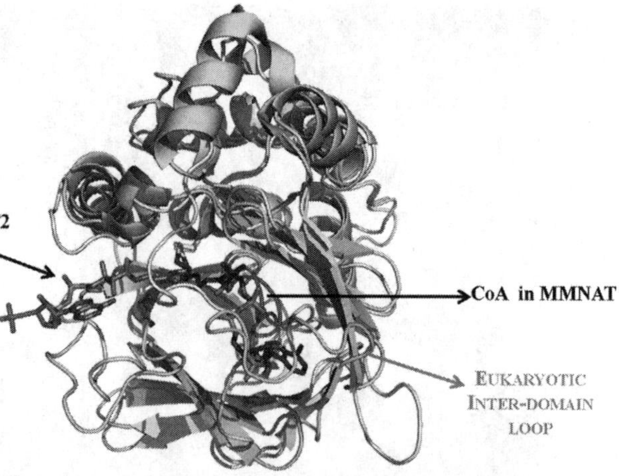

FIGURE 3 Overall structure of human NAT2 and *Mycobacterium marinum* NAT, both with CoA bound. Ribbon diagram showing the overlaid structures of human NAT2 (hNAT2, gray – PDB: 2PFR) and *M. marinum* NAT (MMNAT, turquoise/gray – PDB: 2VFC). The structures were generated and aligned using the program PyMOL. The CoA which was co-crystallized with the appropriate enzyme is shown in stick format and labeled with carbon atoms in gray for human NAT2 and in blue/dark gray for *M. marinum* NAT, nitrogen in blue/black, oxygen in red/medium gray, and sulfur in orange/light gray. The catalytic cysteine residue is shown in stick representation and colored in yellow/white. The sulphydryl group of the active site Cys is suitably positioned for the transfer of the acetyl group from acetyl-CoA. The characteristic eukaryotic loop is colored in green and indicated with an arrow (the reader is advised to view the colored on-line version of this figure for more detail and clarity).

Recent studies with human NAT1 and mouse NAT2, the equivalent enzyme in terms of amino acid sequence identity, tissue expression profile and substrate specificity (Kawamura et al., 2008), suggest that in the presence of folate these enzymes specifically can hydrolyze acetyl-CoA (Dairou et al., 2010) and that raises the question of the NAT enzyme playing a role at the interface between acetyl-CoA homeostasis and folate metabolism. Intriguingly, in the light of the apparently distinct roles of human NAT2 as a drug-metabolizing enzyme and human NAT1 having a role in endogenous metabolism, human NAT2 does not appear to catalyze this hydrolytic reaction (Dairou et al., 2010).

A consistent finding indicating that human NAT1 and its murine counterpart has a role at the interface of folate and acetyl-CoA homeostasis is the acetylation of a breakdown product of folate, *p*-aminobenzoylglutamate, by human NAT1 (Minchin, 1995; Ward et al., 1995) and its mammalian counterparts (Kawamura et al., 2005, 2008), but not by human NAT2.

Recent studies on metabolism of hydralazine have added information to the interaction of the drug with NAT (Abuhammad et al., 2011). The product of the acetylation of hydralazine is a cyclized product methyl triazolophthalazine. From structural studies of the NAT enzyme from *M. marinum* in complex with hydralazine, it is clear that the reaction intermediate is positioned such that the mechanism results in the cyclized product.

III. *NAT* Genes and Pharmacogenetics

NATs have long been recognized as drug-metabolizing enzymes, and have had an important role in establishing the early concept of pharmacogenetics. The enzyme, now known as human NAT2, was demonstrated in 1960 to be responsible for the variation in inactivation of isoniazid, an antitubercular hydrazine still in use today (Evans et al., 1960). The different sub-populations were described as "rapid" (alias "fast") and "slow" acetylators of the drug, and a considerable effort has since been made to understand the biochemical and molecular basis of this phenotypic variability. A twin study confirmed the fast and slow acetylator types as genetically determined (Evans et al., 1960) and showed the inheritance expected of an autosomal recessive trait controlling slow inactivation of isoniazid. The inactivation event was shown to be due to acetylation of a range of substrates – arylamine and arylhydrazines – using the acetyl group of acetyl-CoA. The outstanding initial studies of Jenne (1965) identified that there were likely to be two separable enzymic activities in human liver which could catalyze the acetylation of different substrates. The acetylation of *p*-aminosalicylate and of isoniazid could be separated chromatographically from human liver cytosol. These studies helped explain the pharmacokinetics of *p*-aminosalicylate and isoniazid in tubercular patients (Mitchell & Bell, 1957). The *p*-aminosalicylate acetylating isoenzyme is now known as human NAT1 and the isoniazid-metabolizing enzyme is known as human NAT2 (Hein et al., 2008b for update on nomenclature). Definitive evidence for the existence of two human isoenzymes was established with the cloning of both of these enzymes from liver cDNA (Ohsako & Deguchi, 1990) and genomic DNA (Blum et al., 1990) libraries. These early cloning studies (pre-PCR!) relied on the existence of protein sequence from rabbit (Andres et al., 1987) and chicken (Ohsako et al., 1988).

The fortuitous combination of the approaches taken in these early cloning studies provided an excellent picture of the existence of two functional polymorphic human genes and one pseudogene. The proteins encoded by the two human genes were also demonstrated to have different substrate specificities: human NAT1 having specificity for *p*-aminosalicylate and *p*-aminobenzoic acid, and human NAT2 being specific for isoniazid, sulphamethazine and procainamide (Deguchi et al., 1990; Blum et al., 1991; Kelly & Sim, 1991; Deguchi, 1992; summarized in Weber, 1999). The establishing of a new method for determining enzymic activity of NATs (Brooke et al., 2003), which is universal for all substrates, has allowed the establishing of substrate panel data (Kawamura et al., 2008). Nevertheless, the early enzyme assays (Andres et al., 1983), in which differential quantitative detection of a wide range of arylamines was performed, were used extensively in the early studies and are still in use today. These assays were relatively demanding technically, so the introduction of the simpler plate-format colorimetric assay, based on the hydrolysis of acetyl-CoA and detection of the free CoA, has increased the volume of data available on a range of NAT enzymes (Westwood & Sim, 2007).

It took several decades and the development of cloning techniques for the genetics of arylamine *N*-acetylation to be resolved at the gene level in humans (Ohsako & Deguchi, 1990; Blum et al., 1990; Kelly & Sim, 1991). Cloning the genes for NATs in humans revealed that there was also a third inactive locus, the *NATP1* pseudogene (Blum et al., 1990). The first cloning studies were carried out using human material from different ethnic origins and, again fortuitously, provided evidence suggesting the basis of the pharmacogenetic polymorphism in human NAT2 as SNPs within the *NAT2* gene (Ohsako & Deguchi, 1990; Blum et al., 1990, 1991; Deguchi, 1992). Studies at that time and since, confirmed with site-directed mutagenesis, have identified that several functional SNPs result in unstable NAT protein (Liu et al., 2006; Zang et al., 2007). The combination of studies of Japanese and Caucasian populations resulted in further understanding of the long established geographical differences in the incidence of slow acetylation of isoniazid and sulphamethazine in humans (reviewed by Boukouvala & Fakis, 2005). The commonest polymorphism associated with slow acetylation in Caucasians is rare in Japanese populations (Deguchi et al., 1990; Blum et al., 1991; Sim & Hickman, 1991; Deguchi, 1992).

The localization of the two functional human *NAT* genes and the *NATP1* pseudogene in a small region of the genome, on the short arm of chromosome 8 (Blum et al., 1990; Franke et al., 1994; Hickman et al., 1994; Matas et al., 1997), has allowed haplotype analysis to be carried out. Comparison of genotyping between mothers and babies gave an indication that there was linkage disequilibrium across the region in Caucasian populations (Smelt et al., 1998). Although multiple genotyping methods have been described (Doll & Hein, 2001, 2002; Brans et al., 2004), with the economy of DNA sequencing, the use of sequencing across the region has been described in population genetic studies, and the wealth of SNPs at the *NAT* loci has been useful in anthropological studies. Combining resequencing with the use of advanced bioinformatics tools to analyze data derived from international genome consortia (e.g. HapMap), these studies have been useful in comparing populations of diverse geographical distribution.

In 2006, Patin et al. carried out resequencing and genotyping of the *NAT* loci in 13 populations of diverse origin and suggested a possible selective advantage for the slow acetylator phenotype in Western/Central Euroasians, where the "slow" *NAT2*5B* allele is more common. In this and subsequent genetic population studies, the investigators convincingly argued that the transition of human populations from hunting-gathering to pastoralism and agriculture, about 10,000 years ago, may have provided the environmental stimuli favoring the expansion of "slow" *NAT2* variants in those populations (Patin et al., 2006a, 2006b; Magalon et al., 2008; Luca et al., 2008). Other investigators have supported this hypothesis (Sabbagh et al., 2008, 2011). In contrast with *NAT2,* genetic diversity at the *NAT1* locus is very limited among populations, consistent with its hypothesized role in fundamental cellular functions additional to xenobiotic metabolism (Patin et al., 2006a; Mortensen et al., 2011).

The genetic approaches described above have established the *NAT* gene polymorphisms as useful markers to trace the demographic history of population adaptation to the variable chemical challenges of social environments. In modern societies, genome-wide association studies have demonstrated the synergistic action of "slow" acetylation genotypes and tobacco smoke as risk factors for carcinogenesis of the bladder (Moore et al., 2011; Rothman et al., 2010; García-Closas et al., 2011). These large-scale genotyping studies add to the evidence from a candidate gene approach associating the slow acetylation phenotype with environmental bladder cancer (Cartwright et al., 1982; Risch et al., 1995). An additional challenge of modern lifestyle to xenobiotic biotransformation pathways of humans, including those catalyzed by NATs, is posed by the range of synthetic chemicals administered as drugs. Elucidating the polymorphism patterns of xenobiotic metabolizing enzymes is, therefore, crucial for the development and application of effective personalized therapies (Li et al., 2011).

IV. The Genomic Distribution and Function of NATs

A. Prokaryotic NAT Enzymes

A picture of the distribution amongst organisms and evolutionary history of NATs has emerged recently through a series of comprehensive genomic and phylogenetic investigations across all major clades of the tree of life (Boukouvala & Fakis, 2005; Vagena et al., 2008; Glenn et al., 2010). In bacteria, NATs are found in representatives of most major taxonomic groups, and the study of several such homologs has been of historic significance in the NAT field. A putative *NAT* homolog has also been reported in an archaeon (*Halogeometricum borinquense*), representing a domain of life intermediate between prokaryotes and eukaryotes (Glenn et al., 2010). NAT activity has been identified in many prokaryotic organisms and 5-aminosalicylate was shown to be a particularly potent substrate (Delomenie et al., 2001). The cytosolic enzymes are between 30 and 35 kDa.

Genome analyses have provided a rich seam for identification of NAT homologs in bacteria. These studies were predicated by the role of

S. typhimurium NAT in understanding the structure and functions of the NAT enzymes. The *S. typhimurium* NAT enzyme resolved the controversy as to whether the *O*-acetylation of arylhydroxylamines and the arylamine *N*-acetylation reaction were catalyzed by the same enzyme. The work of Watanabe et al. (1992) showed the enzyme was the same in prokaryotes and paved the way for crystallographic studies. The three-dimensional structure of NAT from *S. typhimurium* (Sinclair et al., 2000) showed for the first time the existence of an active site catalytic triad activating the cysteine through histidine and aspartate residues. This has now been found to be an essential feature of all NAT homologs (Sandy et al., 2005; Wang et al., 2005b).

A separate series of bacterial enzymes which are NAT homologs have also been identified, but which are involved in intramolecular ring formation. Rifamycin amide synthetase is one such enzyme where the function has been identified, although the mode of action has not (Pompeo et al., 2002 for review). The identification of this group of NAT homologs demonstrates that the NAT scaffold, which consists of three domains (Figs. 2 and 3), can be adapted to different functions.

A more extensive identification of NAT enzymes has demonstrated multiple *NAT* genes in bacteria, including *B. anthracis*, *Nocardia farcinica* and also *Mesorhizobium loti*, where the NAT enzyme could play a role in symbiosis between the bacterium in root nodules and its plant host (Martins et al., 2008; Pluvinage et al., 2007; Rodrigues-Lima et al., 2006).

An amino acid loop thought to be specific for the eukaryotic NAT enzymes has been demonstrated to exist in certain bacterial enzymes (Pluvinage et al., 2011). In contrast, in the zebrafish, some of the six *NAT* genes seem to lack this characteristic "eukaryotic loop" (Sim et al., 2008a). The effect of this loop on NAT enzymic activity in the hamster (Kawamura, 2003) and rat (Walraven et al., 2007) has been addressed (see Fig. 3 for position of loop in structure).

1. The Significance of Mycobacterial NATs

The identification of NAT homologs in mycobacteria was particularly intriguing. Isoniazid, which is metabolized in humans by NAT2, is a front line anti-tubercular drug. Isoniazid itself needs to be activated within mycobacterial cells by an oxidative step, catalyzed by katG, and the activated isoniazid inhibits the synthesis of the mycolic acid components of the cell wall. The mycobacterial NAT enzymes were demonstrated to use isoniazid as a substrate (Payton et al., 1999a; Upton et al., 2001; Sandy et al., 2002; Fullam et al., 2008). It was proposed that acetylation would compete with oxidation of isoniazid as a prodrug, and so render the mycobacteria less susceptible to the compound. This was demonstrated to be the case with both *Mycobacterium smegmatis* (Payton et al., 1999a) and *Mycobacterium bovis* BCG (Bhakta et al., 2004).

In a subsequent series of experiments, when the *nat* gene was deleted, other effects on growth and mycobacterial cell morphology were identified. NAT was shown to have a role in controlling growth, as upon deletion of the *nat* gene the mycobacterial cell wall lipids were altered dramatically, the sensitivity to normally non-penetrant antibiotics was increased and, in the case of *M. bovis* BCG, the mycobacterial cells became unable to survive inside macrophage (Payton et al., 2001; Bhakta et al., 2004). This latter effect has since been demonstrated to be closely associated with the deletion of other genes encoded in the same operon as the *nat* gene (Anderton et al., 2006; Yam et al., 2009; Lack et al., 2010). Interestingly, the *nat* gene appears to be part of an operon in *Mycobacterium tuberculosis* (Anderton et al., 2006; Yam et al., 2009), which is essential for survival of the organism inside macrophage (Rengarajan et al., 2005). The novel pathway the operon controls is involved in cholesterol catabolism (Van der Geize et al., 2007) with cholesterol being an essential fuel for *M. tuberculosis* survival within macrophage (Pandey & Sassetti, 2008; Miner et al., 2009 for review). The *nat* operon appears to be part of a major group of genes involved in the metabolism of cholesterol – the so-called Kst Regulon. The functional link between the *nat* gene product with the other four gene products which have a role in the sterol ring degradation (e.g. Lack et al., 2010; Yam et al., 2009), suggest a role through the alkyl chain which is degraded to acetyl and propionyl-CoA, each of which are cofactors for the mycobacterial NATs (Lack et al., 2009).

The NAT proteins from *M. tuberculosis* and *M. bovis* BCG are identical and very similar in amino acid sequence to the NAT enzyme from *M. marinum*. However, enzymological and physical studies show distinct differences (Fullam et al., 2009). The NAT enzyme from *M. tuberculosis* has a much higher melting temperature and is completely folded at temperatures around 42°C. This is also the case for other enzymes encoded by the same operon (HsaD) and this is thought to be related to a protective mechanism during the initial inflammatory response. In contrast, the *M. marinum* enzyme, which is an organism that grows at lower temperatures and infects cold water fish, has a much lower melting temperature (Lack et al., 2009).

It was as a result of these studies that the mycobacterial NATs were included in the panel of recombinant enzymes used to screen a chemical library. Inhibitors of mycobacterial NAT were identified and were demonstrated to have similar effects to the deletion of the *nat* gene (Westwood et al., 2010) which is described in more detail below. The studies on NAT from one mycobacterial organism have also been important in identifying the acetyl-CoA binding site (Fullam et al., 2008), which is distinct albeit sharing some features with the acetyl-CoA binding site in the eukaryotic NATs (Wu et al., 2007) (Fig. 3).

There is also evidence for polymorphism in the *nat* gene from clinical isolates of *M. tuberculosis* and this may contribute to the overall sensitivity of particular strains to isoniazid (Sholto-Douglas-Vernon et al., 2005; Upton et al., 2001; Coelho et al., 2011). In addition, microarray studies of expression of mycobacterial genes inside macrophage and dendritic cells suggest that there is upregulation of the *nat* operon (Tailleux et al., 2008).

B. Eukaryotic NAT Enzymes

1. NATs in Microbial Eukaryotes

A new chapter in NAT research opened with the report of putative NAT homologs in eukaryotic microorganisms, such as the protists and fungi (Vagena et al., 2008; Glenn et al., 2010). The protists (e.g. amoebas, oomycetes, diatoms, ciliates, etc.) are unicellular organisms of polyphyletic origin that inhabit diverse environments. They range from free-living to parasitic (to a divergent spectrum of hosts), and their taxonomic classification and evolutionary history can be uncertain. In most species with putative *NAT* genes, multiple paralogs have been annotated, potentially indicating evolutionary divergence of NAT isoforms with different (specialized) functions. In addition, certain *NAT* paralogs may have found their way into the genomes of protists from bacteria, via horizontal gene transfer. Our analyses have indicated a mixed phylogeny of NATs among bacteria and protists, with clear evidence for horizontal gene transfer between the *Bacillus* bacteria and cellular slime molds (e.g. *Dictyostelium*). NATs are also present in choanoflagellates, a taxonomic group of protists considered to represent the closest unicellular relatives of metazoa (King et al., 2008). A striking finding was also the possible presence of putative NAT homologs in a giant amoeba mimivirus, believed to represent an independent clade of life rooted near the origin of eukaryotes (Glenn et al., 2010).

The phylogeny of fungal NATs is also intriguing. Our survey of 146 fungal genomes identified NATs in chytridiomycetes, basidiomycetes and ascomycetes exclusively from the subphylum of *Pezizomycotina*. Plant pathogenic fungi typically possess multiple *NAT* loci in their genome, in contrast with animal pathogenic species which typically harbor only one *NAT*. Within the monophyletic clade of fungal NATs, paralogy is limited, with about eight distinct lineages of *NAT* ortholog evident, particularly within the plant pathogens (Glenn et al., 2010). Similar results were reported by Martins et al. (2010), who proposed possible evolutionary scenarios of gains and losses of *NAT* genes in sequenced fungal genomes. Moreover, both studies suspected one horizontal gene transfer event from an unknown proteobacterium to the basidiomycete *Malassezia globosa*. A more focused phylogenetic study, analyzing 63 *Fusarium avenaceum* isolates (including wheat pathogenic isolates) for multilocus sequence variability at five genetic loci (*EF1*α, *IGS rDNA*, *RPB2*, *ESYN1* and *NAT2*), reported moderate levels of nucleotide and haplotype diversity at the *NAT* locus, relative to the other loci (Kulik et al., 2011).

The Significance of Fungal NATs

Little is known about the endogenous role of fungal NATs, although interest in the area is accumulating. In 2001, Glenn et al. screened various strains of 11 plant-pathogenic *Fusarium* species for sensitivity to 2-benzoxazolinone (BOA), a potent anti-fungal toxin produced by maize and wheat. Only pathogens associated with these particular hosts demonstrated high tolerance to BOA and the tolerance was linked to the ability of each fungus to metabolize the toxin. Suspecting an endogenous detoxification pathway for BOA in the resistant fungi, the same investigators undertook characterization of the metabolic pathway of BOA in the corn pathogen *Fusarium verticillioides* (Glenn et al., 2002, 2003), followed by refined mapping of the corresponding genetic loci (named *FDB1* and *FDB2*) (Glenn & Bacon, 2009).

The first biotransformation step, converting BOA to the intermediate compound 2-aminophenol (2-AP), is catalyzed by the product of the *FDB1* locus. A malonyl moiety is then attached to the amine group of 2-AP by the enzyme activity encoded at the *FDB2* locus, to generate *N*-(2-hydroxyphenyl) malonamic acid (HPMA) which is non-toxic. Deletion of either or both of the *FDB1* and *FDB2* loci compromised detoxification of BOA, abolishing the ability of *F. verticillioides* to tolerate media supplemented with the toxin. In the *FDB1/fdb2* mutant strains, *N*-acetylation of 2-AP was evident, producing *N*-(2-hydroxyphenyl) acetamide (HPAA) instead of HPMA (Glenn et al., 2002, 2003). Transposon-mediated mutagenesis of 11 open reading frames (ORFs) at the *FDB2* locus identified a *NAT* homologous gene as essential for BOA tolerance by *F. verticillioides*. Moreover, the product of that gene was demonstrated to be responsible for BOA biotransformation to HPMA (Glenn & Bacon, 2009). Two other *NAT*-homologous genes identified in *F. verticillioides* by *in silico* means (Glenn et al., 2010) may encode enzymes with similar functions, e.g. potentially catalyzing the BOA to HPAA secondary biotransformation pathway observed in the *FDB1/fdb2* mutants.

The *F. verticillioides* homologs are representative of three of the eight lineages noted earlier, with the FDB2/NAT1 ortholog forming a well-defined clade consisting of a limited number of plant pathogens often associated with maize and wheat. The work by Dr. Glenn and his colleagues suggests that NAT-mediated detoxification may provide a selective advantage to devastating crop pathogens, like *F. verticillioides*, e.g. by enhancing their virulence or ecological fitness. Our ongoing collaborative investigations to elucidate the role of NATs in plant-pathogenic fungi with variable sensitivities to BOA may potentially enable the design of strategies for more effective management of crops.

Fungal NATs have also been studied from the perspective of bioremediation (Martins et al., 2009). The investigators employed the non-pathogenic ascomycetes *Podospora anserina* as model to investigate the metabolic potential of NATs toward 3,4-dichloroaniline (3,4-DCA), a highly toxic breakdown product of pesticides found in the soil and water. *P. anserina* has two NAT homologs and targeted disruption of the *NAT2* locus compromised the ability of the fungus to grow on arylamine-supplemented media. Moreover, recombinant NAT1 and NAT2 proteins were able to *N*-acetylate typical NAT substrates *in vitro*. Pilot experiments further indicated that, in soils contaminated with 3,4-DCA, the inoculation of *P. anserina* could effectively modulate compound detoxification via *N*-acetylation. The compromised ability of lettuce seeds to germinate in soil with 3,4-DCA was restored when experimentally contaminated soils were also inoculated with the fungus.

Overall, the investigations into the phylogeny and function of NATs in eukaryotic microorganisms promise to uncover the complex nature of organismal adaptation to adverse chemical environments, potentially opening the way for various biotechnological applications of industrial, agro-economic or environmental significance.

2. NATs in Higher Eukaryotes

Genomic surveys have consistently failed to identify *NAT*-homologous sequences in plants, indicating that the entire kingdom may lack *NAT* genes (Boukouvala & Fakis, 2005; Vagena et al., 2008; Glenn et al., 2010). NATs have been predicted in lower animal phyla, including cnidarians, but it is uncertain whether they exist in protostomes (molluscs, worms and arthropods). In contrast, the genomes of most deuterostomes surveyed to date have been demonstrated to possess at least one *NAT*-homolog. Such key, from an evolutionary perspective, organisms include the echinoderm *Strongylocentrotus purpuratus*, the hemichordate *Saccoglossus kowalevskii*, the urochordate *Ciona intestinalis* and the cephalochordate *Branchiostoma floridae* (Glenn et al., 2010). With few exceptions (e.g. the canids, Trepanier et al., 1997), NATs are found in all major taxa of vertebrates, from the primitive sea lamprey to human (Vagena et al., 2008; Glenn et al., 2010).

Historically, the *NAT* genes of animals have been studied by pharmacologists and toxicologists in laboratory models. There is a wealth of literature describing the enzymatic properties of NATs in the chicken, rabbit, mouse, rat and hamster. The presence of genetic polymorphisms affecting the function of NATs in rodents is also well-documented (Martell et al., 1991; Boukouvala et al., 2002; Walraven et al., 2006) and NAT-deficient mice (Cornish et al., 2003; Sugamori et al., 2003), as well as mice carrying human *NAT* transgenes (Leff et al., 1999; Cao et al., 2005; Sugamori et al., 2011) have been developed. The reader is referred to our previous reviews covering these aspects extensively (Boukouvala & Fakis, 2005; Vagena et al., 2008; Sim et al., 2008b).

Various inbred and *Nat*-congenic strains of rodents have been used in the past to study the carcinogenic effects of arylamines (Levy & Weber, 1992; Levy et al., 1994; Hein et al., 2008a; Jefferson et al., 2009). However, the now available transgenic mouse strains have not yet been subjected to long-term toxicological studies employing a range of carcinogenic or therapeutic compounds relevant to NATs. Many of the transgenic models have also been used to investigate the embryonic expression of murine NAT (Loehle et al., 2006), with emphasis on its postulated involvement in the folate cycle and related developmental defects (Wakefield et al., 2007a, b, 2010; Erickson et al., 2008; Cao et al., 2010; Erickson, 2010). The evidence for an *in vivo* role in the folate homeostasis is accumulating. Results are also accumulating suggesting gender-specific effects in mice with *NAT* gene deletions and transgenes (Wakefield et al., 2008a; Sugamori et al., 2011).

Of considerable interest is the study of NATs in primates. A polymorphic variant ($Val^{231}Ile$) of the NAT2-homolog in the Rhesus macaque (*Macaca mulatta*), a primate species used in medical research, has been identified (Fakis et al., 2007). The polymorphism affects substrate selectivity of the enzyme, increasing activity toward typical NAT1 (e.g. *p*-aminobenzoic acid, 5-aminosalicylate) vs. NAT2 (e.g. procainamide, sulphamethazine) substrates. It is likely that polymorphic Ile^{231} affects a serine loop previously reported to determine substrate selectivity of the human NAT2 isoenzyme (Goodfellow et al., 2000). We are currently investigating this hypothesis in the Rhesus and human. Database searches have identified *NAT* homologs in the sequenced genomes of several primate species (Fig. 4) and enzymatic investigations currently underway will shed light on functional differences and similarities.

V. *NAT* Gene Expression and Regulation

A characteristic feature of vertebrate *NAT* genes is that they consist of uninterrupted (intronless) ORFs adjacent to their 3′-untranslated regions (UTRs). Typically, the 5′-UTR of these *NAT* genes is split into one or more short upstream non-coding exons (NCEs), separated from each other and from the coding exon by relatively long introns. This conserved organization of genes for NAT is evident in rodent (Fakis et al., 2000; Abu-Zeid et al., 1991), monkey (Fakis et al., 2007) and human (Boukouvala & Sim, 2005), and is directly linked to transcriptional regulation. To date, *NAT* genes with more than one coding exons have been described only in lower chordates and eukaryotic microorganisms (protists, fungi) (Glenn et al., 2010).

In rodents and humans, transcription is initiated from promoter elements adjacent to one or more NCEs (Boukouvala et al., 2003; Barker et al., 2006; Husain et al., 2007a,b). In human *NAT1*, there are at least eight NCEs and alternative splicing of the introns gives rise to more than one

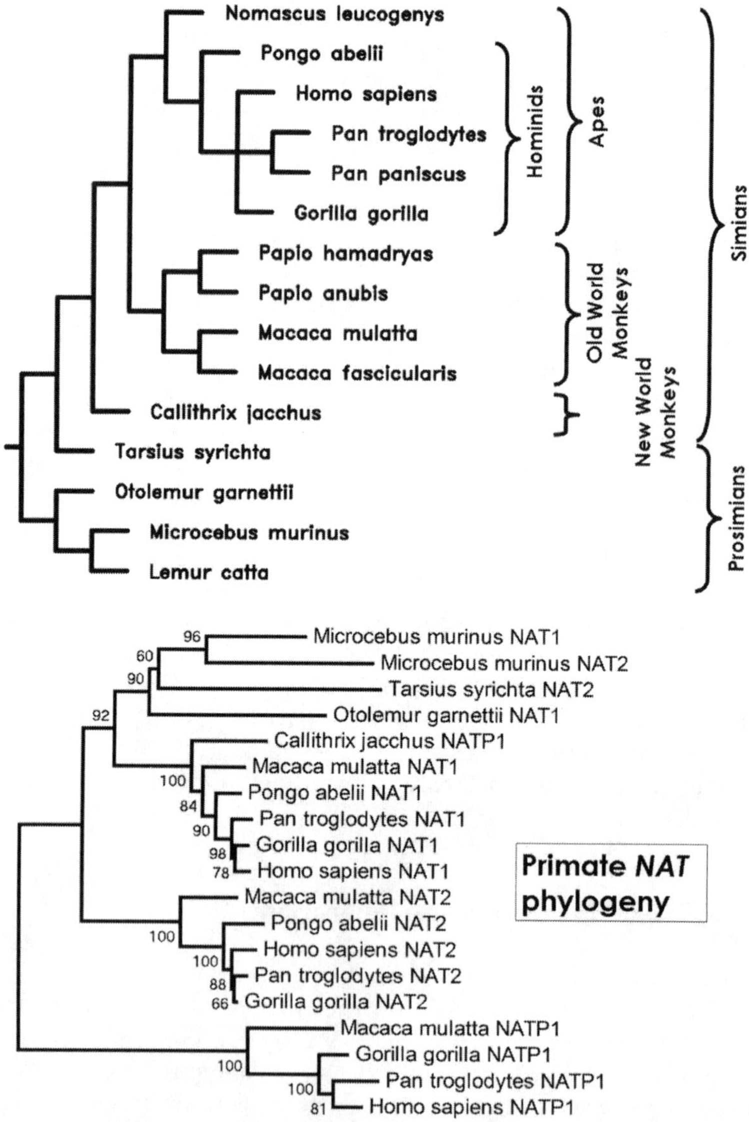

FIGURE 4 **NAT homologs in primates.** The top panel shows the consensus taxonomy of primate species whose genomes have been sequenced. The common taxonomy tree was generated using NCBI's Taxonomy Browser (http://www.ncbi.nlm.nih.gov/Taxonomy/CommonTree/wwwcmt.cgi) and the tree illustration was prepared with Phylip-3.69. The bottom panel shows the phylogeny of *NAT*-homologous sequences in a subset of primate species. Phylogenetic analysis was conducted with MEGA4 using default parameters.

transcript varying at the 5′-UTRs but identical in the coding region (Husain et al., 2004; Boukouvala & Sim, 2005; Butcher et al., 2005). It was been demonstrated recently that transcripts initiated from NCE4 (exons 4, 8 and ORF) are formed at higher levels and generate larger amounts of NAT1 protein, compared with transcripts initiated from NCE1 (exons 1, 2, 3, 8 and ORF). The investigators suggested potential mechanisms for differential regulation of the two transcripts, such as polymerase pausing, microRNA binding and the presence of sequence elements (upstream ORFs and stem-loop structures) delaying expression of the minor *NAT1* transcript. Their speculations were supported by comparative *in silico* inspection of the two 5′-UTR sequences (Millner et al., 2011).

Consistently, the major promoter of human *NAT1* has been mapped approximately 12 kb upstream of the coding region, near NCE4 (Husain et al., 2007a). This promoter consists of an Sp1 box and drives expression of *NAT1* in all tissues. It is conserved in the mouse *Nat2* gene, which is orthologous to human *NAT1* (Boukouvala et al., 2003). A second (minor) promoter is located about 51.5 kb upstream of the coding region (adjacent to NCE1) and drives tissue-specific transcription of human *NAT1* (Barker et al., 2006). Its upregulation has been demonstrated in cancer cell lines derived from estrogen receptor positive breast tumors (Wakefield et al., 2008b). Other regulatory motifs have been predicted for human *NAT1* (reviewed by Sim et al., 2008b), the best validated of which is a heat-shock element for heat-shock factor 1 that modulates prostate-specific induction of *NAT1* expression in response to androgens (Butcher et al., 2007; Butcher & Minchin, 2010).

Elements downstream of *NAT1* ORF may also play a role in control of expression of the gene, as suggested by initial studies assessing the effect of polymorphisms at positions +1088 (rs15561) and +1095 (rs15561) found in the *NAT1*3*, *NAT1*10* and *NAT1*11* alleles (Wang et al., 2011; Zhu et al., 2011). Although the results are as yet inconclusive, the approaches undertaken in these studies may prove useful in elucidating the effects – if any – of 3′-UTR SNPs on human *NAT1* control of expression.

Human *NAT1* has been implicated in various cancers and its involvement is likely to be via deregulation of expression, rather than genetic polymorphism as in the case of *NAT2* (reviewed by Sim et al., 2008b). A series of studies, reported in the Oncomine database, have demonstrated overexpression of human *NAT1* in estrogen/progesterone receptor positive breast tumors, and excessive upregulation of the minor promoter has been reported in the estrogen receptor positive cell line ZR-75-1 (Wakefield et al., 2008b). A recent study (Tiang et al., 2011), undertaking comprehensive phenotypic characterization of *NAT1*-silenced (by shRNA) colon adenocarcinoma cells, observed accelerated cell–cell contact inhibition and decreased cell viability at confluence. On soft agar, the NAT1 knock-downs generated fewer colonies of smaller size, compared with wild type cells. E-cadherin mRNA and protein levels were significantly increased and this outcome was specific to the shRNA-mediated silencing of *NAT1*. Similar observations were made with breast adenocarcinoma cells subjected to chemical inhibition of human NAT1 (Tiang et al., 2010). These studies suggest that suppression of human NAT1 decreases oncogenicity of cancer cell lines, a finding consistent with the results of Oncomine microarray (reviewed in Sim et al., 2008b) and proteomic (Adam et al., 2003) studies, demonstrating *NAT1* overexpression in tumors. Selective small-molecule inhibitors of human NAT1 have been generated by high-throughput compound screening and the application of combinatorial chemistry (Russell et al., 2009; Laurieri et al., 2010). In the future, these compounds may be optimized as putative anti-cancer drugs or developed as potential diagnostic tests to monitor NAT1 biomarker levels in tumors (Laurieri et al., 2010).

Apart from its suspected implication in carcinogenesis, human *NAT1* (and its murine ortholog *Nat2*) have been postulated to act as putative modulators of folate catabolism (reviewed by Boukouvala & Fakis, 2005). Recent studies with knock-out and transgenic mouse models have investigated this hypothesis, particularly in relation with developmental defects potentially attributed to deregulation of the folate cycle. Previous studies have detected the *N*-acetylated derivative of *p*-aminobenzoylglutamate (a folate catabolite) in the urine of *Nat2* wild type mice given folate supplement, but not in the urine of *Nat2* null mice (Wakefield et al., 2007a). In transgenic mice expressing human *NAT1*, higher NAT activities were associated with lower folate levels (Cao et al., 2010). Murine NAT2 expression has been demonstrated in the neural tube, around the period of neural tube closure (Stanley et al., 1998; Wakefield et al., 2008a), and higher incidence of neural tube defects has been reported in heterozygous *Nat2* null offspring of C57Bl/6J background (Wakefield et al., 2007a). Sporadic ocular defects in knock-out offspring have been observed too (Wakefield et al., 2007b), and the murine *Nat2* locus has been confirmed to influence teratogen-induced orofacial clefting in the slow acetylator A/J mouse strain (Erickson et al., 2008).

Folate is essential for the synthesis of S-adenosylmethionine, the methyl donor for CpG methylation of cellular DNA. Abnormal expression of *Nat2* in transgenic mice might potentially affect the availability of folate, consequently modifying the epigenetic regulation of specific loci. We have shown variable, but moderate (<20%), methylation levels at the *Nat2* promoter (Sp1 box) in different mouse tissues. These increased upon dietary supplementation with folate (Wakefield et al., 2010). Other investigators have assessed CpG methylation in the region immediately upstream of the human *NAT1* gene, which is unlikely to harbor basal promoter elements but contains other regulatory sites. Decreased methylation of this genomic region was observed in malignant vs. non-malignant mammary tissue (Kim et al., 2008), while tamoxifen resistance was linked to hypermethylation (Kim et al., 2010). The role of histone deacetylation in controlling human NAT1 expression has also been investigated (Paterson et al., 2011).

In our recent study (Wakefield et al., 2010), the mouse *Nat2* promoter demonstrated highest methylation levels in the heart. This is consistent with our earlier observation that the cardiac activity of the mouse *Nat2* basal (Sp1) promoter appears to be relatively low (Boukouvala et al., 2002). Cardiac NAT2 expression has been demonstrated at various stages of development and is particularly evident in clusters of cells within the atria and pulmonary artery (Wakefield et al., 2005, 2008a). The ontogenic origin of these *Nat2*-expressing foci is currently unknown and it should be interesting to investigate whether these might coincide with the embryonic stem (ES) cell derived multipotent *Isl1*$^{+}$ cardiovascular progenitors responsible for the generation of the different cardiovascular cell types *in vivo* (Moretti et al., 2006). Expression of the mouse *Nat2* gene, as well as of its human ortholog *NAT1*, has been demonstrated in ES cells (Payton et al., 1999b; Smelt et al., 2000), thus, investigation of the transcriptional signature of the cardiac cells expressing murine *Nat2* might prove useful.

VI. Development of NAT Inhibitors

Inhibitors of the NAT enzymes were important in establishing the existence of an active site substrate and were also important in determining the structure of the first NAT enzyme (Sinclair et al., 2000) and also of the first eukaryotic NAT (Wu et al., 2007). In each case, a bromacetanilide inhibitor was used to alkylate the active site cysteine. Other studies have demonstrated that tamoxifen is also an inhibitor of human NAT1. This appears particularly important in view of the observation that human NAT1 is overexpressed in estrogen receptor positive breast cancer (Adam et al., 2003) and also in estrogen receptor positive breast cancer cell lines (Wakefield et al., 2008b), as described above. These studies have been followed up further with the observation that bisphenol A which is an estrogen-like molecule has also been demonstrated to bind to the mouse equivalent of human NAT1 – the mouse NAT2 protein (Kawamura et al., 2008). These particular studies used ^{15}N NMR to establish the amino acid residues which appeared to be involved in the interaction with bisphenol A.

A more extensive series of studies was carried out, designed to look specifically for small-molecule inhibitors of NAT enzymes. These studies were possible as a result of the availability of pure recombinant NAT proteins. The enzymes which were used in the high-throughput screen were from a range of sources and the screening was carried out for several reasons:

1. To establish small-molecule inhibitors of the NAT enzymes from mycobacteria, since it had been demonstrated that gene deletion resulted in the loss of the ability of *M. bovis* BCG (a model for *M. tuberculosis*) to survive inside macrophage (Bhakta et al., 2004).

2. To ensure that any compounds identified as inhibiting mycobacterial NATs, and which might subsequently be developed as anti-tubercular agents, would not inhibit human NATs.
3. To establish a panel of ligands for human NATs, in relation to observations that expression of human NAT1 appeared to control proliferation of cells (Adam et al., 2003; Tiang et al., 2011).
4. To develop potential diagnostic probes for identification of human NAT1 in breast cancer cells.

High-throughput screening using a customized chemical library was carried out (Russell et al., 2009; Westwood et al., 2011), against a range of recombinant NAT enzymes which were relatively easy to produce in sufficient quantities for such a screen which requires approximately 100 mg of each enzyme. Therefore, enzymes were chosen which were appropriate for the end purpose and also which were stable, easy to produce and store. The initial screening was carried out with NATs from *S. typhimurium*, *M. smegmatis*, *P. aeruginosa* and also with mouse NAT2 and hamster NAT2. Subsequent screening of hits was carried out using human NAT1, human NAT2, mouse NAT1 and also NAT from *M. marinum*. The enzyme from *M. marinum* is readily generated as a recombinant enzyme, whereas the enzyme for which it is a close model, i.e. *M. tuberculosis* NAT, is much more difficult to generate as a recombinant protein. Interestingly, the enzyme from *M. tuberculosis* has a much higher melting temperature and this property appears to reside in the two C-terminal domains of the *M. tuberculosis* enzyme (Lack et al., 2009). More recent attempts have greatly improved the yield of NAT from *M. tuberculosis* as a recombinant protein (Abuhammad et al., 2011).

From the above screens, small molecules were identified which bound specifically to prokaryotic NAT enzymes (Westwood et al., 2011; Fullam et al., 2011) or to eukaryotic NAT enzymes (Laurieri et al., 2010; Russell et al., 2009) (Figs. 5–7).

Of the classes of compounds identified as inhibitors of prokaryotic NAT enzymes in the screen two have so far been analyzed in detail (Fig. 5A and D) and have been reported on Fullam et al. (2011) and Westwood et al. (2010). Compound A is a beta-amino alcohol. The hit compound did not have strong anti-tubercular activity, although analysis of a series of analogs has allowed identification of the interaction with the prokaryotic NAT enzymes (Fullam et al., 2011).

In the case of the compounds of the 1,2,4-triazole class, analysis of the effects on inhibition of growth of mycobacteria and the effects on cell wall lipids demonstrated very similar results to the effects of deleting the *nat* gene from *M. bovis* BCG (Westwood et al., 2010; Bhakta et al., 2004). Structure–activity relationships following synthesis of a panel of analogs of the triazoles, coupled with enzymological analysis and modeling of protein–ligand interaction, demonstrated the fit of the inhibitor into the active site of the

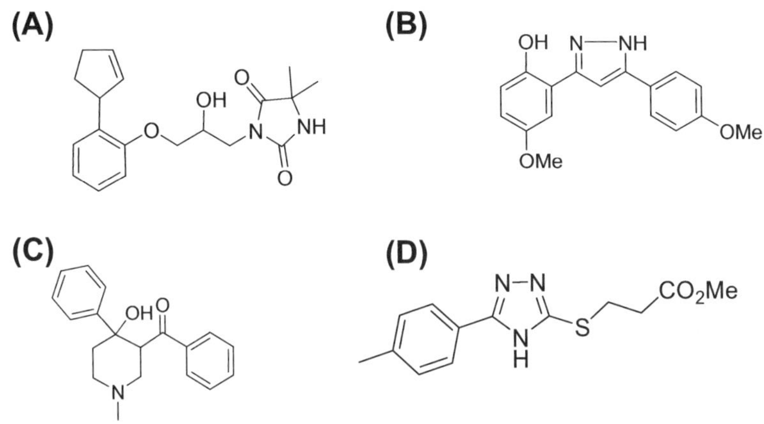

FIGURE 5 Compounds identified as inhibitors of prokaryotic NATs following high-throughput screening. NAT inhibitors were identified through a high-throughput screen of a 5000-strong small-molecule library of drug-like molecules (Russell et al., 2009; Westwood et al., 2010, 2011) using a panel of recombinant NAT enzymes from prokaryotes and eukaryotes. The prokaryote-specific compounds do not inhibit the eukaryotic enzymes at 100 μM, but showed 50% inhibition of bacterial NATs at less than 20 μM apart from A which was less potent. The classes of compounds identified as NAT inhibitors belong to distinct chemical classes and were subsequently tested for anti-tubercular activity. "A" was the weakest inhibitor with "B" and "D" showing most promise.

NAT enzyme from *M. tuberculosis* (Westwood et al., 2010). These studies have formed the basis for subsequent commercial screening for anti-tuberculars with NAT from *M. marinum* as a target.

In the initial high-throughput screen of over 5000 compounds two mammalian NATs were included which were the most stable as recombinant proteins – mouse NAT2 and hamster NAT2 – both of which resemble human NAT1 in terms of specificity and functional activity (Kawamura et al., 2005, 2008). Of the 50 compounds which were identified as specific inhibitors of these eukaryotic NAT proteins, a secondary screen was carried out to establish isoenzyme specificity by using a panel of mammalian isoenzymes which included human NAT1, human NAT2, mouse NAT2, and mouse NAT1 as well as two prokaryotic NATs for comparison: *P. aeruginosa* NAT and *M. marinum* NAT (Russell et al., 2009). Of the 50 compounds tested, six compounds showed selectivity for human NAT1 and mouse NAT2 over the other isoenzymes, and were further investigated for their effects on the inhibition of human NAT1 activity in a breast cancer cell (ZR-75-1) lysate overexpressing the protein (Wakefield et al., 2008b): only two compounds, namely a rhodanine and a naphthoquinone (Fig. 6) inhibited human NAT1 activity in ZR-75-1 cell lysate. The reduced activity of the remaining four compounds was considered to be a consequence of increased binding of these species to other proteins within the lysate (Russell et al., 2009). These two compound classes of specific human NAT1

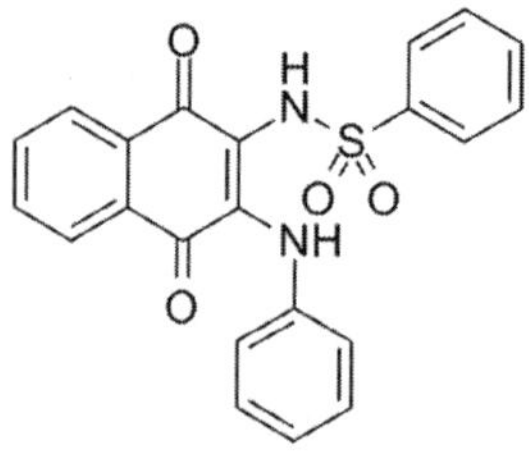

Compound 1
(a naphthoquinone)

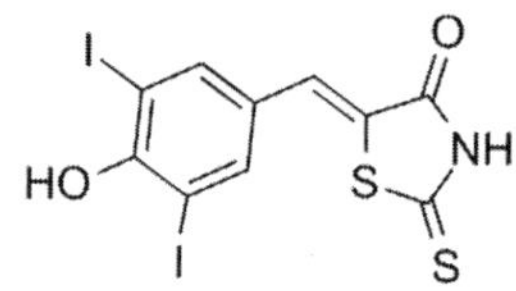

Compound 5
(a rhodanine)

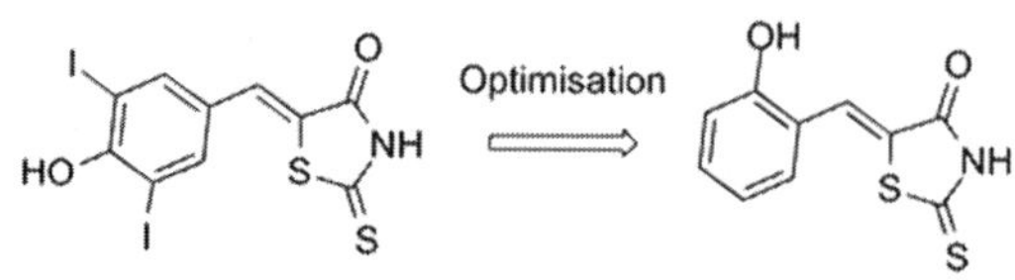

Rhodanine 5 **Rhod-o-hp**

FIGURE 6 Compounds identified as inhibitors of pure human NAT1 and its murine equivalent mouse NAT2 following high-throughput screening. Naphthoquinone (designated compound 1) and rhodanine (designated compound 5) were identified following high-throughput screening of a 5000 drug-like molecule library (Russell et al., 2009; Westwood et al., 2010, 2011) and testing as human NAT1 inhibitors in lysates of ZR-75-1 cells (Russell et al., 2009; Kawamura et al., 2008). The cytotoxic rhodanine has been modified to minimize cytotoxic effects and the analog Rhod-o-hp has been demonstrated to inhibit tumorigenic properties of MDA-MB-231 breast cancer cells (after Tiang et al., 2010), such as concentration-dependent reduction of colony formation on soft agar and concentration-dependent reduction in cell invasiveness. It also demonstrated an inverse correlation between human NAT1 inhibition and cell number.

inhibitors (Fig. 6) have been the subject of further studies (Russell et al., 2009; Tiang et al., 2010).

Rhodanine (designated compound 5) was illustrated to be a competitive inhibitor of mouse NAT2, a good analog of the less stable human NAT1. The compound class is well known as showing cytotoxicity and non-specific cytotoxicity with one series of analogs has proved a problem, although optimization studies appear to have generated a rhodanine derivative which inhibits the tumorigenic properties of a breast cancer cell line showing similar concentration dependence in a similar manner to inhibition of human NAT1. These studies together with evidence for human NAT1 having a role in growth make a good spring-board for further research in this area.

The naphthoquinone designated as compound 1 (Fig. 6) is a selective competitive inhibitor of human NAT1 and mouse NAT2 (Laurieri et al., 2010) showing a single binding site following Scatchard analysis with mouse

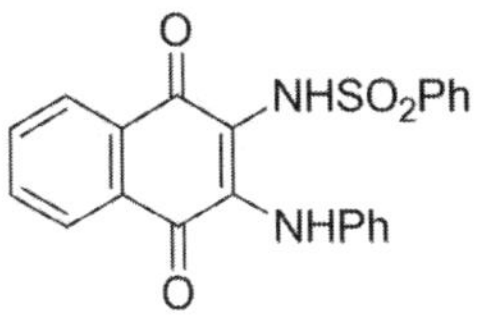
Naphthoquinone **1**

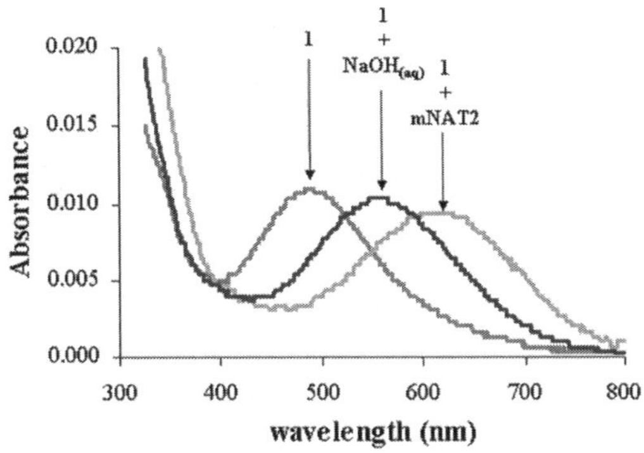

FIGURE 7 Colorimetric properties of naphthoquinone 1, specific human NAT1 inhibitor. (left) Chemical structure of naphthoquinone 1. (Right) Visible spectra of 1 (10 μM) in aq. Tris–HCl (pH 8.0, red line/dark gray λ_{max} = 489 nm), 1 in aq. NaOH solution (dark blue/black line, λ_{max} = 561 nm), and 1 with 2 eq. of mouse NAT2 in aq. Tris–HCl (pH 8.0, light blue/light gray line, λ_{max} = 610 nm); (after Laurieri et al., 2010). The conditions are noted above each spectrum.

NAT2. In addition, compound 1 shows the remarkable quality of changing color from red to blue on binding specifically to human NAT1 or mouse NAT2 (Fig. 7). It did not change color on binding to other isoenzymes – in particular human NAT2. These studies are consistent with the different substrate specificity patterns which have been observed for these isoenzymes (e.g. Kawamura et al., 2008). The color change is likely to be associated with a protonation step as pH also induces a red-blue color change but the wavelength shift is less marked than occurs on binding of the naphthoquinone to human NAT1 or mouse NAT2 (Fig. 7).

As well as high-throughput screening with NAT proteins as targets, *in silico* methods have also been exploited to open up possibilities for identifying novel chemical entities as NAT inhibitors. Results with virtual screening have in general been mixed (Sneider, 2010). Nevertheless, Ultrafast Shape Recognition (USR) (Ballester et al., 2010), a method which allows small molecules to be compared in three-dimensional space with a panel of almost 700 million molecular conformers, has been used to interrogate all purchasable chemical space with the human NAT1 specific inhibitor naphthoquinone (compound 1) (Fig. 6) for "shapemers". Of the 23 compounds randomly selected amongst the eligible molecules with the best USR score, more than 10 were found to be inhibitors with an IC50 of between 1 and 10μM and each of the molecules had a distinct chemical scaffold from the query molecule (Fig. 8). Although none of the these new bioactive mouse NAT2 inhibitors were more potent than naphthoquinone 1, they are likely to be useful as alternative starting points for a lead optimization process (Ballester et al., 2010).

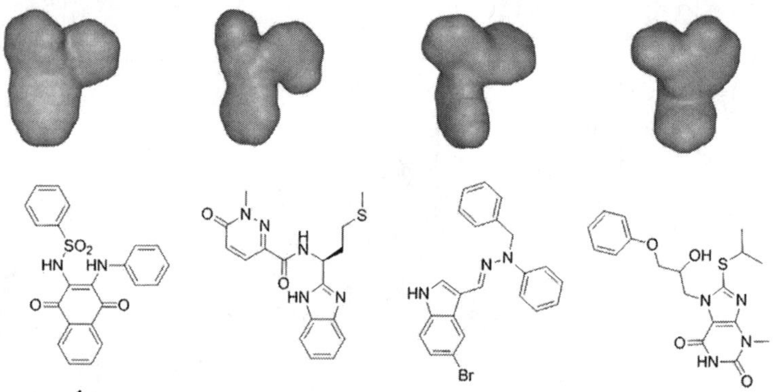

1

IC_{50} (μM)	1.10	1.17	2.05	2.33

FIGURE 8 Comparison of Ultrafast Shape Recognition (USR) query molecule naphthoquinone 1 and three molecules which were identified as having the closest shape. Shapes, chemical structure and IC_{50} values against pure recombinant mouse NAT2 for the query molecule and the three most potent active molecules found by USR are shown (from left to right: $S_0^{USR} = 1.000$, $S_1^{USR} = 0.969$, $S_3^{USR} = 0.966$ and $S_{17}^{USR} = 0.950$) (after Ballester et al., 2010).

VII. Conclusion

Starting from understanding of drug metabolism, insight into the biology of the NAT enzymes has developed hand in hand with an increase in understanding of fundamental cell functions. This trend is continuing apace with comparative genomics, now involving thousands of genomes, putting together the pieces of NAT evolution. Investigation of NAT homologs from representatives of divergent domains of life (especially prokaryotic and eukaryotic microbes) is revealing new diverse roles for these enzymes, with relevance beyond drug metabolism, for biotechnology, agriculture, environmental sciences as well as pharmacology, pharmacogenetics and understanding disease susceptibility. Large-scale molecular anthropological studies, employing high-throughput genotyping technologies and advanced bioinformatics, are writing a parallel story about the evolution of *NAT* allelic distribution in human populations worldwide. These investigations are broadening our understanding of adaptation to the ever-changing chemical environment of everyday life throughout the history of mankind, revealing a new dimension of xenogenomics in addition to the well-established pharmacogenomics and cancer toxicogenomics.

Earlier and current efforts to understand the molecular structure and function of the NAT enzymes in a range of organisms has opened the way toward intervention with new compounds as potential diagnostics and therapeutics. Investigation of the expression and regulation of genes for NAT in humans and animal models is allowing insights into the role of the enzymes in embryonic development and carcinogenesis. As the field integrates new tools for research – ranging from genomics to high-speed chemistry and *in silico* methods – more fundamental questions will be answered with regard to the role of NATs in pharmacology and more widely in cell biology.

Acknowledgments

We wish to thank our many colleagues, both local and international, who have contributed to the development of ideas, including James Sandy and Isaac Westwood, Akane Kawamura, Angela Russell and all our colleagues in the NAT community. We also thank Dr. Anthony Glenn (Toxicology and Mycotoxin Research Unit, Agricultural Research Service, US Department of Agriculture, Athens, GA, USA) for his comments on the manuscript.

Conflict of Interest: The authors have no conflicts of interest to declare.

Abbreviations

2-AP	2-aminophenol
BOA	2-benzoxazolinone
3,4-DCA	3,4-dichloroaniline
NAT	arylamine *N*-acetyltransferase
CoA	coenzyme A
ES cells	embryonic stem cells
HPAA	*N*-(2-hydroxyphenyl) acetamide
HPMA	*N*-(2-hydroxyphenyl) malonamic acid
NCE	non-coding exon
ORF	open reading frame
pNPA	*p*-nitrophenyl acetate
SNP	single nucleotide polymorphism
USR	ultrafast shape recognition
UTR	untranslated region

References

Abuhammad, A., Lack, N., Schweichler, J., Staunton, D., Sim, R. B., & Sim, E. (2011). Improvement of the expression and purification of *Mycobacterium tuberculosis* arylamine *N*-acetyltransferase (TBNAT) a potential target for novel anti-tubercular agents. *Protein Expression and Purification*, *80*, 246–252.

Abu-Zeid, M., Nagata, K., Miyata, M., Ozawa, S., Fukuhara, M., Yamazoe, Y., et al. (1991). An arylamine acetyltransferase (AT-I) from Syrian golden hamster liver: cloning, complete nucleotide sequence, and expression in mammalian cells. *Molecular Carcinogenesis*, *4*, 81–88.

Adam, P. J., Berry, J., Loader, J. A., Tyson, K. L., Craggs, G., Smith, P. , et al. (2003). Arylamine *N*-acetyltransferase-1 is highly expressed in breast cancers and conveys enhanced growth and resistance to etoposide *in vitro*. *Molecular Cancer Research*, *1*, 826–835.

Anderton, M. C., Bhakta, S., Besra, G. S., Jeavons, P., Eltis, L. D., & Sim, E. (2006). Characterization of the putative operon containing arylamine *N*-acetyltransferase (NAT) in Mycobacterium bovis BCG. *Molecular Microbiology*, *59*, 181–192.

Andres, H. H., Klem, A. J., Schopfer, L. M., Harrison, J. K., & Weber, W. W. (1988). On the active site of liver acetyl-CoA. Arylamine *N*-acetyltransferase from rapid acetylator rabbits (iii/j). *Journal of Biological Chemistry*, *263*, 7521–7527.

Andres, H. H., Kolb, H. J., Schreiber, R. J., & Weiss, L. (1983). Characterization of the active site, substrate specificity and kinetic properties of acetyl-CoA:arylamine *N*-acetyltransferase from pigeon liver. *Biochimica et Biophysica Acta*, *746*, 193–201.

Andres, H. H., Vogel, R. S., Tarr, G. E., Johnson, L., & Weber, W. W. (1987). Purification, physicochemical, and kinetic properties of liver acetyl-CoA:arylamine *N*-acetyltransferase from rapid acetylator rabbits. *Molecular Pharmacology*, *31*, 446–456.

Ballester, P. J., Westwood, I., Laurieri, N., Sim, E., & Richards, W. G. (2010). Prospective virtual screening with Ultrafast Shape Recognition: the identification of novel inhibitors of arylamine *N*-acetyltransferases. *Journal of the Royal Society Interface*, *7*, 335–342.

Barker, D. F., Husain, A., Neale, J. R., Martini, B. D., Zhang, X., Doll, M. A., et al. (2006). Functional properties of an alternative, tissue-specific promoter for human arylamine *N*-acetyltransferase 1. *Pharmacogenetics and Genomics*, *16*, 515–525.

Bhakta, S., Besra, G. S., Upton, A. M., Parish, T., Sholto-Douglas-Vernon, C., Gibson, K. J., et al. (2004). Arylamine *N*-acetyltransferase is required for synthesis of mycolic acids and complex lipids in Mycobacterium bovis BCG and represents a novel drug target. *Journal of Experimental Medicine*, *199*, 1191.

Blum, M., Demierre, A., Grant, D. M., Heim, M., & Meyer, U. A. (1991). Molecular mechanism of slow acetylation of drugs and carcinogens in humans. *Proceedings of the National Academy of Sciences of the USA*, *88*, 5237–5241.

Blum, M., Grant, D. M., McBride, W., Heim, M., & Meyer, U. A. (1990). Human arylamine *N*-acetyltransferase genes: Isolation, chromosomal localization, and functional expression. *DNA and Cell Biology*, *9*, 193–203.

Boukouvala, S., & Fakis, G. (2005). Arylamine *N*-acetyltransferases: what we learn from genes and genomes. *Drug Metabolism Reviews*, *37*, 511–564.

Boukouvala, S., & Sim, E. (2005). Structural analysis of the genes for human arylamine *N*-acetyltransferases and characterization of alternative transcripts. *Basic and Clinical Pharmacology and Toxicology*, *96*, 343–351.

Boukouvala, S., Price, N., Plant, K. E., & Sim, E. (2003). Structure and transcriptional regulation of the Nat2 gene encoding for the drug-metabolising enzyme arylamine *N*-acetyltransferase type 2 in mice. *Biochemical Journal*, *375*, 593–602.

Boukouvala, S., Price, N., & Sim, E. (2002). Identification and functional characterization of novel polymorphisms associated with the genes for arylamine *N*-acetyltransferases in mice. *Pharmacogenetics*, *12*, 385–394.

Boukouvala, S., Westwood, I. M., Butcher, N. J., & Fakis, G. (2008). Current trends in *N*-acetyltransferase research arising from the 2007 International NAT workshop. *Pharmacogenomics*, *9*, 765–771.

Brans, R., Laizane, D., Khan, A., & Blömeke, B. (2004). *N*-acetyltransferase 2 genotyping: an accurate and feasible approach for simultaneous detection of the most common NAT2 alleles. *Clinical Chemistry*, *50*, 1264–1266.

Brooke, E. W., Davies, S. G., Mulvaney, A. W., Pompeo, F., Sim, E., & Vickers, R. J. (2003). An approach to identifying novel substrates of bacterial arylamine *N*-acetyltransferases. *Bioorganic and Medicinal Chemistry*, *11*, 1227–1234.

Butcher, N. J., & Minchin, R. F. (2010). Arylamine *N*-acetyltransferase 1 gene regulation by androgens requires a conserved heat shock element for heat shock factor-1. *Carcinogenesis*, *31*, 820–826.

Butcher, N. J., Arulpragasam, A., Goh, H. L., Davey, T., & Minchin, R. F. (2005). Genomic organization of human arylamine *N*-acetyltransferase type I reveals alternative promoters that generate different 5'-UTR splice variants with altered translational activities. *Biochemical Journal*, *387*, 119–127.

Butcher, N. J., Tetlow, N. L., Cheung, C., Broadhurst, G. M., & Minchin, R. F. (2007). Induction of human arylamine *N*-acetyltransferase type I by androgens in human prostate cancer cells. *Cancer Research*, *67*, 85–92.

Butcher, N. J., Tiang, J., & Minchin, R. F. (2008). Regulation of arylamine *N*-acetyltransferases. *Current Drug Metabolism*, *9*, 498–504.

Cao, W., Chau, B., Hunter, R., Strnatka, D., McQueenm, C. A., & Erickson, R. P. (2005). Only low levels of exogenous *N*-acetyltransferase can be achieved in transgenic mice. *Pharmacogenomics Journal*, *5*, 255–261.

Cao, W., Strnatka, D., McQueen, C. A., Hunter, R. J., & Erickson, R. P. (2010). *N*-acetyltransferase 2 activity and folate levels. *Life Sciences*, *86*, 103–106.

Cartwright, R. A., Glasham, R. W., Rogers, H. J., Ahmad, R. A., Barham-Hall, D., Higgins, E., et al. (1982). Role of *N*-acetyltransferase phenotypes in bladder carcinogenesis:a pharmacogenetic epidemiological approach to bladder cancer. *Lancet*, *2*, 842–845.

Coelho, M. B., Costa, E. R., Vasconcellos, S. E., Linck, N., Ramos, R. M., Amorim, H. L., et al. (2011). Sequence and structural characterization of tbNAT gene in isoniazid-resistant *Mycobacterium tuberculosis*: identification of new mutations. *Mutation Research*, *712*, 33–39.

Cornish, V. A., Pinter, K., Boukouvala, S., Johnson, N., Labrousse, C., Payton, M., et al. (2003). Generation and analysis of mice with a targeted disruption of the arylamine *N*-acetyltransferase type 2 gene. *Pharmacogenomics Journal*, *3*, 169–177.

Dairou, J., Laurieri, N., Sim, E., & Rodriges-Lima, F. (2010). *Uncoupled reaction of N-acetylation and AcCoA hydrolysis*. Paris, France: International NAT Workshop.

Dairou, J., Malecaze, F., Dupret, J. M., & Rodrigues-Lima, F. (2005). The xenobiotic-metabolizing enzymes arylamine *N*-acetyltransferases in human lens epithelial cells: inactivation by cellular oxidants and UVB-induced oxidative stress. *Molecular Pharmacology*, *67*, 1299–1306.

Dairou, J., Petit, E., Ragunathan, N., Baeza-Squiban, A., Marana, F., Dupret, J. -M., et al. (2009). Arylamine *N*-acetyltransferase activity in bronchial epithelial cells and its inhibition by cellular oxidants. *Toxicology and Applied Pharmacology*, *236*, 366–371.

Deguchi, T. (1992). Sequences and expression of alleles of polymorphic arylamine *N*-acetyltransferase of human liver. *Journal of Biological Chemistry*, *267*, 18,140–18,147.

Deguchi, T., Mashimo, M., & Suzuki, T. (1990). Correlation between acetylator phenotypes and genotypes of polymorphic arylamine *N*-acetyltransferase in human liver. *Journal of Biological Chemistry*, *265*, 12,757–12,760.

Delgoda, R., Lian, L. Y., Sandy, J., & Sim, E. (2003). NMR investigation of the catalytic mechanism of arylamine *N*-acetyltransferase from *Salmonella typhimurium*. *Biochimicaet Biophysica Acta*, *1620*, 8–14.

Delomenie, C., Fouix, S., Longuemaux, S., Brahimi, N., Bizet, C., Picard, B., et al. (2001). Identification and functional characterization of arylamine *N*-acetyltransferases in eubacteria: evidence for highly selective acetylation of 5-aminosalicylic acid. *Journal of Bacteriology*, *183*, 3417–3427.

Doll, M. A., & Hein, D. W.. (2001). Comprehensive human NAT2 genotype method using single nucleotide polymorphism-specific polymerase chain reaction primers and fluorogenic probes. *Analytical Biochemistry*, *288*, 106–108.

Doll, M. A., & Hein, D. W. (2002). Rapid genotype method to distinguish frequent and/or functional polymorphisms in human *N*-acetyltransferase-1. *Analytical Biochemicstry*, *301*, 328–332.

Dupret, J. M., & Grant, D. M. (1992). Site-directed mutagenesis of recombinant human arylamine *N*-acetyltransferase expressed in *Escherichia coli*. Evidence for direct involvement of Cys68 in the catalytic mechanism of polymorphic human NAT2. *Journal of Biological Chemistry*, *267*, 7381–7385.

Erickson, R. P. (2010). Genes, environment, and orofacial clefting: *N*-acetyltransferase and folic acid. *Journal of Craniofacial Surgery*, *21*, 1384–1387.

Erickson, R. P., Cao, W., Acuña, D. K., Strnatka, D. W., Hunter, R. J., Chau, B. T., et al. (2008). Confirmation of the role of *N*-acetyltransferase 2 in teratogen-induced cleft palate using transgenics and knockouts. *Molecular Reproduction and Development*, *75*, 1071–1076.

Evans, D. A., Manley, K. A., & McKuisick, V. A. (1960). Genetic control of isoniazid acetylation in man. *British Medical Journal*, *2*, 485–491.

Fakis, G., Boukouvala, S., Buckle, V., Payton, M., Denning, C., & Sim, E. (2000). Chromosomal localisation and mapping of the genes for murine arylamine *N*-acetyltransferases (NATs), enzymes involved in the metabolism of carcinogens: Identification of a novel upstream non-coding exon for murine Nat2. *Cytogenetics and Cell Genetics*, *90*, 134–138.

Fakis, G., Boukouvala, S., Kawamura, A., & Kennedy, S. (2007). Description of a novel polymorphic gene encoding for arylamine *N*-acetyltransferase in the rhesus macaque (Macaca mulatta), a model animal for endometriosis. *Pharmacogenetics and Genomics*, *17*, 181–188.

Franke, S., Klowitz, I., Schnakenberg, E., Rommel, B., van den Ven, W., Bullerdiek, J. et al. (1994). Isolation and mapping of a cosmid clone containing the human NAT2 gene. *Biochemical and Biophysical Research Communications*, *199*, 1672–1675.

Fullam, E., Abuhammad, A., Wilson, D. L., Anderton, M. C., Davies, S. G., Russell, A. J., et al. (2011). Analysis of β-amino alcohols as inhibitors of the potential anti-tubercular target *N*-acetyltransferase. *Bioorganic and Medicinal Chemistry Letters*, *21*, 1185–1190.

Fullam, E., Kawamura, A., Wilkinson, H., Abuhammad, A., Westwood, I., & Sim, E. (2009). Comparison of the arylamine *N*-acetyltransferase from *Mycobacterium marinum* and *Mycobacterium tuberculosis*. *Protein Journal*, *28*, 281–293.

Fullam, E., Westwood, I. M., Anderton, M. C., Lowe, E. D., Sim, E., & Noble, M. E. (2008). Divergence of cofactor recognition across evolution: Coenzyme A binding in a prokaryotic arylamine *N*-acetyltransferase. *Journal of Molecular Biology*, *375*, 178–191.

García-Closas, M., Hein, D. W., Silverman, D., Malats, N., Yeager, M., Jacobs, K. et al. (2011). A single nucleotide polymorphism tags variation in the arylamine *N*-acetyltransferase 2 phenotype in populations of European background. *Pharmacogenetics and Genomics*, *21*, 231–236.

Glenn, A. E., & Bacon, C. W. (2009). FDB2 encodes a member of the arylamine *N*-acetyltransferase family and is necessary for biotransformation of benzoxazolinones by Fusarium verticillioides. *Journal of Applied Microbiology*, *107*, 657–671.

Glenn, A. E., Gold, S. E., & Bacon, C. W. (2002). Fdb1 and Fdb2, Fusarium verticillioides loci necessary for detoxification of preformed antimicrobials from corn. *Molecular Plant–Microbe Interactions*, *15*, 91–101.

Glenn, A. E., Hinton, D. M., Yates, I. E., & Bacon, C. W. (2001). Detoxification of corn antimicrobial compounds as the basis for isolating Fusarium verticillioides and some other Fusarium species from corn. *Applied and Environmental Microbiology*, *67*, 2973–2981.

Glenn, A. E., Karagianni, E. P., Ulndreaj, A., & Boukouvala, S. (2010). Comparative genomic and phylogenetic investigation of the xenobiotic metabolizing arylamine *N*-acetyltransferase enzyme family. *FEBS Letters*, *584*, 3158–3164.

Glenn, A. E., Meredith, F. I., Morrison, W. H., III, & Bacon, C. W. (2003). Identification of intermediate and branch metabolites resulting from biotransformation of 2-benzoxazolinone by Fusarium verticillioides. *Applied and Environmental Microbiology*, *69*, 3165–3169.

Goodfellow, G. H., Dupret, J. M., & Grant, D. M. (2000). Identification of amino acids imparting acceptor substrate selectivity to human arylamine acetyltransferases NAT1 and NAT2. *Biochemical Journal*, *348*, 159–166.

Hein, D. W., Bendaly, J., Neale, J. R., & Doll, M. A. (2008a). Systemic functional expression of *N*-acetyltransferase polymorphism in the F344 Nat2 congenic rat. *Drug Metabolism and Disposition*, *36*, 2452–2459.

Hein, D. W., Boukouvala, S., Grant, D. M., Minchin, R. F., & Sim, E. (2008b). Changes in consensus arylamine *N*-acetyltransferase gene nomenclature. *Pharmacogenetics and Genomics*, *18*, 367–368.

Hickman, D., Risch, A., Buckle, V., Spurr, N. K., Jeremiah, S. J., McCarthy, A., et al. (1994). Chromosomal localisation of human genes for arylamine *N*-acetyltransferase. *Biochemical Journal*, *297*, 441–445.

Holton, S. J., Dairou, J., Sandy, J., Rodrigues-Lima, F., Dupret, J. M., Noble, M. E., et al. (2005). Structure of Mesorhizobium loti arylamine *N*-acetyltransferase 1. *Acta Crystallographica Section F: Structural Biology and Crystallization Communincations*, *61*, 14–16.

Husain, A., Barker, D. F., States, J. C., Doll, M. A., & Hein, D. W.. (2004). Identification of the major promoter and non-coding exons of the human arylamine *N*-acetyltransferase 1 gene (NAT1). *Pharmacogenetics*, *14*, 397–406.

Husain, A., Zhang, X., Doll, M. A., States, J. C., Barker, D. F., & Hein, D. W. (2007a). Functional analysis of the human *N*-acetyltransferase 1 major promoter: quantitation of tissue expression and identification of critical sequence elements. *Drug Metabolism and Disposition*, *35*, 1649–1656.

Husain, A., Zhang, X., Doll, M. A., States, J. C., Barker, D. F., & Hein, D. W. (2007b). Identification of *N*-acetyltransferase 2 (NAT2) transcription start sites and quantitation of NAT2-specific mRNA in human tissues. *Drug Metabolism and Disposition*, *35*, 721–727.

Ilett, K. F., Kadlubar, F. F., & Minchin, R. F. (1999). 1998 International Meeting on the arylamine *N*-Acetyltransferases: synopsis of the workshop on nomenclature, biochemistry, molecular biology, interspecies comparisons, and role in human disease risk. *Drug Metabolism and Disposition*, *27*, 957–959.

Jefferson, F. A., Xiao, G. H., & Hein, D. W. (2009). 4-Aminobiphenyl downregulation of NAT2 acetylator genotype-dependent *N*- and O-acetylation of aromatic and heterocyclic amine carcinogens in primary mammary epithelial cell cultures from rapid and slow acetylator rats. *Toxicological Science*, *107*, 293–297.

Jencks, W. P., Gresser, M., Valenzuela, M. S., & Huneeus, F. C. (1972). Acetyl-Coenzyme A: Arylamine acetyltransferase measurement of the steady state concentration of the acetyl-enzyme intermediate. *Journal of Biological Chemistry*, *247*, 3756–3760.

Jenne, J. W. (1965). Partial purification and properties of the isoniazid transacetylase in human liver. Its relationship to the acetylation of *p*-aminosalicylic acid. *Journal of Clinical Investigation*, *44*, 1992–2002.

Kawamura, A. (2003). *Studies on Hamster Arylamine N-acetyltransferase*. D. Phil. thesis, UK: University of Oxford.

Kawamura, A., Graham, J., Mushtaq, A., Tsiftsoglou, S. A., Vath, G. M., Hanna, P. E., et al. (2005). Eukaryotic arylamine *N*-acetyltransferase. Investigation of substrate specificity by high-throughput screening. *Biochemical Pharmacology*, *69*, 347–359.

Kawamura, A., Westwood, I., Wakefield, L., Long, H., Zhang, N., Walters, K., et al. (2008). Mouse *N*-acetyltransferase type 2, the homologue of human *N*-acetyltransferase type 1. *Biochemical Pharmacology*, *LL75*, 1550–1560.

Kelly, S. L., & Sim, E. (1991). Expression of *N*-acetyltransferase in a human monocytic cell line, U937. *Human and Experimental Toxicology*, *10*, 33–38.

Kim, S. J., Kang, H. S., Chang, H. L., Jung, Y. C., Sim, H. B., Lee, K. S., et al. (2008). Promoter hypomethylation of the *N*-acetyltransferase 1 gene in breast cancer. *Oncology Reports*, *19*, 663–668.

Kim, S. J., Kang, H. S., Jung, S. Y., Min, S. Y., Lee, S., Kim, S. W., et al. (2010). Methylation patterns of genes coding for drug-metabolizing enzymes in tamoxifen-resistant breast cancer tissues. *Journal of Molecular Medicine (Berlin)*, *88*, 1123–1131.

King, N., Westbrook, M. J., Young, S. L., Kuo, A., Abedin, M., Chapman, J., et al. (2008). The genome of the choanoflagellate Monosiga brevicollis and the origin of metazoans. *Nature*, *451*, 783–788.

Kulik, T., Pszczółkowska, A., & Lojko, M. (2011). Multilocus phylogenetics show high intraspecific variability within *Fusarium avenaceum*. *International Journal of Molecular Science*, *12*, 5626–5640.

Lack, N., Kawamura, A., Fullam, E., Laurieri, N., Beard, S., Russell, A. J., et al. (2009). Temperature stability of proteins essential for the intracellular survival of *Mycobacterium tuberculosis*. *Biochemical Journal*, *418*, 369–378.

Lack, N. A., Yam, K. C., Lowe, E. D., Horsman, G. P., Owen, R. L., Sim, E., et al. (2010). Characterization of a carbon-carbon hydrolase from *Mycobacterium tuberculosis* involved in cholesterol metabolism. *Journal of Biological Chemistry*, *285*, 434–443.

Laurieri, N., Crawford, M. H., Kawamura, A., Westwood, I. M., Robinson, J., Fletcher, A. M., et al. (2010). Small molecule colorimetric probes for specific detection of human arylamine *N*-acetyltransferase 1, a potential breast cancer biomarker. *Journal of the American Chemical Society*, *132*, 3238–3239.

Leff, M. A., Epstein, P. N., Doll, M. A., Fretland, A. J., Devanboyina, U. S., Rustan, T. D., et al. (1999). Prostate-specific human *N*-acetyltransferase 2 (NAT2) expression in the mouse. *Journal of Pharmacology and Experimental Therapeutics*, *290*, 182–187.

Levy, G. N., & Weber, W. W. (1992). 2-Aminofluorene-DNA adducts in mouse urinary bladder: effect of age, sex and acetylator phenotype. *Carcinogenesis*, *13*, 159–164.

Levy, G. N., Chung, J. G., & Weber, W. W. (1994). 2-Aminofluorene metabolism and DNA adduct formation by mononuclear leukocytes from rapid and slow acetylator mouse strains. *Carcinogenesis*, *15*, 353–357.

Li, J., Zhang, L., Zhou, H., Stoneking, M., & Tang, K. (2011). Global patterns of genetic diversity and signals of natural selection for human ADME genes. *Human Molecular Genetics*, *20*, 528–540.

Lipmann, F. (1945). Acetylation of sulfanilamide by liver homogenates and extracts. *Journal of Biological Chemistry*, *160*, 173–190.

Liu, F., Zhang, N., Zhou, X., Hanna, P. E., Wagner, C. R., Koepp, D. M., et al. (2006). Arylamine *N*-acetyltransferase aggregation and constitutive ubiquitylation. *Journal of Molecular Biology*, *361*, 482–492.

Liu, L., Wagner, C. R., & Hanna, P. E. (2009). Isoform-selective inactivation of human arylamine *N*-acetyltransferases by reactive metabolites of carcinogenic arylamines. *Chemical Research in Toxicology*, 22, 1962–1974.

Loehle, J. A., Cornish, V., Wakefield, L., Doll, M. A., Neale, J. R., Zang, Y., et al. (2006). *N*-acetyltransferase (NAT) 1 and 2 expression in Nat2 knockout mice. *Journal of Pharmacology and Experimental Therapeutics*, *319*, 724–728.

Luca, F., Bubba, G., Basile, M., Brdicka, R., Michalodimitrakis, E., Rickards, O., et al. (2008). Multiple advantageous amino acid variants in the NAT2 gene in human populations. *PLoS One*, *3*(9), e3136.

Magalon, H., Patin, E., Austerlitz, F., Hegay, T., Aldashev, A., Quintana-Murci, L., et al. (2008). Population genetic diversity of the NAT2 gene supports a role of acetylation in human adaptation to farming in Central Asia. *European Journal of Human Genetics*, *16*, 243–251.

Malka, F., Dairou, J., Ragunathan, N., Dupret, J. M., & Rodrigues-Lima, F. (2009). Mechanisms and kinetics of human arylamine *N*-acetyltransferase 1 inhibition by disulfiram. *FEBS Journal*, *276*, 4900–4908.

Martell, K. J., Vatsis, K. P., & Weber, W. W. (1991). Molecular genetic basis of rapid and slow acetylation in mice. *Molecular Pharmacology*, *40*, 218–227.

Martins, M., Dairou, J., Rodrigues-Lima, F., Dupret, J. M., & Silar, P. (2010). Insights into the phylogeny or arylamine *N*-acetyltransferases in fungi. *Journal of Molecular Evolution*, *71*, 141–152.

Martins, M., Pluvinage, B., Li de la Sierra-Gallay, I., Barbault, F., Dairou, J., Dupret, J. M., et al. (2008). Functional and structural characterization of the arylamine *N*-acetyltransferase from the opportunistic pathogen Nocardia farcinica. *Journal of Molecular Biology*, *383*, 549–560.

Martins, M., Rodrigues-Lima, F., Dairou, J., Lamouri, A., Malagnac, F., Silar, P., et al. (2009). An acetyltransferase conferring tolerance to toxic aromatic amine chemicals: molecular and functional studies. *Journal of Biological Chemistry*, *284*, 18,726–18,733.

Matas, N., Thygesen, P., Stacey, M., Risch, A., & Sim, E. (1997). Mapping AAC1, AAC2 and AACP, the genes for arylamine *N*-acetyltransferases, carcinogen metabolising enzymes on human chromosome 8p22, a region frequently deleted in tumours. *Cytogenetics and Cell Genetics*, *77*, 290–295.

McQueen, C. A. (2004). Summary of the third workshop on arylamine *N*-acetyltransferases. *ISSX Newsletter*, *24*(3), 13.

Millner, L. M., Doll, M. A., Cai, J., States, J. C., & Hein, D. W. (2011). NATb/NAT1*4 promotes greater arylamine *N*-acetyltransferase 1 mediated DNA adducts and mutations than NATa/NAT1*4 following exposure to 4-aminobiphenyl. *Molecular Carcinogenesis*10.1002/mc.20836. [Epub ahead of print].

Minchin, R. F. (1995). Acetylation of *p*-aminobenzoylglutamate, a folic acid catabolite, by recombinant human arylamine *N*-acetyltransferase and U937 cells. *Biochemical Journal*, *307*, 1–3.

Minchin, R. F., Hanna, P. E., Dupret, J. M., Wagner, C. R., Rodrigues-Lima, F., & Butcher, N. J. (2007). Arylamine *N*-acetyltransferase I. *International Journal of Biochemistry and Cell Biology*, *39*, 1999–2005.

Miner, M. D., Chang, J. C., Pandey, A. K., Sassetti, C. M., & Sherman, D. R. (2009). Role of cholesterol in *Mycobacterium tuberculosis* infection. *Indian Journal of Experimental Biology*, *47*, 407–411.

Mitchell, R. S., & Bell, J. C. (1957). Clinical implications of isoniazid, PAS and streptomycin blood levels in pulmonary tuberculosis. *Transactions of the American Clinical and Climatological Association*, *69*, 98–102.

Moore, L. E., Baris, D. R., Figueroa, J. D., Garcia-Closas, M., Karagas, M. R., Schwenn, M. R., et al. (2011). GSTM1 null and NAT2 slow acetylation genotypes, smoking intensity and bladder cancer risk: results from the New England bladder cancer study and NAT2 meta-analysis. *Carcinogenesis*, *32*, 182–189.

Moretti, A., Caron, L., Nakano, A., Lam, J. T., Bernshausen, A., Chen, Y., et al. (2006). Multipotent embryonic isl1+ progenitor cells lead to cardiac, smooth muscle, and endothelial cell diversification. *Cell*, *127*, 1151–1165.

Mortensen, H. M., Froment, A., Lema, G., Bodo, J. M., Ibrahim, M., Nyambo, T. B., et al. (2011). Characterization of genetic variation and natural selection at the arylamine *N*-acetyltransferase genes in global human populations. *Pharmacogenomics*, *12*, 1545–1558.

Mushtaq, A., Payton, M., & Sim, E. (2002). The COOH terminus of arylamine *N*-acetyltransferase from *Salmonella typhimurium* controls enzymic activity. *Journal of Biological Chemistry*, *277*, 12,175–12,181.

Ohsako, S., & Deguchi, T. (1990). Cloning and expression of cDNAs for polymorphic and monomorphic arylamine *N*-acetyltransferases from human liver. *Journal of Biological Chemistry*, *265*, 4630–4634.

Ohsako, S., Ohtomi, M., Sakamoto, Y., Uyemura, K., & Deguchi, T. (1988). Arylamine *N*-acetyltransferase from chicken liver ii. Cloning of cDNA and expression in chinese hamster ovary cells. *Journal of Biological Chemistry*, *263*, 7534–7538.

Pandey, A. K., & Sassetti, C. M. (2008). Mycobacterial persistence requires the utilization of host cholesterol. *Proceedings of the National Academy of Sciences of the USA*, *105*, 4376–4380.

Paterson, S., Sin, K. L., Tiang, J. M., Minchin, R. F., & Butcher, N. J. (2011). Histone deacetylase inhibitors increase human arylamine *N*-acetyltransferase-1 expression in human tumor cells. *Drug Metabolism and Disposition*, *39*, 77–82.

Patin, E., Barreiro, L. B., Sabeti, P. C., Austerlitz, F., Luca, F., Sajantila, A., et al. (2006a). Deciphering the ancient and complex evolutionary history of human arylamine *N*-acetyltransferase genes. *American Journal of Human Genetics*, *78*, 423–436.

Patin, E., Harmant, C., Kidd, K. K., Kidd, J., Froment, A., Mehdi, S. Q., et al. (2006b). Sub-Saharan African coding sequence variation and haplotype diversity at the NAT2 gene. *Human Mutation*, *27*, 720.

Payton, M., Auty, R., Delgoda, R., Everett, M., & Sim, E. (1999a). Cloning and characterization of arylamine *N*-acetyltransferase genes from mycobacterium smegmatis and *Mycobacterium tuberculosis*: Increased expression results in isoniazid resistance. *Journal of Bacteriology*, *181*, 1343–1347.

Payton, M., Gifford, C., Schartau, P., Hagemeier, C., Mushtaq, A., Lucas, S., et al. (2001). Evidence towards the role of arylamine *N*-acetyltransferase in *Mycobacterium smegmatis* and development of a specific antiserum against the homologous enzyme of *Mycobacterium tuberculosis*. *Microbiology*, *147*, 3295–3302.

Payton, M., Smelt, V., Upton, A., & Sim, E. (1999b). A method for genotyping murine arylamine *N*-acetyltransferase type 2 (NAT2): A gene expressed in preimplantation embryonic stem cells encoding an enzyme acetylating the folate catabolite *p*-aminobenzoylglutamate. *Biochemical Pharmacology*, *58*, 779–785.

Pluvinage, B., Dairou, J., Possot, O. M., Martins, M., Fouet, A., Dupret, J. M., et al. (2007). Cloning and molecular characterization of three arylamine *N*-acetyltransferase genes from Bacillus anthracis: identification of unusual enzymatic properties and their contribution to sulfamethoxazole resistance. *Biochemistry*, *46*, 7069–7078.

Pluvinage, B., Sierra-Gallay, I. L., Kubiak, X., Xu, X., Dairou, J., Dupret, J. M., et al. (2011). The Bacillus anthracis arylamine *N*-acetyltransferase ((BACAN)NAT1) that inactivates sulfamethoxazole, reveals unusual structural features compared with the other NAT isoenzymes. *FEBS Letters*, *585*, 3947–3952.

Pompeo, F., Brooke, E. W., Kawamura, A., Mushtaq, A., & Sim, E. (2002). The pharmacogenetics of NAT: structural aspects. *Pharmacogenomics*, *3*, 19–30.

Ragunathan, N., Busi, F., Pluvinage, B., Sanfins, E., Dupret, J. M., Rodrigues-Lima, F., et al. (2010). The human xenobiotic-metabolizing enzyme arylamine *N*-acetyltransferase 1 (NAT1) is irreversibly inhibited by inorganic (Hg2+) and organic mercury (CH3Hg+): mechanism and kinetics. *FEBS Letters*, *584*, 3366–3369.

Rengarajan, J., Bloom, B. R., & Rubin, E. J. (2005). Genome wide requirements for *Mycobacterium tuberculosis* adaptation and survival in macrophages. *Proceedings of the National Academy of Sciences of the USA*, *102*, 8327–8332.

Riddle, B., & Jencks, W. P.. (1971). Acetyl-coenzyme A: Arylamine *N*-acetyltransferase. Role of the acetyl-enzyme intermediate and the effects of substituents on the rate. *Journal of Biological Chemistry*, *246*, 3250–3258.

Risch, A., Wallace, D. M., Bathers, S., & Sim, E. (1995). Slow N-acetylation genotype is a susceptibility factor in occupational and smoking related bladder cancer. *Human Molecular Genetics*, *4*, 231–236.

Rodrigues-Lima, F., Blömeke, B., Sim, E., & Dupret, J. M. (2002). NAT – from bugs to brains. An overview of the 2nd International Workshop on the arylamine Nacetyltransferases. *Pharmacogenomics Journal*, *2*, 152–155.

Rodrigues-Lima, F., Dairou, J., Diaz, C. L., Rubio, M. C., Sim, E., Spaink, H. P., et al. (2006). Cloning, functional expression and characterization of *Mesorhizobium loti* arylamine *N*-acetyltransferases: rhizobial symbiosis supplies leguminous plants with the xenobiotic N-acetylation pathway. *Molecular Microbiology*, *60*, 505–512.

Rodrigues-Lima, F., Dairou, J., Laurieri, N., Busi, F., & Dupret, J. M. (2011). Fifth international workshop on arylamine *N*-acetyltransferases. University Paris Diderot, Paris, France, 1–3 September 2010. *Pharmacogenomics*, *12*, 1091–1093.

Rothman, N., Garcia-Closas, M., Chatterjee, N., Malats, N., Wu, X., Figueroa, J. D., et al. (2010). A multi-stage genome-wide association study of bladder cancer identifies multiple susceptibility loci. *Nature Genetics*, *42*, 978–984.

Russell, A. J., Westwood, I. M., Crawford, M. H., Robinson, J., Kawamura, A., Redfield, C., et al. (2009). Selective small molecule inhibitors of the potential breast cancer marker, human arylamine *N*-acetyltransferase 1, and its murine homologue, mouse arylamine *N*-acetyltransferase 2. *Bioorganic and Medicinal Chemistry*, *17*, 905–918.

Sabbagh, A., Darlu, P., Crouau-Roy, B., & Poloni, E. S. (2011). Arylamine *N*-acetyltransferase 2 (NAT2) genetic diversity and traditional subsistence: a worldwide population survey. *PLoS One*, *6*(4), e18507.

Sabbagh, A., Langaney, A., Darlu, P., Gérard, N., Krishnamoorthy, R., & Poloni, E. S. (2008). Worldwide distribution of NAT2 diversity: implications for NAT2 evolutionary history. *BMC Genetics*, *9*, 21.

Sandy, J., Mushtaq, A., Holton, S. J., Schartau, P., Noble, M. E., & Sim, E. (2005). Investigation of the catalytic triad of arylamine *N*-acetyltransferases: Essential residues required for acetyl transfer to arylamines. *Biochemical Journal*, *390*, 115–123.

Sandy, J., Mushtaq, A., Kawamura, A., Sinclair, J., Noble, M., & Sim, E. (2002). The structure of arylamine *N*-acetyltransferase from Mycobacterium smegmatis – an enzyme which inactivates the anti-tubercular drug, isoniazid. *Journal of Molecular Biology*, *318*, 1071–1083.

Sholto-Douglas-Vernon, C., Sandy, J., Victor, T. C., Sim, E., & Helden, P. D. (2005). Mutational and expression analysis of tbNAT and its response to isoniazid. *Journal of Medical Microbiology*, *54*, 1189–1197.

Sim, E., & Hickman, D. (1991). Polymorphism in human *N*-acetyltransferase – the case of the missing allele. *Trends in Pharmacological Science*, *12*, 211–213.

Sim, E., Lack, N., Wang, C. J., Long, H., Westwood, I., Fullam, E., et al. (2008a). Arylamine *N*-acetyltransferases: structural and functional implications of polymorphisms. *Toxicology*, *254*, 170–183.

Sim, E., Walters, K., & Boukouvala, S. (2008b). Arylamine *N*-acetyltransferases: from structure to function. *Drug Metabolism Reviews*, *40*, 479–510.

Sinclair, J. C., Sandy, J., Delgoda, R., Sim, E., & Noble, M. E. (2000). Structure of arylamine *N*-acetyltransferase reveals a catalytic triad. *Nature Structural Biology*, *7*, 560–564.

Smelt, V. A., Mardon, H. J., & Sim, E. (1998). Placental expression of arylamine *N*-acetyltransferases: evidence for linkage disequilibrium between NAT1*10 and NAT2*4 alleles of the two human arylamine *N*-acetyltransferase loci NAT1 and NAT2. *Pharmacology and Toxicology*, *83*, 149–157.

Smelt, V. A., Upton, A., Adjaye, J., Payton, M. A., Boukouvala, S., Johnson, N., et al. (2000). Expression of arylamine *N*-acetyltransferases in pre-term placentas and in human preimplantation embryos. *Human Molecular Genetics*, *9*, 1101–1107.

Sneider, G. (2010). Virtual screening: an endless staircase? *Nature Reviews Drug Discovery*, *9*, 273–276.

Stanley, L. A., Copp, A. J., Pope, J., Rolls, S., Smelt, V., Perry, V. H., et al. (1998). Immunochemical detection of arylamine *N*-acetyltransferase during mouse embryonic development and in adult mouse brain. *Teratology*, *58*, 174–182.

Sugamori, K. S., Brenneman, D., & Grant, D. M. (2011). Liver-selective expression of human arylamine *N*-acetyltransferase NAT2 in transgenic mice. *Drug Metabolism and Disposition*, *39*, 882–890.

Sugamori, K. S., Wong, S., Gaedigk, A., Yu, V., Abramovici, H., Rozmahel, R., et al. (2003). Generation and functional characterization of arylamine *N*-acetyltransferase Nat1/Nat2 double-knockout mice. *Molecular Pharmacology*, *64*, 170–179.

Tailleux, L., Waddell, S. J., Pelizzola, M., Mortellaro, A., Withers, M., Tanne, A., et al. (2008). Probing host pathogen cross-talk by transcriptional profiling of both *Mycobacterium tuberculosis* and infected human dendritic cells and macrophages. *PLoS One*, *3*(1), e1403.

Tiang, J. M., Butcher, N. J., Cullinane, C., Humbert, P. O., & Minchin, R. F. (2011). RNAi-mediated knock-down of arylamine *N*-acetyltransferase-1 expression induces E-cadherin up-regulation and cell-cell contact growth inhibition. *PLoS One*, 6(2), e17031.

Tiang, J. M., Butcher, N. J., & Minchin, R. F. (2010). Small molecule inhibition of arylamine *N*-acetyltransferase Type I inhibits proliferation and invasiveness of MDA-MB-231 breast cancer cells. *Biochemical and Biophysical Research Communications*, *393*, 95–100.

Trepanier, L. A., Ray, K., Winand, N. J., Spielberg, S. P., & Cribb, A. E. (1997). Cytosolic arylamine *N*-acetyltransferase (NAT) deficiency in the dog and other canids due to an absence of NAT genes. *Biochemical Pharmacology*, *54*, 73–80.

Upton, A. M., Mushtaq, A., Victor, T. C., Sampson, S. L., Sandy, J., Smith, D. M., et al. (2001). Arylamine *N*-acetyltransferase of *Mycobacterium tuberculosis* is a polymorphic enzyme and a site of isoniazid metabolism. *Molecular Microbiology*, *42*, 309–317.

Vagena, E., Fakis, G., & Boukouvala, S. (2008). Arylamine *N*-acetyltransferases in prokaryotic and eukaryotic genomes: a survey of public databases. *Current Drug Metabolism*, *9*, 628–660.

Van der Geize, R., Heuser, T., Yam, K., Wilbrink, M. H., Hara, H., Anderton, M. C., et al. (2007). A gene cluster encoding cholesterol catabolism in a soil actinomycete provides insight into *Mycobacterium tuberculosis* survival in macrophages. *Proceedings of the National Academy of Sciences of the USA*, *104*, 1947–1952.

Wakefield, L., Boukouvala, S., & Sim, E. (2010). Characterisation of CpG methylation in the upstream control region of mouse Nat2: evidence for a gene–environment interaction in a polymorphic gene implicated in folate metabolism. *Gene*, *452*, 16–21.

Wakefield, L., Cornish, V., Broackes-Carter, F., & Sim, E. (2005). Arylamine *N*-acetyltransferase 2 expression in the developing heart. *Journal of Histochemistry and Cytochemistry*, *53*, 583–592.

Wakefield, L., Cornish, V., Long, H., Griffiths, W. J., & Sim, E. (2007a). Deletion of a xenobiotic metabolizing gene in mice affects folate metabolism. *Biochemical and Biophysical Research Communications*, *364*, 556–560.

Wakefield, L., Cornish, V., Long, H., Kawamura, A., Zhang, X., Hein, D. W., et al. (2008a). Mouse arylamine *N*-acetyltransferase 2 (NAT2) expression during embryogenesis: A potential marker for the developing neuroendocrine system. *Biomarkers*, *13*, 106–118.

Wakefield, L., Long, H., Lack, N., & Sim, E. (2007b). Ocular defects associated with a null mutation in the mouse arylamine *N*-acetyltransferase 2 gene. *Mammalian Genome*, *18*, 270–276.

Wakefield, L., Robinson, J., Long, H., Ibbit, J. C., Cooke, S., Hurst, H. C., et al. (2008b). Arylamine *N*-acetyltransferase I expression in breast cancer cell lines: A potential marker in estrogen receptor-positive tumors. *Genes Chromosomes and Cancer*, *47*, 118–126.

Walraven, J. M., Doll, M. A., & Hein, D. W. (2006). Identification and characterization of functional rat arylamine *N*-acetyltransferase 3: comparisons with rat arylamine *N*-acetyltransferases 1 and 2. *Journal of Pharmacology and Experimental Therapeutics*, *319*, 369–375.

Walraven, J. M., Trent, J. O., & Hein, D. W. (2007). Computational and experimental analyses of mammalian arylamine *N*-acetyltransferase structure and function. *Drug Metabolism and Disposition*, *35*, 1001–1007.

Wang, D., Para, M. F., Koletar, S. L., & Sadee, W. (2011). Human *N*-acetyltransferase 1*10 and *11 alleles increase protein expression through distinct mechanisms and associate with sulfamethoxazole-induced hypersensitivity. *Pharmacogenetics and Genomics*, *21*, 652–664.

Wang, H., Liu, L., Hanna, P. E., & Wagner, C. R. (2005a). Catalytic mechanism of hamster arylamine *N*-acetyltransferase 2. *Biochemistry*, *44*, 11,295–11,306.

Wang, H., Vath, G. M., Gleason, K. J., Hanna, P. E., & Wagner, C. R. (2004). Probing the mechanism of hamster arylamine *N*-acetyltransferase 2 acetylation by active site modification, site-directed mutagenesis, and pre-steady state and steady state kinetic studies. *Biochemistry*, *43*, 8234–8246.

Wang, H., Wagner, C. R., & Hanna, P. E. (2005b). Irreversible inactivation of arylamine *N*-acetyltransferases in the presence of N-hydroxy-4-acetylaminobiphenyl: a comparison of human and hamster enzymes. *Chemical Research in Toxicology*, *18*, 183–197.

Ward, A., Summers, M. J., & Sim, E. (1995). Purification of recombinant human *N*-acetyltransferase type 1 (NAT1) expressed in *E. coli* and characterization of its potential role in folate metabolism. *Biochemical Pharmacology*, *49*, 1759–1767.

Watanabe, M., Sofuni, T., & Nohmi, T. (1992). Involvement of cys69 residue in the catalytic mechanism of N-hydroxyarylamine *O*-acetyltransferase of *Salmonella typhimurium*. Sequence similarity at the amino acid level suggests a common catalytic mechanism of acetyltransferase for *S. typhimurium* and higher organisms. *Journal of Biological Chemistry*, *267*, 8429–8436.

Watson, A. P., Wang, P. D., & Sim, E. (1990). Arylamine *N*-acetyltransferase from fast (C57BL6) and slow (A/J) N-acetylating strains of mice. *Biochemical Pharmacology*, *39*, 647–654.

Weber, W. W. (1999). Populations and genetic polymorphisms. *Molecular Diagnostics*, *4*, 299–307.

Westwood, I. M., & Sim, E. (2007). Kinetic characterisation of arylamine *N*-acetyltransferase from *Pseudomonas aeruginosa*. *BMC Biochemistry*, *8*, 3.

Westwood, I. M., Bhakta, S., Russell, A. J., Fullam, E., Anderton, M. C., Kawamura, A., et al. (2010). Identification of arylamine *N*-acetyltransferase inhibitors as an approach towards novel anti-tuberculars. *Protein Cell*, *1*, 82–95.

Westwood, I. M., Holton, S. J., Rodrigues-Lima, F., Dupret, J. M., Bhakta, S., Noble, M. E., et al. (2005). Expression, purification, characterization and structure of *Pseudomonas aeruginosa* arylamine *N*-acetyltransferase. *Biochemical Journal*, *385*, 605–612.

Westwood, I. M., Kawamura, A., Fullam, E., Russell, A., Davies, S. G., & Sim, E. (2006). Structure and mechanism of arylamine *N*-acetyltransferases. *Current Topics in Medicinal Chemistry*, 6, 1641–1654.

Westwood, I. M., Kawamura, A., Russell, A. J., Sandy, J., Davies, S. G., & Sim, E. (2011). Novel small-molecule inhibitors of arylamine *N*-acetyltransferases: drug discovery by high-throughput screening. *Combinatorial Chemistry and High Throughput Screening*, *14*, 117–124.

Wu, H., Dombrovsky, L., Tempel, W., Martin, F., Loppnau, P., Goodfellow, G. H., et al. (2007). Structural basis of substrate-binding specificity of human arylamine *N*-acetyltransferases. *Journal of Biological Chemistry*, *282*, 30,189–30,197.

Yam, K. C., D'Angelo, I., Kalscheuer, R., Zhu, H., Wang, J. X., Snieckus, V., et al. (2009). Studies of a ring-cleaving dioxygenase illuminate the role of cholesterol metabolism in the pathogenesis of *Mycobacterium tuberculosis*. *PLoS Pathogens*, *5*, e1000344.

Zang, Y., Doll, M. A., Zhao, S., States, J. C., & Hein, D. W. (2007). Functional characterization of single-nucleotide polymorphisms and haplotypes of human *N*-acetyltransferase 2. *Carcinogenesis*, *28*, 1665–1671.

Zhu, Y., States, J. C., Wang, Y., & Hein, D. W. (2011). Functional effects of genetic polymorphisms in the *N*-acetyltransferase 1 coding and 3' untranslated regions. *Birth Defects Research A: Clinical and Molecular Teratology*, *91*, 77–84.

R. L. C. Sison-Young[1,2,4], R. Kia[1,4], J. Heslop[1], L. Kelly[1,2], C. Rowe[1,2], M. J. Cross[1], N. R. Kitteringham[1,2], N. Hanley[2,3], B. K. Park[1,2] and C. E. P. Goldring[1,2]

[1]MRC Centre for Drug Safety Science, Department of Molecular and Clinical Pharmacology, University of Liverpool, Liverpool, United Kingdom
[2]Stem Cells for Safer Medicine, Department of Molecular and Clinical Pharmacology, University of Liverpool, Liverpool, United Kingdom
[3]Manchester Academic Health Science Centre, University of Manchester, Manchester, United Kingdom
[4]These authors contributed equally

Human Pluripotent Stem Cells for Modeling Toxicity

Abstract

The development of xenobiotics, driven by the demand for therapeutic, domestic and industrial uses continues to grow. However, along with this increasing demand is the risk of xenobiotic-induced toxicity. Currently, safety screening of xenobiotics uses a plethora of animal and *in vitro* model systems which have over the decades proven useful during compound development and for application in mechanistic studies of xenobiotic-induced toxicity. However, these assessments have proven to be animal-intensive and costly. More importantly, the prevalence of xenobiotic-induced toxicity is still significantly high, causing patient morbidity and mortality, and a costly impediment during drug development. This suggests that the current models for drug safety screening are not reliable in toxicity prediction, and the results not easily translatable to the clinic due to insensitive assays that do not recapitulate fully the complex phenotype of a functional cell type *in vivo*.

Recent advances in the field of stem cell research have potentially allowed for a readily available source of metabolically competent cells for toxicity studies, derived using human pluripotent stem cells harnessed from embryos or reprogrammed from mature somatic cells. Pluripotent stem cell-derived cell types also allow for potential disease modeling *in vitro* for the purposes of drug toxicology and safety pharmacology, making this model possibly more predictive of drug toxicity compared with existing models. This article will review the advances and challenges of using human pluripotent stem cells for modeling metabolism and toxicity, and offer some perspectives as to where its future may lie.

Advances in Pharmacology, Volume 63

1054-3589/12 $35.00
http://dx.doi.org/10.1016/B978-0-12-398339-8.00006-9

I. Introduction

The development of xenobiotics, driven by the demand for therapeutic, domestic and industrial uses continues to grow. However, along with this increasing demand is the risk of xenobiotic-induced toxicity. To address this issue, regulatory requirements for mandatory toxicological safety assessments have been implemented by the government to ensure that hazard and safety risks are identified and preventative measures are put in place during the development of xenobiotics (EC1907/2006). This is particularly challenging in the pharmaceutical industry where therapeutic efficacy and the toxic effects of drugs must be carefully balanced to ensure that safe and effective therapy is provided and wasteful drug developmental costs are reduced.

To date, safety screening of xenobiotics uses a plethora of model systems including wild-type and transgenic animals, freshly-isolated cells and established cell lines, which over the decades have proven highly useful during compound development and for application in mechanistic studies of xenobiotic-induced toxicity (Guguen-Guillouzo & Guillouzo, 2010). However, despite rigorous safety screening protocols, there is still a significantly high prevalence of xenobiotic-induced toxicity (Andrade et al., 2005; Lazarou et al., 1998; Pirmohamed et al., 2004). Factors involved have been reported to include genetic polymorphisms (Singh et al., 2011; Tekin et al., 2011; Wilffert et al., 2011), gender (Nicolson et al., 2010; Renaud et al., 2011), age (Espandiari et al., 2010; Maddrey, 2005; Mitchell et al., 2011) and environmental factors (Elsaesser & Howard, 2011; Sudakin & Stone, 2011), which the current models are not able to fully account for. Furthermore, extrapolation of *in vitro* data to *in vivo* conditions and the clinical setting has proved challenging. A major factor is inter-species differences (Celander et al., 2011; Lee et al., 2006; Saldana-Ruiz et al., 2011), especially with toxicology data generated using animal models, demonstrating the complexity in undertaking the design and development of protocols for safety assessment studies on xenobiotics. An example of such complexity is embryotoxicity testing where it is essential for the assays to represent a particular stage in the mammalian developmental process to enable identification of the exact developmental stage at which the compound is toxic (de Jong et al., 2011; Schmidt et al., 2001).

Furthermore, many drugs withdrawn in recent years were due to unforeseen effects, particularly cardiotoxicity, which is one of the major causes for late-stage drug attrition post-licensing (Wobus & Loser, 2011). Many drugs with cardiac adverse effects had non-cardiovascular applications – the most prominent example being rofecoxib used as a selective COX2 inhibitor for its analgesic properties, but voluntarily withdrawn from the market in 2004 due to higher risks of patients on chronic usage suffering myocardial infarctions and stroke (Topol, 2004). Effects of the circadian rhythm on cellular defense mechanisms of hepatocytes such as the antioxidant glutathione (GSH), and therefore the susceptibility of organisms to xenobiotic-induced toxicity have also been demonstrated (Gachon & Firsov, 2011). Many current assays for drug toxicology have not so far taken this effect into account, further illustrating the challenges that are faced in toxicology research.

Clinical cases of xenobiotic-induced toxicity are common in drug therapy. In particular, adverse drug reactions (ADRs) have long been recognized as the leading cause of patient morbidity and mortality (Andrade et al., 2005; Lazarou et al., 1998; Pirmohamed et al., 2004), costing the NHS £466 million a year (Pirmohamed et al., 2004) and accounting for 6.5% of all hospital admissions to two NHS secondary care hospitals in the North West between 2002 and 2003. Furthermore, ADRs have also proven to be a costly impediment in drug development, resulting in the withdrawal of a number of approved drugs (Lee, 2003; Pirmohamed et al., 2004; Smith & Schmid, 2006).

The majority of ADRs are often dose-dependent (on-target); therefore toxicity can be ameliorated, by adjustment of the dose as classically demonstrated during paracetamol toxicity (Gokhale & Martin, 2011; Roth & Ganey, 2010). ADRs can also be idiosyncratic in nature, although the mechanisms underlying these are yet to be uncovered (Edwards & Aronson, 2000; Park et al., 2005). Research into ADRs, particularly the idiosyncratic type, is hampered by the lack of model systems that directly reflect the clinical situation.

There has been a huge weight of expectation that progress will be made in bridging this gap in toxicology research through research in the field of human embryonic stem cells (hESC). The main attractions of embryonic stem cells (ESC) in regenerative medicine and toxicological studies are their ability to continually divide in an undifferentiated state in culture, and potential to differentiate into multiple cell lineages (Bielby et al., 2004; Hamazaki et al., 2001; Lumelsky et al., 2001; Vittet et al., 1996; Wobus et al., 2002). hESC also have potential as a readily available source of metabolically competent cells, such as hepatocytes and cardiomyocytes for toxicity studies. Well-established animal-derived pluripotent stem cell (PSC) models are available and are routinely used in a wide variety of applications. In contrast, the use of hESC (Thomson et al., 1998) has been delayed due to the complex and highly technical culture and maintenance methods required for these cells (Kusuda Furue et al., 2010; Lin & Talbot, 2011). To address this, maintenance and differentiation protocols of hESC are continually being optimized allowing the use of these cells for toxicology studies, as will be described in the following sections. More recently, PSC have also been produced through the reprogramming of mature somatic cells, termed as induced pluripotent stem cells (iPSC). This approach would negate the controversies surrounding the usage of human embryonic tissue and may allow for modeling of normal and pathologic phenotypes and disease modeling *in vitro* for the purposes of drug toxicology and safety pharmacology. In view of their potential, it is not surprising that many pharmaceutical companies in recent years have also invested and/or developed joint collaborations with academia, to develop hPSC-based *in vitro* systems for drug toxicology and safety pharmacology (Bahadur & Morrison, 2010; Prescott, 2011) . This review will discuss the advances and challenges of using human pluripotent stem cells (hPSC) in the arena of drug toxicology and safety pharmacology, and aims to provide an insight as to where its future may lie.

II. The Use of Human Stem Cells in Developmental Toxicity

Among the many reported adverse side effects of xenobiotics, embryotoxicity is one of the most severe. In an effort to reduce the incidence of developmental toxicity, mandatory toxicological safety assessment of xenobiotics has been implemented along with official guidelines set up by the Organization for Economic Co-operation and Development (OECD). However, these assessments have proven to be animal-intensive, costly and time consuming. Indeed it has been estimated that the toxicological safety screening of one compound requires 3200 animals (Hofer et al., 2004) with an estimated cost of more than €300,000 (Fleischer, 2007). Several reports have estimated that of the total number of animals used in *in vivo* toxicology studies, 70% are used in reproductive and developmental toxicology testing, particularly with the implementation of the US High Production Volume Challenge programme and the new EU REACH legislation (Hartung & Rovida, 2009; Spielmann & Vogel, 2006; van der Jagt et al., 2004).

A. *In vivo* Models of Developmental Toxicity Studies

The mammalian reproductive cycle is a complex process. It comprises several stages of embryonic and fetal development, all of which are potential for xenobiotic-induced toxicity. As such, model systems and tests developed to screen compounds for reproductive and developmental toxicity should be carefully and specifically designed for the particular stage of the reproductive cycle that is being simulated in the laboratory, ensuring the inclusion of specific molecular targets and a set of informative endpoints to assist in elucidating the reproductive and developmental toxic mechanism(s) of compounds. A selection of *in vivo* investigative methods are available including multi-generation studies that look for a number of well-defined toxic effects of compounds including teratogenicity and neurotoxicity as well as estrogenic and androgenic modulations. However, with such rigorous requirements, it is envisaged that the number of animals used in these experiments will continue to be significant. Therefore, there is a pressing need for the development of alternative non-animal methods that will not only significantly improve animal welfare, but also reduce costs.

B. Alternative Developmental Toxicity Testing Methods

In response, a wide array of alternative *in vitro* tests have been developed for reproductive and developmental toxicity studies (Piersma, 2006; Spielmann, 2005) (Table I), three of which have been commissioned for validation by the European Centre for Validation of Alternative Methods (ECVAM). The rat limb bud micromass (MM) test is a validated *in vitro* test for embryotoxicity. It is designed to evaluate the effect of a compound on cell differentiation and proliferation of MM cultures of rat embryonic limb buds or in combination with rat embryo midbrain (Flint, 1984). The whole-embryo culture (WEC) test uses isolated and cultured early post-implantation rat embryos to assess malformations or developmental delays in certain organs at the end of a 48 h culture period (Flick & Klug, 2006; Piersma et al., 2004). Although both the MM and WEC tests are considered alternative methods to conventional *in vivo* tests, neither provides a true animal-free protocol as both rely on a constant source of embryonic tissues or whole embryos from pregnant animals.

However, the advent of stem cell technology has resulted in the development of a third fully validated alternative method, the mouse embryonic stem cell test (EST). EST was first introduced more than 10 years ago by Spielmann et al. (1997) which was designed to measure the embryotoxicity of compounds during the differentiation process through the use of two specific mouse cell lines, the pluripotent ESC line (D3) and the differentiated 3T3 fibroblasts. The EST consists of three measurements, two of which [$IC_{50}D3$ and $IC_{50}3T3$] define the concentration at which the compound causes a 50% reduction in cell viability of the respective cell lines, and one which defines the concentration at which the compound inhibits 50% of D3 cells differentiating in fetal bovine serum (FBS) into cardiomyocytes [ID_{50}] (Genschow et al., 2002). Combined with a biostatistical prediction model (PM), the EST-PM has also been fully validated in an ECVAM study (Genschow et al., 2000, 2004, 2002), where results were interrogated using a linear discriminant analysis. Using this approach, the embryotoxic potency of compounds *in vivo* can then be categorized as non-embryotoxic, weakly embryotoxic or strongly embryotoxic. Indeed, a vast number of reproductive and developmental toxicity studies have been published using this method on various compounds including drugs (Eckardt & Stahlmann, 2010; Tian et al., 2011), cosmetics (Chen et al., 2010), heavy metals, dental materials (Imai & Nakamura, 2006; Schwengberg et al., 2005), nanoparticles (Di Guglielmo et al., 2010) and other industrial chemicals. The EST test has a reported 78% accuracy in predicting the embryotoxic potency of 20 selected compounds of known varying embryotoxic potencies during its

TABLE 1 Summary of Reviewed *In vitro* Models for Toxicity Testing

Area of Toxicity	*Application for Toxicity*
Developmental toxicity	
Rat embryonic limb bud micromass test (MM) – rat	Cell differentiation and proliferation
Whole-embryo culture (WEC) – rat	Organ malformations or developmental delays.
Mouse embryonic stem cell test (mEST)	IC_{50} for looking at cytotoxicity, differentiation, teratogenicity, genomic perturbations
Human neural rosettes	Morphology changes and genetic perturbations
Cardiotoxicity	
Aneuploid cell lines with overexpression of single ion channels	Function modification
Isolated cardiac tissues	
Purkinje fibres	Effect on cardiac ion channels
Primary cardiomyocytes	Cardiac action potential and ion channel activities
Explanted hearts	Cardiac functions
hESC-cardiomyocytes	Electrophysiological properties, necrosis
hiPSC-cardiomyocytes	Electrophysiological properties
Hepatotoxicity	
Primary human hepatocytes	Non-specific toxicity, metabolism, genomic perturbations, mechanism/function
Hepatocellular carcinoma-derived cell lines	Non-specific toxicity, metabolism, genomic perturbations, mechanism/function
hESC-derived hepatocyte-like cells	Non-specific toxicity
hiPSC-derived hepatocyte-like cells	Non-specific toxicity, disease modeling
Neurotoxicity	
NT2 cell line	Non-specific cytotoxicity, morphological changes
ReNcell CX	Proliferation and cell viability
Human umbilical cord blood neural stem cells (HUCB-NSC)	Non-specific cytotoxicity, apoptosis (nuclear chromatin staining), Proliferation and differentation
SH-SY neuroblastoma cells	Cell viability and differentiation
hESC-derived neurospheres	Electrical activity (using microelectrode array), genomic perturbation, proliferation, differentation and culture morphology
hN2 cell line	Neurite outgrowth
Neural-committed stem cells	High-throughput cytotoxicity, pathway, analysis
hESC-derived neural stem cells	Cytotoxicity, apoptosis, reactive oxygen species formation

validation, compared with 70% and 68% reported accuracy for the MM and WEC tests respectively (Genschow et al., 2002). The EST test also conforms to a true *in vitro* model with no animals used after the establishment of the cell lines (Seiler & Spielmann, 2011).

Despite significant advances that the EST has over *in vivo* assays, the original EST protocol was time consuming, requiring a 10 day exposure of the cells to the compound of interest; technically complex, involving monolayer cell cultures for cytotoxicity measurements and culture of 'hanging drop' embryoid bodies (EBs) for differentiation observations; and highly laborious (Seiler & Spielmann, 2011). As such, various optimizations of the original EST protocol have been proposed. These include a reduction in exposure time of the cells to the compound from 10 to 5 days without compromising data quality (Romero et al., 2011), automated imaging analysis of contractile cardiomyocyte-like cells which was proposed to have the potential for high-throughput application (Peters et al., 2008), additional cytotoxicity measurement and cardiac muscle foci counts at specific time points to differentiate between the effect of compounds undergoing cell proliferation or differentiation (van Dartel et al., 2009), and optimization of cell cultivation methods to improve on the yield of strong beating myocardial cells (De Smedt et al., 2008; Greenlee et al., 2005). Furthermore, as the cell lines used in the EST have no or very limited metabolic capacity, Hettwer et al. (2010) have devised a combined approach by incubating compounds that require bioactivation using primary mouse hepatocytes first, after which the media is then added to the mouse ESC (mESC) to determine the embryotoxic effect of the bioactivation of the test compound. However, despite these improvements, the general consensus from various research groups applying EST in embryotoxicity studies is that the information obtained is still limited, as the results refer to only one stage of the highly complex reproductive cycle where various stages can become targets of xenobiotic-induced toxicity. Modifications to this test using various analytical techniques such as microarray (Bigot et al., 1999; Pellizzer et al., 2004; Suzuki et al., 2011; van Dartel et al., 2011) and proteomic analyses (Groebe et al., 2010a, 2010b; Osman et al., 2010) have been applied to increase the data output as well as the predictive power and accuracy of the EST (currently at 78%) (Baek et al., 2011; Romero et al., 2011; Suzuki et al., 2011).

Despite the advances made in the development of alternative *in vitro* tests, particularly the EST which has shown great potential in its adaptability to a wide array of applications, rodent model systems do not address inter-species differences. In a recent study, the role of the neurotoxic viral protein tat in HIV-positive individuals with neuronal dysfunction was investigated using rat and human-derived neuronal cell models. Eugenin et al. (2011) reported that tat-mediated neuronal apoptosis as measured by the expression of *N*-methyl-D-aspartate receptor, differed between primary cultures of rat and human neurons, in corresponding developmental stages. In another study, differential expression of the multidrug transporter ABCG2 in the cell membranes of mouse and human ESC demonstrated that the absence of ABCG2 is a distinguishable feature of hPSC which may be a contributing factor to their sensitivity to xenobiotic toxins at suboptimal culture conditions (Zeng et al., 2009). As such, the use of hPSC in *in vitro* toxicology studies offers additional benefit in avoiding misclassification of compounds. This issue was addressed by Adler et al. (2008a) where a modified version of the EST using hESC was developed with additional marker genes reported to be promising endpoints for a developmental toxicity test. In a different study, the same group (Adler et al., 2008b) also suggested the use of three hESC lines at different developmental stages to determine stage-specific embryotoxicity of compounds. Zhu et al. (2011) also adapted the murine EST using hESC in investigating the embryotoxic potential of cyclophosphamide.

Metabolomic analysis on a blinded subset of 11 chemicals selected from the chemical library of the United States Environmental Protection Agency's (EPA) ToxCast™ chemical screening prioritization research project identified a number of human specific metabolic pathways including nicotinate and nicotinamide metabolism, pantothenate and CoA biosynthesis as well as GSH metabolism, processes proposed to be involved in the adaptive responses of hESC upon exposure (Kleinstreuer et al., 2011). Toxicogenomic studies in hESC also offer a sensitive *in vitro* developmental toxicity model that could provide invaluable information during pathway analysis, as was the case in a study that looked at the teratogenic effect of cytosine arabinoside. Through the use of gene expression microarrays, dysregulation in expression of multi-lineage markers in response to Ara-C treatment were identified including MAP2, TUBBIII, PAX6 and nestin for the induction of the ectoderm, whilst HAND2, PITX2, GATA5, MYL4, TNNT2, COL1A1 and COL1A2 were used to monitor inhibition of the mesoderm (Jagtap et al., 2011).

To date, developmental toxicity screening using hESC has predominantly focused on developmental neurotoxicity (DNT) (Callihan et al., 2011; Eugenin et al., 2011; Stummann et al., 2009). Colleoni et al. (2011) have developed a neural teratogenicity test by generating neural rosettes using hESC that represent the developing neural plate and neural tube. Using the teratogenic agent retinoic acid (RA), this group has demonstrated concentration-dependent morphological and gene expression changes that concord with *in vivo* data. This human cell model of neural rosettes was therefore proposed as a promising alternative test for human prenatal developmental toxicity. Another hESC-based model for screening compounds for DNT was derived from umbilical cord blood. Through the use of a number of known neurotoxicants and non-neurotoxicants, this model system has been demonstrated to have potential as an *in vitro* model of DNT (Buzanska et al., 2009).

Much improvement has been made in the development of experimental protocols for the screening of developmentally toxic compounds and the elucidation of toxic mechanisms underlying this effect. From animal-intensive, expensive and highly laborious *in vivo* tests, we are today equipped with a rich source of human-derived materials, particularly hESC, which continues to show great potential in replacing the conventional *in vivo* methods through the development of *in vitro* methods such as the EST that can be adapted to a wide array of applications. What research in this field should strive for now is to harmonize and fully validate these protocols in order to bring us closer in achieving the ultimate goal within the context of developmental toxicity research, which is to significantly reduce or replace the conventional *in vivo* tests that over the years have raised problematic issues which, with the availability of hESC, we are now equipped to address.

III. The Use of Human Stem Cells in Cardiotoxicity

Robust and detailed assessment for subclinical cardiotoxicity of new chemical entities (NCE) is now required by regulatory authorities (The International Conference on Harmonisation, 2011), while early detection of cardiac toxicity in pre-clinical stages is critical for the pharmaceutical industry as it remains one of the leading causes of drug failure (Fermini & Fossa, 2003). Accurate and early detection of these toxic effects in pre-clinical stages, and also the high attrition rate of NCE drug candidates seen during screening and early development is hampered by insensitive assays that do not recapitulate fully the complex phenotype of a functional cardiomyocyte *in vivo*.

One of the most common cardiotoxic effect from drugs is delayed repolarization of the ventricular action potential due to transmembrane ion flux, which is then detected electrophysiologically as a prolonged QT interval. This can lead to life-threatening ventricular tachyarrhythmia such as torsade de pointes (TdP) (Pouton & Haynes, 2007). Although questions remain as to whether a prolonged QT interval is an accurate marker for TdP (Lee et al., 2010), safety assessment of NCE drug candidates dictates that the QT interval is not prolonged at therapeutic and supra-therapeutic doses (The International Conference on Harmonisation, 2011).

A common assay used in the early stages of the drug development process to test for QT prolongation involves using aneuploid cell lines with overexpression of single ion channels to investigate channel-modulating activity. However, this approach does not reflect the functional cardiomyocyte with complex multi-channel interactions (Pouton & Haynes, 2007). This was best shown by *in vitro* studies of verapamil using Chinese-hamster ovary (CHO) cells overexpressing human ether-a-go-go-related gene (HERG), which predicted a prolongation of the QT interval due to blocking of the I_{Kr} channel. However, the QT interval in a functional cardiomyocyte is in fact unaffected due to concomitant blockage of the L-type calcium channel, resulting in a net zero effect on the potassium current flowing through the cell (Meyer et al., 2004).

Other models applied in pre-clinical drug safety assessment include isolated cardiac tissues such as Purkinje fibers, primary cardiomyocytes and explanted hearts from animals (Kettenhofen & Bohlen, 2008; Skrzypiec-Spring et al., 2007). However, these approaches are expensive, labor-intensive, highly variable inter-experimentally, unethical due to large numbers of animals required and importantly, the relationship between the drug responses observed in these animal models and their human equivalents is not always clear due to inter-species variation (Terrar et al., 2007). Human cardiomyocytes would be the preferred cellular model for drug safety screening, but harvesting mature cardiomyocytes is limited by availability, low proliferative capacity and variability in disease state, especially when harvested from cadavers (Kettenhofen & Bohlen, 2008; Pouton & Haynes, 2007). Recent advances in stem cell technology have allowed the creation of a renewable source of cardiomyocytes derived from hPSC, as an alternative *in vitro* screening system for cardiotoxicity.

A. Production and Characterization of Cardiomyocytes from hPSC

A high volume of work has been and continues to be dedicated to the research and development of PSC-based cardiac models for cardiac toxicity applications (Table I). Studies using mESC-derived cardiomyocytes have previously suggested their utility in drug safety screening and toxicology (Wobus & Boheler, 2005). However, the use of mESC for drug safety testing in humans is again limited due to inter-species variation (Terrar et al., 2007).

Cardiomyocytes derived from hESC were first reported in 2000 (Itskovitz-Eldor et al., 2000) and from human iPSC (hiPSC) in 2009 (Zhang et al., 2009). These pluripotent cells are most commonly differentiated into cardiomyocytes by forming three-dimensional (3-D) spheroids, better known as EBs, either spontaneously in suspension culture (He et al., 2003), or by forced aggregation using centrifugation which also allows for control of the size of EBs (Burridge et al., 2007; Ungrin et al., 2008). A protocol employing co-culture of the undifferentiated pluripotent cells with END2 cells has also been used (Mummery et al., 2007; Xu et al., 2008a). $ISLI^+$ multipotent cardiac progenitor cells isolated from iPSC were also used as a source to differentiate into cardiac cells (Moretti et al., 2010). The number of beating EBs produced generally ranges from 0 to 70% of EBs at a rate of 30–130 beats per minute, with contractions commencing between days 6 and 24 of differentiation (Dick et al., 2010). The composition of the beating EBs is also highly variable, with cardiomyocytes comprising <25% of the total cells with the rest comprising fibroblasts of endodermal lineage. This huge heterogeneity is postulated to be due to differences in the hESC lines, differentiation protocols and also the culture media used (Anderson et al., 2007; Braam et al., 2010). Interestingly, an efficient, cost-effective non-viral protocol of cardiac differentiation from hiPSC was recently described, with a reported production efficiency of beating EBs of 94.7% in 9 days with up to 89% of cardiac troponin I-positive cells detected (Burridge et al., 2011). However, to the best of our knowledge, no other centers have replicated this success so far. Previous strategies to improve the cardiomyocyte differentiation efficiencies by inducing cardiomyogenesis, have included using small molecules (Graichen et al., 2008; Xu et al., 2002) and growth factors (Burridge et al., 2007; Yang et al., 2008) with reported efficiencies of up to 50% (Yang et al., 2008) (see Fig. 1).

Another approach to generate pure cardiomyocyte populations is by application of selection procedures. Early attempts include manual dissection of contracting cells (Kehat et al., 2001) and separation by centrifugation (Xu et al., 2006), both of which were labor-intensive and non-scalable. A different approach using identified endogenous cardiomyocyte surface markers for cell sorting was also limited by either low abundance of cardiac-specific proteins and/or poor antibody avidity (Mummery, 2010; Rust et al.,

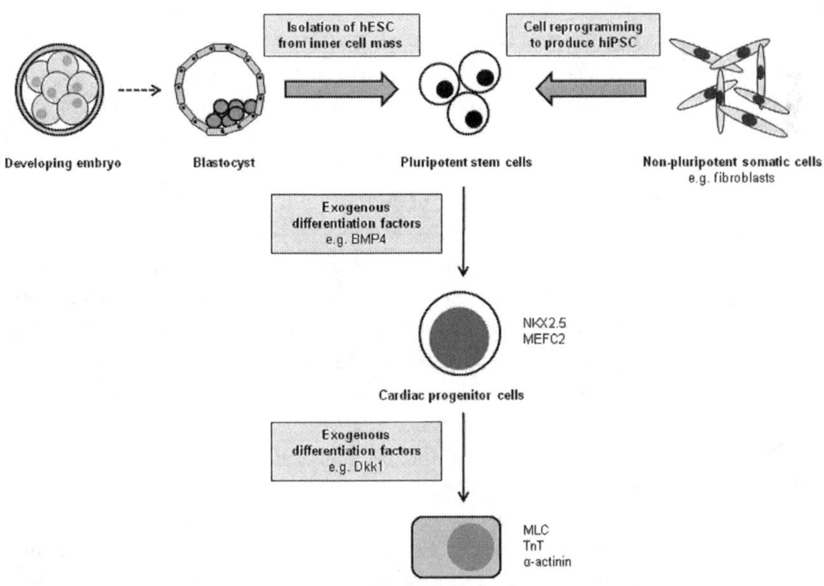

FIGURE 1 Differentiation of human pluripotent stem cells into cardiomyocytes with expression of stage-specific transcription factors. BMP4, bone morphogenetic protein; Dkk1, dickkopf homolog 1; MLC, myosin light chain; TnT, troponin T.

2009; Van Hoof et al., 2010), though the recently identified cardiomyocyte-specific cell surface marker, signal-regulatory protein alpha (SIRPA), is a promising candidate resulting in isolated populations of up to 98% cardiac troponin T-positive cells (Dubois et al., 2011). Another method of cardiomyocyte enrichment uses genetic modification of hESC to positively select for cardiomyocytes with expressed reporter and/or marker genes or negatively select against non-cardiomyocyte proliferating cells within the EBs using a suicide gene (Andersson et al., 2010). Combination of both positive and negative selections resulted in an enrichment of cardiomyocytes to nearly 100% (Xu et al., 2008b). A simpler non-genetic method uses fluorescence-activated cell sorting (FACS) of differentiating EBs stained with a reversible mitochondrial dye, as cardiomyocytes have much more mitochondria than non-cardiac cells (Hattori et al., 2010). This resulted in a purity of hPSC-derived cardiomyocytes (hPSC-CM) of more than 99%.

Studies directly comparing the characteristics of cardiomyocytes differentiated from hESC and hiPSC have reported close similarities in gene expression profile, electrophysiological properties and response to cardioactive drugs (Yokoo et al., 2009; Zhang et al., 2009), although hiPSC generally have a more impaired differentiation potential compared with hESC (Yoshida & Yamanaka, 2011).

The differentiation of hPSC into beating cardiomyocytes in terms of gene expression have been shown to be similar to the developing heart *in vivo*, with down-regulation of pluripotency markers such as Oct4 and Nanog, and up-regulation of cardiac transcription factors such as NK2 transcription factor-related (NKX2.5) and myocyte enhancer factor 2C (MEFC2C), genes encoding structural proteins such as myosin heavy polypeptide 7 (MYH7) (Anderson et al., 2007; Beqqali et al., 2006) and cardiac ion channels (Honda et al., 2011). Immunofluorescence studies also show the presence of cardiac structural proteins such as α-actinin and myosin light chain but the cardiomyocytes have relatively disorganized sarcomeric striations with multi-angular appearance, similar to the human fetal cardiac phenotype (Xu et al., 2002). In contrast, adult cardiomyocytes have a rod-shaped morphology and organized sarcomeric striations (Mummery et al., 2007; Snir et al., 2003; Xu et al., 2002). hESC-CM also lack a developed T tubule system, typically found in the mature phenotype (Snir et al., 2003). Additionally, they have been shown electrophysiologically to behave like 16-week-old fetal human ventricular cardiomyocytes (Mummery et al., 2003), have a low resting membrane potential (Braam et al., 2010) and display immaturity of intracellular calcium handling (Satin et al., 2008).

However, as hPSC-CM can be maintained in culture for at least 5 months, maturation of the cardiomyocytes can be induced if required. It has been shown that the number and organization of myofibrils increases with time, and beyond day 50 of culture, a high degree of sarcomeric organization is seen, with occasional formation of a T tubule system, indicating a phenotype compatible with a mature cardiomyocyte (Baharvand et al., 2004; Snir et al., 2003). It has been postulated that discrepancies of recorded upstroke velocities in hESC-CM may be caused by increasing contribution from the developing cardiac sodium channel, as a consequence of increasing time in culture (Mummery et al., 2003; Sartiani et al., 2007; Satin et al., 2004). Similarly, calcium handling by the sarcoplasmic reticulum (SR) also increases with maturation (Tohse et al., 2004), which may account for reported differences in the pharmacologic response of hESC-CM to SR modulators of caffeine, ryanodine and thapsigargin. However, the discrepancies are likely to be secondary to differences in the hESC lines used, differentiation and culture protocols employed and the architecture of the cardiomyocytes being assessed (Dick et al., 2010).

The relative immaturity of the hPSC-CM may ultimately not matter, as long as the cellular model is able to predict clinical outcome. Two recent reviews which neatly summarize the pharmacological tests performed on both hESC- and hiPSC-derived cardiomyocytes, show the potential utility of hPSC-CM in drug toxicology and safety pharmacology (Dick et al., 2010; Laposa, 2011).

B. Application of hPSC-CM in Cardiotoxicity Studies

Forty-three compounds, representing a variety of pharmacologic classes have been shown to affect hESC-CM as expected based on microscopic evaluations of beat alterations and electrophysiological changes detected using microelectrode arrays (MEAs) and patch clamp (Dick et al., 2010). Although there are fewer studies using hiPSC-CM for pharmacological research, at least 19 compounds have clinically correlated chronotropic and electrophysiological responses (Laposa, 2011). The drugs evaluated span a variety of pharmacologic classes including adrenoceptor agonists and antagonists, muscarinic receptor agonists, acetylcholine inhibitors, calcium channel inhibitors, hERG potassium channel inhibitor, phosphodiesterase inhibitor, sodium channel inhibitors and multiple ion channel blockers, amongst others (Dick et al., 2010; Laposa, 2011). Therefore, although derived *in vitro*, hPSC-CM show good predictivity of clinically observed cardiotoxicity that make them useful tools in drug discovery and safety pharmacology.

To fully assess the potential of hPSC-CM in their utility for drug toxicology, a few critical comparisons are required (Wobus & Loser, 2011), including sophisticated dose–response studies, examining the drug responses on hPSC-CM at concentrations measured in patients under treatment. Direct comparisons with currently used *in vitro* and *in vivo* models are also required to demonstrate its competency. One such detailed dose–response analysis study showed that the serum levels in patients of drugs with known QT interval effects corresponded to prolonged field potential duration in hESC-CM as detected by MEAs (Braam et al., 2010). Although more such studies are required, the potential wider application of hPSC-CM has already attracted the attention of the pharmaceutical industry with a commercially prepared hiPSC-CM product available from Cellular Dynamics International. A recent proof-of-concept study also highlighted the potential application of hPSC-CM for drug screening in a high-throughput format (Guo et al., 2011). A functional assay employing a monolayer of beating hiPSC-CM in 96-well plates with interdigitated electrode arrays was used to assess the electrophysiological changes induced by 28 different compounds with known cardiac effects. The results from the set of compounds tested were then used to construct an index of drug-induced arrhythmias, enabling potential assessment of an NCE drug candidate's proarrythmic potential.

An advantage of hiPSC-CM compared with hESC-CM is the potential use in safety pharmacology for selecting optimal medication for specific patients or patient cohorts. This was shown in a recent study where hiPSC-CM carrying a congenital long QT syndrome type 2 mutation developed early after depolarizations to the clinically used stressor isoprenaline, and reversed by the β-blocker nadolol, which was used as the patient's therapy (Matsa et al., 2011). The authors concluded that the patient's hiPSC-CM responded appropriately to clinically relevant pharmacology, and will be a valuable human *in vitro* model for disease modeling and individualizing drug testing. From the drug screening perspective, the possibility of generating a library of hiPSC-CM reflecting the pharmacogenetic variation of the human population is a very attractive proposition.

Another potential application of hiPSC-CM is in unraveling the mechanisms of a cardiac disorder. hiPSC-CM from patients with the rare autosomal dominant LEOPARD syndrome were used to study its pathophysiology with the cardiomyocytes *in vitro* showing characteristic hypertrophy, consistent with cardiac hypertrophy commonly encountered in this patient group (Carvajal-Vergara et al., 2010). Through its ability to model these genetically characterized diseases *in vitro*, patient-specific hiPSC-CM may allow deeper understanding of disease mechanisms, and hence potential novel drug targets.

Most studies on cardiotoxicity using hPSC-CM have so far focused largely on detection of electrophysiological changes. However, cardiac toxicity is an important complication of many drugs, including high-dose chemotherapy (Albini et al., 2010). The mechanisms in cardiac damage induced by anti-cancer drugs include direct damage to the cardiomyocytes through alterations of cellular signaling, stimulation of free radical production or conduction alterations secondary to massive histamine release (Albini et al., 2010). One such example of anti-cancer drug-induced cardiac damage is trastuzumab (Herceptin), used as a monoclonal antibody therapy against the HER-2 membrane protein that is overexpressed in certain breast cancers. Its use resulted in cardiac failure in 4% of patients, with a higher incidence in patients given anthracyclines concurrently (Chien, 2006). Although the exact target of the cardiac effects of trastuzumab is unclear, its cardiotoxicity was not detected before phase III clinical trials, again emphasizing the paucity of reliable predictive models for cardiotoxicity. The evaluation of non-electrophysiological cardiac side effects has also been hampered by a lack of agreed surrogate endpoints and the lack of adequate pre-clinical test systems (Wobus & Loser, 2011). There have been recent efforts to address these issues. Human cardiac troponins and cardiac natriuretic peptides have been proposed as biomarkers of cardiac damage induced by chemotherapeutic agents (Dolci et al., 2008), while an hESC-CM-based assay to detect release of troponin T and fatty acid binding protein 3 from doxorubicin-induced cardiac necrosis, has been described (Andersson et al., 2010). However, more studies evaluating the utility of hPSC-CM for the detection and quantification of non-electrophysiological cardiomyocyte derangements are needed.

hPSC-CM show great potential as a tool for drug safety evaluation and toxicology studies, with hiPSC-CM increasingly used for disease modeling and to aid understanding of pathophysiology with potential new therapeutic targets identified as a consequence. Preliminary studies on the application of hPSC-CM specifically for drug safety evaluation have largely shown them to have high clinical prediction of cardiotoxicity effects, though more sophisticated dose–response studies are needed to confirm this. However, some practical issues remain to be resolved. Firstly, efficient differentiation and enrichment protocols are needed to routinely obtain pure populations of hPSC-CM, though recently reported methods are highly encouraging (Burridge et al., 2011; Hattori et al., 2010). Secondly, their application in drug safety evaluation and drug toxicology needs to be scalable using a robust high-throughput format. A recent proof-of-concept study is encouraging (Guo et al., 2011), but unless scalability can be achieved, any refinement of the hPSC-CM as a cellular model for drug safety testing is unlikely to be widely applicable, especially in the pharmaceutical industry.

IV. The Use of Human Stem Cells in Hepatotoxicity

Current research in hepatic toxicology and safety pharmacology is focused on improving the existing *in vitro* cellular models with a view to enhancing their reliability in toxicity prediction and metabolic pathway delineations (Table I). In part, the demand for these improvements stems from ADRs as a consequence of the liver's role in drug metabolism and excretion. As such, ADRs are commonly caused by toxicity as a result of drug-induced liver injury (DILI) (Baillie & Rettie, 2011) (see Fig. 2).

The liver is a highly complex multicellular organ with a wide range of interacting cell types *in vivo*. Whilst drugs are tested pre-clinically using

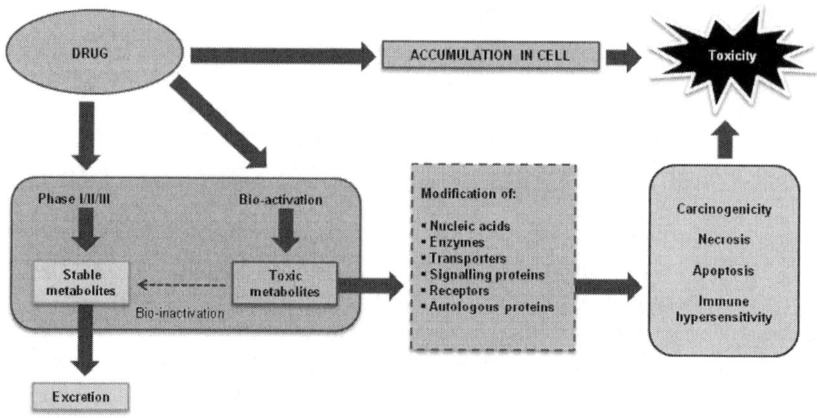

FIGURE 2 Schematic diagram of drug-induced liver injury.

established *in vitro* and *in vivo* models derived from either human or rodent sources, there are well-understood inter-species differences in liver metabolism with consequent difficulties in accurately extrapolating pre-clinical data to the clinic, making current investigative models sub-optimal in predicting ADRs as a result of DILI (Olson et al., 2000). Many drugs fail once human trials are initiated, or have to be removed from the market post-licensing following the identification of hepatotoxicity.

A. Current Models of Hepatotoxicity

The current human cellular system of choice for most drug safety screening is the primary human hepatocyte (PHH). This offers a more physiologically relevant model of a human liver cell, allowing for increased reliability in metabolic and toxicity testing. This model has benefited from recent advances in cryopreservation and culture techniques which have improved human hepatocyte availability for testing (Hang et al., 2011). Other enhancements have included co-culture of hepatocytes with other cells forming multi-cellular models, in an attempt to emulate physiological interactions of hepatocytes with other cells *in vivo*, some of which are implicated in DILI, as well as to improve on hepatocyte quality and longevity (Salerno et al., 2011). However, despite these efforts, PHH remains a sub-optimal system for drug safety screening. Phenotypic changes of PHH during cell culture result in the loss of differentiated features associated with hepatocytes (Elaut et al., 2006), particularly the loss of inducible cytochrome P450 (CYP) enzymes (Park et al., 1996). The cell therefore has a reduced capacity to be induced by transcription factors and nuclear receptors, compromising drug metabolism and diminishing model effectiveness (Goldring et al., 2004, 2006; Itoh et al., 1995, 1997). The difficulties in maintaining PHH in culture over a long term also means that drug exposure over greater lengths of time cannot be carried out, which is problematic as long exposure times are thought to be one of the main causes of drug toxicity (Elaut et al., 2006). Fresh PHH are also not readily accessible and can suffer from a lack of quality when obtainable (Baxter et al., 2010). Additionally, an inability to represent more than one stage of hepatocyte maturity and the diversity of phenotypes in the population make the PHH model inadequate (Ponsoda et al., 2001). One example of this is the CYP3A isoforms, along with other CYP enzymes, which are differentially expressed throughout the population. Therefore PHH from one individual would be unable to capture all these phenotypic variations in culture (Ingelman-Sundberg et al., 2007).

Hepatocellular carcinoma-derived cell lines are also commonly used as hepatic models. They offer advantages over PHH due to possessing clonal characteristics, making culture comparatively easy (Baxter et al., 2010; Castell et al., 2006). These cell lines are readily available and are popular for examining specific isotopes of enzymes and for simple transfection (Aoyama et al., 2009; Goldring et al., 2006). However, due to a combination of cellular abnormalities, the loss of complete metabolic pathways including CYP enzymes, and up-regulation of tumor associated genes, results taken from these lineages can be unreliable (Baxter et al., 2010). These cell lines also suffer from a lack of genomic variation (Anson et al., 2011). Recent work investigating the differences between PHH and hepatocellular carcinoma lineages has revealed differences in the activity of growth factor receptors and intracellular kinase cascades in response to different ligands, particularly IR, PI3K, AKT, and NF-κB (Saez-Rodriguez et al., 2011). This is especially relevant for safety pharmacology as these pathways are related to inflammation and cytokine release; therefore using hepatocellular carcinoma cell lines which display different responses to the human condition for screening ADRs, provide obvious concerns (Birrell et al., 2005; Podolin et al., 2005).

B. Production and Characterization of Hepatocyte-like Cells from hPSC

Whilst the aforementioned models reflect the best currently available systems for screening ADRs caused by NCE, there have been huge efforts to develop new models from PSC in order to improve the lead optimization of new compounds and to counteract the disadvantages associated with PHH and hepatocellular carcinoma cell lines.

Of the two forms of hPSC, the hESC have been available for longer and thus a greater body of work in relation to hepatocyte-like cell generation. Studies into deriving hepatocytes from hESC have been based around existing knowledge of cascades in normal liver development. This is split into three main stages – definitive endoderm differentiation, hepatocyte progenitor specification and hepatocyte maturation. The first technique established utilized the formation of EBs (Hamazaki et al., 2001). Once plated, this can act to imitate gastrulation, followed by the differentiation of hESC and commitment to a cell type. This process is, however, random and thus suffers from low efficiency (Kubo et al., 2004; Momose et al., 2009; Soto-Gutiérrez et al., 2006). To combat this, studies have examined numerous avenues of research including the replacement of EBs with direct stimulation of hESC in culture and increasing the specificity of cell lineage differentiation. This is augmented by the addition of exogenous factors associated with each of the stages of hepatic development to stimulate the cells toward a hepatocyte lineage (see Fig. 3). During initial definitive endoderm differentiation, cells have been subjected to the addition of Wnt3a and activin A to imitate Wnt and Nodal signalings, whilst PI3K inhibitors are also added to prevent PI3K-associated endoderm differentiation inhibition (Cai et al., 2007; McLean et al., 2007; Nakanishi et al., 2009; Zhao et al., 2009). A recent paper has suggested that rapid hepatocyte-like cell induction can be achieved through the addition of HGF (hepatocyte growth factor) at this stage, although further examination regarding the functional ability of these cells must be obtained (Chen et al., 2011). Following the expression of GATA4, FOXA2 and SOX17, hepatocyte specification is induced via the addition of fibroblast growth factor 4 (FGF2/4) and bone morphogenetic protein 4 (BMP2/4), dependent upon the protocol used (Cai et al., 2007; Chung et al., 2008; D'Amour et al., 2005; Gouon-Evans et al., 2006). These factors are commonly found during hepatic development from the septum transversum and the cardiac mesoderm and are thought to induce alpha-fetoprotein

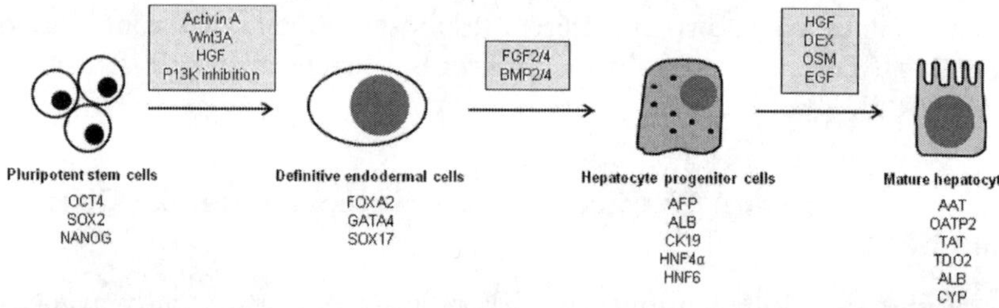

FIGURE 3 Schematic diagram of the differentiation of human pluripotent stem cells into hepatocyte-like cells, including the typical exogenous differentiation factors required (in shaded boxes) and gene expressions associated with each stage of development. OCT4, octamer-binding transcription factor 4; SOX2, sex determining region Y-box 2; NANOG, homeobox protein nanOg; FOXA2, forkhead box protein 2; SOX17, sex determining region Y-box 17; AFP, alpha-fetoprotein; ALB, albumin; CK19, cytokeratin-19; HNF4α, hepatocyte nuclear factor 4 alpha; HNF6, hepatocyte nuclear factor 6; AAT, alpha-1-antitrypsin; OATP2, organic anion transporting polypeptide 2; TAT, tyrosine transaminase; TDO2, tryptophan 2,3-dioxygenase; CYP, cytochrome P450s; HGF, hepatocyte growth factor; FGF, fibroblast growth factor; BMP, bone morphogenetic protein; DEX, dexamethasone; OSM, oncostatin M; EGF, epidermal growth factor.

(AFP), albumin, cytokeratin-19 (CK19), HNF4α and HNF6 (hepatocyte nuclear factor) gene expression (Baxter et al., 2010; Lavon & Benvenisty, 2005; Soto-Gutierrez et al., 2007; Tanimizu & Miyajima, 2004). The final step in inducing hepatocytes from hepatocyte progenitor cells is the addition of HGF, oncostatin M (OSM) and dexamethasone (DEX), which act to induce maturation and stimulate expression of metabolic enzymes associated with a mature hepatocyte (Duanmu et al., 2002; Kamiya et al., 2001). A mature hepatocyte-like phenotype can be distinguished through CYP, albumin, alpha-1-antitrypsin (AAT), organic anion transporting polypeptide 2 (OATP2), tyrosine transaminase (TAT) and tryptophan 2,3-dioxygenase (TDO2) gene expression (Basma et al., 2009; Cai et al., 2007; Chiao et al., 2008; Duan et al., 2007; Ishii et al., 2008; Zhao et al., 2009). More recently, the use of the small molecule 1m, a glycogen synthase kinase 3 inhibitor, was shown to be an effective inducer of ESC toward a population of hepatocyte-like cells (Burridge et al., 2011). In this study, alpha-fetoprotein and HNF4α expressions were observed indicating a hepatocyte progenitor phenotype, with the capacity to differentiate further into hepatocyte-like cells capable of producing albumin.

In addition to exogenous factors, other techniques have been employed in order to improve differentiation efficiency. Co-culture with various cell types has been implemented to replicate the *in vivo* condition. Studies have shown this approach to be possible with cardiac cells, various mesoderm cell lineages, non-parenchymal liver lineages and feeder cells which produce growth factors required for hepatocyte differentiation (Chung et al., 2008; Fair et al., 2003; Kang et al., 2004; Lavon et al., 2004; Pei et al., 2009). This is also particularly important as cell-to-cell interactions are now widely accepted to have an important role in the manifestation of DILI (Salerno et al., 2011). The utility of extracellular matrix has also been identified in various studies. Three-dimensional (3-D) models using collagen scaffolds, which mimic the *in vivo* condition of the collagen-filled septum transversum, have been shown to be an improvement to two-dimensional (2-D) matrix models (Baharvand et al., 2006; Hamazaki et al., 2001).

The relatively recent discovery of the functions of small non-coding micro RNA (miRNA) species (Lagos-Quintana et al., 2001) in governing cellular behavior is also important in this field. miRNA is thought to bind to the seed sequence of the untranslated 3′ region of the messenger RNA (mRNA) (Hafner et al., 2010; Karginov et al., 2007; Tan et al., 2007), to inhibit translation by inducing its degradation as part of a genome regulatory complex (Lin, 2011; Zhang & Su, 2009). They are also considered to be vital in maintaining ESC pluripotency (Li et al., 2009). miR-10a, miR-122 and miR-21 have all been shown to be abundant in hESC-derived hepatocytes, whilst miR-122 has also been described as relatively liver-specific and has been shown to be down-regulated in human hepatocellular carcinoma as it loses its hepatic phenotype with cancer progression (Coulouarn et al., 2009; Kim et al., 2011). This has sparked interest in the ability of miR-122 to induce and maintain a hepatic phenotype. A recent study has suggested that this miRNA interacts with liver-enriched transcription factors (LETFs), specifically HNF6, forming a positive feedback loop (Laudadio et al., 2011). HNF4 has also been found to regulate miR-122 expression in Huh7 cells (a well-differentiated hepatocellular carcinoma cell line) and mouse hepatocytes (Li et al., 2011). These studies demonstrate a huge untapped area for improved knowledge of hepatic differentiation, especially in the context of directed differentiation of hPSC toward functional hepatocytes.

Through transcriptomic analysis, Jozefczuk et al. (2011) have reported highly comparable metabolic and phenotypic characteristics between hepatocyte-like cells derived from hESC or hiPSC. However, they also differ in expression of CYP isoforms. Hepatocytes induced from hESC demonstrated enriched CYP19A1, CYP1A1, and CYP11A1 expression, whilst hiPSC-derived cells had enriched CYP46A1 and CYP26A1. Studies such as this are highly useful particularly when comparing the utility and efficiency between hESC- and iPSC-derived hepatocyte-like cells. However, it is imperative that for any given differentiation experiment using either sources, a full characterization of the resulting 'differentiated' hepatocyte-like cells should be carried out, particularly by analysis of hepatic phenotype markers through gene expression analysis, functional assays and activity analyses, against PHH which is currently considered as the 'gold standard' of hepatic model systems, as this will determine the 'success' of a hepatic differentiation experiment. Several groups have over the years reported differentiation protocols that they claim to have yielded hepatocyte-like cells that were able to simulate DILI *in vivo*, though full characterization against relevant controls and comparators such as PHH are often missing (Yildirimman et al., 2011), making it difficult to determine whether these hepatocyte-like cells are better than the current 'gold standard'. It is therefore important to map where these hepatocyte-like cells fit within the hepatic model systems now available, with the human hepatocarcinoma cell line HepG2 being one of the most metabolically redundant and the PHH being the most physiologically relevant *in vitro* model of a hepatocyte so far (see Fig. 4).

With regards to using iPSC, the differentiation of hiPSC into hepatocyte-like cells is still a relatively new process. However, it has been achieved by several groups, using similar mechanisms with comparable efficiency of differentiation to using hESC, with only slight differences in genotypic and functional characteristics (Si-Tayeb et al., 2010; Song et al., 2009; Sullivan et al., 2010). However, recent studies have also reported ESC to possess multiple self-replicating genes whilst iPSC contain fewer tumor suppressing genes along with duplications of genes associated with tumorigenesis (Laurent et al., 2011), demonstrating imperfections in both cell types. This reiterates the need for work to continue in refining differentiation protocols

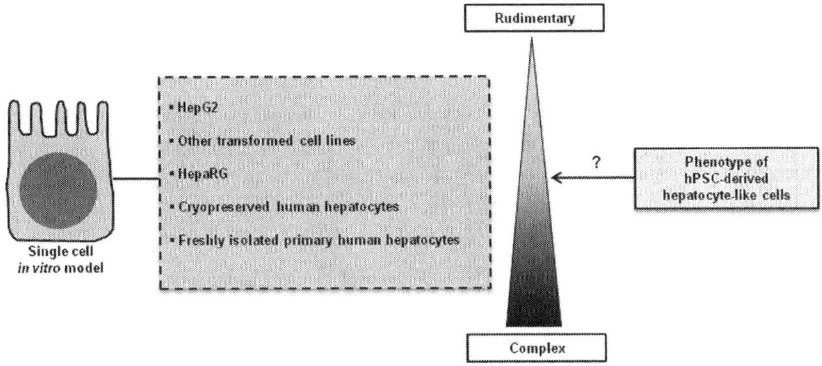

FIGURE 4 It is important to map where hepatocyte-like cells lie amongst the available hepatic model systems, with the human hepatocarcinoma cell line HepG2 being one of the most metabolically redundant and the PHH being the most physiologically relevant in vitro model of a hepatocyte.

using hESC or iPSC to achieve the most accurate hepatocyte-like phenotype possible.

hiPSC offer a unique ability to model metabolic disorders and as such, is a hugely exciting prospect for hepatotoxicity screening. In order to recognize the validity of hiPSC for use in drug safety, metabolic studies and clinical use, it is important to understand the mechanisms used to induce pluripotency from somatic cells. The first iPSC were developed in 2006 through retroviral insertion of the pluripotency genes Oct4, Sox2, Klf4 and c-Myc (Takahashi & Yamanaka, 2006). However, this approach was limited by the relatively low colony forming efficiency of 0.2–0.8% (Huangfu et al., 2008), along with tumorigenic potential due to genomic insertions close to oncogenes (González et al., 2011). Since then, several different approaches have been developed for inducing pluripotency by attempting to modify and adapt the original technique through the use of different delivery methods. These methods are however still limited by low efficiency rates, the use of viral vectors, the need for genome insertion and highly complex protocols and therefore have remained sub-optimal (Miyoshi et al., 2011). This is especially important with regards to the demands of high-throughput screening of compounds, which would require high yields of genetically uncompromised cells with a high purity for reliable investigations.

An alternative technique with the hope of addressing these concerns is the expression of miRNAs to induce pluripotency. The use of the miRNA cluster miR302/367 has been shown to induce pluripotency in embryonic mouse fibroblasts with a two-order of magnitude increase in efficiency when compared with the Yamanaka technique (Anokye-Danso et al., 2011; Takahashi & Yamanaka, 2006). Whilst these results demonstrate large improvements in optimal efficiency, the technique still uses a viral vector for delivery. A direct approach using miRNAs without any viral vector has since been reported by utilizing repeated transfection of human adipose stromal cells and dermal fibroblasts with mir-200c, mir-302s and mir-369s to produce hiPSC (Miyoshi et al., 2011). However, they describe efficiency levels close to that of the Yamanaka technique (Miyoshi et al., 2011; Takahashi & Yamanaka, 2006). This represents a small step forward in hiPSC generation as it allows a relatively simple protocol to be used without the use of a viral vector, allowing for genomic stability. However, it remains to be seen whether this technique can be optimized to improve efficiency, with a view to scaling up production of hiPSC-derived hepatocytes for use in drug toxicology.

Both techniques using miRNAs are thought to induce pluripotency in somatic cells through the use of both acceleration of mesenchymal-to-epithelial transition through inhibition of the TGF-β signaling pathway, and the inhibition of mRNAs associated with epigenetic regulation (Liao et al., 2011; Subramanyam et al., 2011). These epigenetic regulators include Meox2, AOF2/1, LSD1/2, KDM1/1B, DNMT1 and MECP1/2 (Lin et al., 2011; Pfaff et al., 2011; Subramanyam et al., 2011). However, whilst this process causes demethylation of the genome and 'resetting' of the epigenetic clock, these derived cells may still retain an epigenetic memory (Barrilleaux & Knoepfler, 2011), perhaps due to incomplete reprogramming during transformation from a differentiated somatic state to iPSC. During this time, CpG dinucleotides accounting for DNA methylation, fall from nearly 100% to 20–30% of the total in iPSC (Lister et al., 2011). Incomplete reprogramming is particularly common during early derivation and in some cases may lead to improper differentiation into unrelated cell lineages (Lister et al., 2011; Pick et al., 2009; Polo et al., 2010; Stadtfeld et al., 2010). One theory suggests that isolated genes are less efficient at engaging silencing mechanisms during early passage, resulting in incomplete reprogramming (Ohi et al., 2011). However, whilst this remains possible, epigenetic faults have been found following differentiation and may possibly persist in re-differentiated cell types from iPSC (Lister et al., 2011). Despite the mechanisms remaining incompletely explained, this phenomenon paradoxically raises the possibility of utilizing the incomplete reprogramming to improve the efficiency, quality and purity of iPSC differentiation (Barrilleaux & Knoepfler, 2011). This has been demonstrated in pancreatic β cells, with improved efficiency of differentiation into the parental cell type (Bar-Nur et al., 2011). Thus, it has been postulated that this approach may be applied to create hepatocytes with desired phenotypes at a much greater efficiency, purity and quality (Wobus & Loser, 2011).

In relation to disease modeling, a recent study has demonstrated that it is possible to take a parental hepatocyte with a metabolic disorder, induce pluripotency and re-differentiate into a hepatocyte-like cell with the retained diseased phenotype. This has been shown in alpha-1-antitrypsin (AAT) deficiency, familial hypercholesterolemia, glycogen storage disease type 1α, tyrosinemia, progressive familial hereditary cholestasis and Crigler–Najjar syndrome, which points toward the exciting possibility of modeling specific disease phenotypes for new therapeutic targets (Ghodsizadeh et al., 2010; Rashid et al., 2010). In support of the therapeutic potential of hiPSC in liver diseases, zinc-finger nucleases (ZFN) and piggyBac technology in hiPSC can correct a point mutation in the AAT gene, with subsequent restoration of function using hepatocytes derived from these cells. This demonstrates the clinical benefits that hiPSC can potentially offer in future medicine (Yusa et al., 2011).

C. Application of hPSC-Derived Hepatocyte-like Cells in Hepatotoxicity Studies

These developments offer real hope for the use of hPSC in hepatotoxicity studies to produce hepatocyte-like cells representing the phenotypic variations of the population. However, it is important to firstly examine the differentiated cells' ability to behave like a primary hepatocyte, particularly in the metabolism of drug compounds. Specific markers of differentiation to a hepatic lineage need to be present. These include functional abilities such as urea and albumin secretion along with markers such as CYPs, tyrosine amino-transferase (TAT) and tryptophan-oxygenase (TO) amongst others (Snykers et al., 2009). Indocyanine green can also be used as a hepatocyte-specific dye-marker as this should only be taken up and secreted by hepatocytes (Cooke et al., 1963).

Hepatic metabolic enzymes can be split into two main groups, phase I and phase II. The most common phase I enzyme group is the CYP family which has been associated with the formation of reactive metabolites and is therefore linked to DILI, making the presence of CYP enzymes vitally important for drug metabolism studies. Studies of CYP in hPSC have produced varied results. For example, transcripts of certain isoforms of CYP3A4 have been shown to vary in comparison to primary hepatocytes by over 300% between studies (Basma et al., 2009; Brolén et al., 2010; Ek et al., 2007; Shiraki et al., 2008). Whilst these studies exhibit CYP3A4 expression below that of a primary hepatocyte, several different factors are likely to be responsible. A recent review suggested that the quality of primary hepatocytes, being used as reference cells, may be one of the causes of large variations between studies (Wobus & Loser, 2011). CYP3A4 activity have been demonstrated in hepatocyte-like cells derived from hESC in further studies, through the conversion of testosterone to 6-beta-hydroxytestosterone, suggesting this pathway to be active. Stimulation with rifampin and midazolam has been shown to induce CYP3A4 levels close to that of HepG2 cells (Agarwal et al., 2008). A large body of research has focused upon the ability of CYP in hepatocyte-like cells to metabolize known compounds, with results suggesting detectable metabolic activity despite variations in results (Basma et al., 2009; Hay et al., 2008; Moore & Moghe, 2009; Touboul et al., 2010). These studies have included the use of the pentoxyresorufin-O-dealkylase assays (Cai et al., 2007), whereas other groups have demonstrated CYP activity with mRNA expression, specific proteins and drug transporters (Ek et al., 2007). Using ultra performance liquid chromatography tandem mass spectrometry (UPLC–MS–MS), Duan et al. (2010) measured the activity of four well-established human CYPs (CYP1A2, CYP2C9, CYP3A4 and CYP2D6) and also carried out a metabolite profiling study based on the known metabolism of bufuralol (BF), a non-selective β-adrenoceptor blocking agent. Results from these experiments indicated comparable metabolic activity of ESC-derived hepatocyte-like cells compared with PHH. Furthermore, four new metabolic pathways of BF in addition to the three that have been previously reported were identified, demonstrating as well the effectiveness of the differentiation protocol employed in this study. Other research has found active glutathione-S-transferases (GSTs), which have been shown to have an overall comparable activity to that of PHH, though examination of subunits have shown differential expression, including much lower expression of GSTM-1 (Söderdahl et al., 2007).

Very few studies have attempted to culture hepatocyte-like cells over a longer time period. This is an area which needs to be improved as many DILI are as a result of long term use of drug compounds. Of those relatively few studies, the results are varied. Hepatocyte-like cells undergo further maturation displaying increased AAT secretion, but still less than that of PHH (Shirahashi et al., 2004). Similar results were also found with albumin and CYP3A4 levels (Shiraki et al., 2008). However, there is concern that the cells may de-differentiate if cultured over long periods, and work must continue in order to fully understand the differentiation patterns of hepatocytes *in vitro* (Wobus & Loser, 2011).

ADRs, particularly the idiosyncratic type, are often due to inter-individual susceptibility to DILI. This is an important factor to consider when developing these model systems as hESC- or hiPSC-derived hepatocyte-like cells would have originated from one donor, thereby encapsulating genetic polymorphisms of that particular individual only. A panel or bank of hepatocyte-like cells from a randomly selected population of donors could be one possible strategy in addressing this but this will certainly require a significant amount of resource to investigate further.

V. The Use of Human Stem Cells in Neurotoxicity

Modeling of neurotoxicity is vital, since damage to neuronal cells during development often results in lifelong learning disabilities or mental retardation. Once developed, models of functional neurons can be used to screen NCE for their ability to cause damage to mature or developing neuronal tissue. Current models of neurotoxicity often involve immortalized or cancer-derived cell lines, although there is extensive work in animals and primary animal cell cultures (de Groot et al., 2005; Kang et al., 2001; Meamar et al., 2010; Park et al., 2010; Xu et al., 2010; Zimmer et al., 2011) (Table I). Primary human material is difficult to obtain since brain tissue does not regenerate in the same way as liver tissue after surgical resection. Fetal tissue can be used instead, but this raises ethical issues as well as problems with availability. Nevertheless, normal human neural progenitor cells are commercially available as a source of primary human fetal tissue, and have been shown to differentiate into functional and metabolically active neurons, astrocytes and oligodendrocytes in culture (Fritsche et al., 2005). Prior to the development of protocols to differentiate stem cells into specific neuronal cell types, the majority of neurotoxicity screening was carried out using immortalized cell lines taken from neuroblastomas and embryocarcinomas, or derived from primary neural tissue using a variety of techniques.

SK-N-SH and SK-N-MC cells were generated from a human neuroblastoma in 1973, which can be kept in culture for 1–2 years. SK-N-SH cells have been found to possess high dopamine-β-hydroxylase activity, the enzyme responsible for converting dopamine to norepinephrine in functional neuronal cells (Biedler et al., 1973; Weinshilboum, 1978). NTera2 (NT2) cells, which are similar to neural progenitor cells, are a commercially available cell line derived from an embryocarcinoma. They can be differentiated into dopaminergic neurons using RA, and have been shown to share a similar gene expression profile to hESC (Misiuta et al., 2006; Schwartz et al., 2005). NT2 cells have been used to screen for DNT using various established assays such as the MTT cell proliferation assay (Tada et al., 1986), assessment of their change in morphology and expression of specific transcription factors, using known teratogens and neurotoxins such as lithium, acrylamide, valproic acid and hydroxyurea (Johnson, 1998; LoPachin, 2004; Phiel et al., 2001; Yarbro, 1992). Another commercially available human neural progenitor cell line, ReNcell CX, derived from a 14-week gestation human fetal cortex, has also been used to develop a high-throughput screening assay for potential developmental neurotoxicants using proliferation and cell viability assays (Breier et al., 2008).

A. Application of Human Stem Cell-Derived Neuronal Cells for Neurotoxicity Studies

Significant progress has been made in the differentiation of stem cells to neuronal cells, particularly with an application in neurotoxicity studies. Protocols have been developed whereby hESC, human umbilical cord blood stem cells and human fetal tissue can be differentiated into progenitor and mature neuronal cells, whilst differentiated neural progenitor cells can now be maintained in culture for long periods (Buzanska et al., 2005; Vescovi et al., 1999). Further refinement of the differentiation protocol using neurotrophic growth factors NT3 and NT4, and also by maintaining cell contacts, have also been reported (Caldwell et al., 2001).

Though demonstration of toxicity using these models with typical neurotoxins is still in its early stages, some progress has been achieved. The human umbilical cord blood neural stem cell line (HUCB-NSC) developed by Buzanska et al. (2005) has been tested for its ability to model neurotoxicity at three stages of differentiation – undifferentiated, committed (2 weeks in culture in the absence of RA) and lineage-directed (2 weeks in culture in the presence of RA). The group used a panel of compounds including six known neurotoxins and two non-neurotoxins and analyzed the toxicity of these compounds on the cells using live/dead viability/cytotoxicity fluorescence assay (staining for markers of metabolic activity and plasma membrane integrity), MTT assay, resazurin reduction cell viability assay as well as nuclear chromatin staining and immunocytochemical labeling for markers of cell proliferation, apoptotic cell death and neural differentiation. This model was shown to be able to discriminate between neurotoxic and non-neurotoxic compounds, and the responses to the compounds correlated well with published observations of these compounds on PC12 cells (cell line derived from pheochromocytoma) and cerebellar granule cells. The study concluded that HUCB-NSCs are as sensitive as current models of neurotoxicity (Buzanska et al., 2009).

Several groups have also differentiated hESC into neuronal cells for toxicity screening (see Fig. 5). A common model neurotoxin, methylmercury

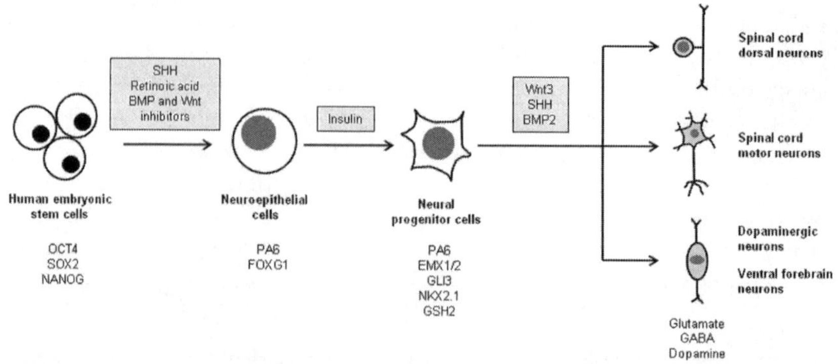

FIGURE 5 Schematic diagram of the differentiation of embryonic stem cells into defined neuronal cell types, including the typical exogenous differentiation factors required (in shaded boxes) and gene expressions associated with each stage of development. OCT4, octamer-binding transcription factor 4; SOX2, sex determining region Y-box 2; NANOG, homeobox protein nanOg; FOXG1, forkhead box protein G1; EMX1/2, homeobox transcription factors; GLI3, zinc-finger protein transcription factor; TTF1, thyroid transcription factor 1; GSH2, GS homeobox 2; SHH, sonic hedgehog; BMP, bone morphogenetic protein; GABA, γ-aminobutyric acid.

(MeHg) is used to test the predictivity of several differentiated neuronal cell lines. MeHg is an environmental toxin found in freshwater fish, which may cause toxicity through increased membrane lipoperoxidation and depletion of GSH. MeHg also increases *N*-methyl-D-aspartate receptors on SH-SY 5Y neuroblastoma cells (Clarkson, 1997; Ndountse & Chan, 2008; Sarafian & Verity, 1991). H1 cells (a hESC line) were differentiated to neuronal cells using a three-step differentiation protocol which involves plating derived progenitor cells on fibronectin in medium containing N-2 supplement, followed by a two-step maturation protocol using human recombinant glial-derived neurotrophic factor (Zhang et al., 2001). MeHg toxicity was tested using the resazurin cell viability assay and rtPCR of key neuronal cell markers nestin, NCAM1, NEUROD1 and MAP2. The study improved on a previously reported differentiation protocol (Zhang et al., 2001), and importantly showed that the use of cellular markers is more sensitive than a cytotoxicity assay alone. This study was also the first to show how MeHg affects different stages of differentiation to different degrees (Stummann et al., 2009). Another study by Yla-Outinen made use of the MEA to assay spontaneous electrical activity in neurospheres differentiated from hESC (Lappalainen et al., 2010). Use of this MEA technology is novel in this context. The assay is highly sensitive to changes in function before cell perturbation is seen, compared with the cytotoxicity assays (Yla-Outinen et al., 2010). However, the assay is plating-dependent so batch-to-batch variation is expected. Alongside the MEA assay, other toxicity endpoints used include rtPCR for the neuronal cell markers musashi and NF68, time-lapse imaging of cultures during exposure, ELISA for BrdU and Wst1 (cell proliferation assays), and immunocytochemistry for MAP2 and TUBBIII for neurons, GFAP for astrocytes and GALC for oligodendrites.

Following on from the early promise of using stem cell-derived neuronal cells for DNT, an hESC-derived cell line, hN2, is now commercially available as fully differentiated neuronal cells for toxicity screening. Harrill et al., (2010) tested the application of these cells using known neurite outgrowth inhibitors such as bisindolylmaleimide I, U0126, lithium, sodium orthovanadate and brefeldin A, and concluded that the hN2 model is as predictive of neurotoxicity as other animal models and human immortalized cell lines. The authors also opined that cell viability endpoints alone may not successfully predict a neurotoxicant, and should be coupled with other functional endpoints such as neurite outgrowth (Harrill et al., 2010).

Stem cell-derived neuronal cells have also been tested for their ability to predict neurotoxicity in a range of compounds for which neurotoxicity has not yet been established. Neural-committed stem cells were differentiated from hESC lines I6 and H9 using a five-step protocol which employed neural growth factors NEAA and N2. Differentiation to dopaminergic neurons was then carried out using medium conditioned on the PA6 stromal cell line. A collection of 720 FDA-approved drugs was tested in high-throughput format using an ATP assay. Potential hits such as amiodarone were assayed further, using a full dose–response curve and gene set enrichment analysis to identify pathways, molecular functions and biological processes perturbed by the administration of amiodarone. Pathway analysis was consistent with what is currently known about the mechanism of action of amiodarone (Han et al., 2009).

Another major benefit of the use of stem cell-derived neuronal cells is the ability to model diseases of neuronal dysfunction. A study using hESC lines BG01 and I6 differentiated to neuronal cells using mouse stromal P6 cells as feeder cells has attempted to model the features of Parkinson's disease (PD) using 1-methyl-4-phenylpyridinium (MPP^+), a drug which depletes dopaminergic neurons, mimicking the disease process in PD. It has also been suggested that PD may be caused by environmental toxins. The endpoints for cytotoxicity used in this study included LDH activity, immunocytochemistry for the apoptosis marker caspase-3 and formation of reactive oxygen species. Though this study is of value for the development of treatments for PD and other diseases associated with neuronal loss in the brain rather than toxicity screening of NCE, its findings may be applicable in predicting environmental toxins that cause damage to neuronal tissues and simulate mechanistic features of PD (Zeng et al., 2006).

In summary, development of the use of human stem cells as models for neurotoxicity is progressing using different starting cell types including hESC, HUCB-NSC and neural progenitor cell lines, and also by using newer model neurotoxicants. These *in vitro* models are also being tested for their capacity to predict neurotoxicity of drugs whose risk to neuronal tissue is not yet defined. Cell viability assays which are routinely used as an endpoint of neurotoxicity are still limited in their predictive capabilities. Combination of viability assays and analysis of other markers of cell health (functional markers, markers of apoptosis and cell death) is a more useful way of monitoring the effects of test compounds, as are functional assays such as neurite outgrowth and MEA to test for spontaneous electrical activity.

VI. Conclusion

The application of PSC in drug toxicology and safety pharmacology has enabled significant progress to be made in this area. In particular, the availability of hPSC brings us closer to bridging the gap when translating preclinical data to the clinical setting, an issue that has and continues to play a key role in the development of ADRs. Much work have demonstrated such progress through the use of these novel model systems, with some good correlations between *in vitro*, *in vivo* and clinical data, providing greater confidence in the predictive power of these novel stem cell-based model systems. Furthermore, the application of iPSC for disease modeling is an attractive proposition, while its potential as an alternative source of undifferentiated stem cells for use in mechanistic studies of disease states will serve to reduce derivation of hPSC from embryos.

Recently, the ability to directly convert from one cell lineage to another through lineage reprogramming or transcription factor-based trans-differentiation has been demonstrated in a number of studies. Reports include the direct conversion of human fibroblasts (Vierbuchen et al., 2010) and hepatocytes (Marro et al., 2011) into neuronal cells, the bi-directional trans-differentiation of pancreatic cells into hepatocytes (Eberhard et al., 2010; Shen & Tosh, 2010), and HepG2 cells into pancreatic-like cells which have been shown to produce insulin (Peran et al., 2011) . This technique is particularly advantageous over the traditional method of inducing pluripotency in somatic cells initially before differentiation into a different lineage, as it avoids the potentially tumorigenic state of PSC, as well as contamination within the reprogrammed population of cells by residual undifferentiated PSC (Wobus & Loser, 2011). As described earlier, this approach also provides an alternative source of human cell types which could ultimately reduce significantly or remove the need for sourcing ESC from human and animal embryos (Vierbuchen & Wernig, 2011).

The advent of PSC in combination with state-of-the-art analytical techniques have provided drug toxicology and safety pharmacology an incredibly rich resource and a large window of opportunity to carry out experiments that a decade or two ago would have been deemed unimaginable. These new systems require further refinement and optimization but most importantly, should be fully validated. Limitations of these systems should also be identified. Current and future validations of *in vitro* models for drug toxicity are likely to differ in accordance with the demands of which they are designed to meet. Within the area of developmental toxicity, attempts to validate the EST by several working groups that have been established solely for this purpose such as ReproTech (Genschow et al., 2004; Hareng et al., 2005; Marx-Stoelting et al., 2009) have collectively demonstrated that further refinement of this test for the screening of xenobiotic-induced developmental toxicity is required. Independent assessments of reference compounds with known toxicities using the EST have shown varying predictive accuracies of the EST method between laboratories. As such, there is yet no fully validated EST protocol that has been approved for regulatory registrations and risk assessments of NCE. However, modified versions of the EST according to the requirements of the user have been developed and are routinely used within the pharmaceutical industry as a tool to facilitate in the decision making on compounds during the early stages of drug discovery and development (Paquette et al., 2008). There is still however great interest in the development of a fully validated EST that is suitable for regulatory registrations and risk assessments. To assist in achieving this, a number of optimization strategies has been suggested by the pharmaceutical industry, academia and regulatory authorities. One such suggestion with reference to the original EST protocol is to drive the differentiation process from ESC into different lineages instead of generically driving the differentiation process toward a cardiac phenotype. Through this, the predictive power of the EST could be increased as the endpoint during the differentiation process will have more relevance depending on the compound(s) being tested as previously demonstrated with Thalidomide (Marx-Stoelting et al., 2009).

Similar to the current situation in the developmental toxicity arena, no hPSC-based *in vitro* cardiotoxicity assay has been formally validated yet, as some of the official test development criteria, such as the biological relevance of the hPSC-CM model, is not fulfilled (OECD). Although the hPSC-CM model with its fetal phenotype has been shown to predict the electrophysiological alterations similar to clinically detected electrocardiographic changes, the full impact on the toxicological response to cardiotoxicants, especially non-electrophysiological cellular cardiotoxicity, is not ascertained. A full characterization of the hPSC-CM against the gold standard of human primary cardiomyocytes in terms of functional assessment, as well as standardization of an agreed and reproducible differentiation protocol are still needed before formal validation of models using hPSC-CM can be considered. Similarly, for the purposes of toxicology research and screening of NCE by the pharmaceutical industry using hPSC-CM, reproducibility of the expressed phenotype is important and the detection of a panel of agreed markers will serve as internal validation of the hPSC-CM-based assay.

Given the difficulties which currently prevent the development of HLC from fully representing a model close to a PHH phenotype, choosing the correct assays to validate the HLCs' relevance for purpose is essential. Whilst not currently in use, it will be important for models used for the regulatory registration and risk assessment of new compounds in the pharmaceutical industry to be as metabolically similar to PHHs as possible particularly in regards to drug metabolism. Toxicity assays would therefore need to be thorough, examining major CYP and phase II metabolic pathways for signs of active metabolite formation over an extended culture period in comparison to an industry standard PHH, enabling acute and chronic modeling which are essential when attempting to simulate the clinical setting. Identification of resulting metabolites from modeled compounds would also need to be examined as, if reactive, may lead to DILI. Furthermore, the aforementioned panel representing the major variations in population phenotype would be required to provide additional toxicity assays for potential idiosyncratic ADRs to new compounds (Wobus & Löser, 2011). Conversely, similar but less thorough assays could be used in order to make quick internal decisions in regards to the initial development of the compound, with more emphasis being placed on functional endpoints rather than toxicity.

Thus far, the hPSC-derived models for neurotoxicity described above are not being used beyond proof-of-principle stage to model and predict neurotoxicity in an industrial setting. There is no consensus on differentiation protocols or endpoint assays, and there is evidence that plating variation between differentiated and partially differentiated cultures may impact on these models' utility.

Despite the advantages that both hESC and hiPSC provide, the unicellular *in vitro* models still do not fully recapitulate the most accurate and physiologically relevant conditions of the cells *in vivo*. Indeed, it is now becoming widely accepted that simple one-dimensional *in vitro* cell cultures are not fully representative of the physiological, biological and molecular interactions of a cell type with other surrounding cells within its environment. The liver for instance is a multi-cellular organ that is composed of a heterogenous population of cells including hepatocytes and non-parenchymal cells (NPCs). Mechanistic investigations on DILI have demonstrated the important role of multi-cellular interactions in the manifestation of liver injury such as that in inflammatory ADRs (Bourdi et al., 2002; Luyendyk et al., 2003), demonstrating that a single population of cells is not enough to detect ADRs for all drugs. This is a particularly important factor to consider during drug development as certain compounds requiring complex multi-cellular interactions to produce toxicity may be misclassified as 'safe'. Furthermore, the distribution of oxygen, defense molecules such as the antioxidant GSH, the expression of CYP and matrix interactions are just some of the many important factors to consider when assessing, understanding and predicting the toxic potential of an NCE. To address this specific concern, a new field to develop more relevant model systems replicating the *in vivo* environment has emerged.

2-D and 3-D cell culture systems have been developed to push the boundaries of the currently available models. 2-D cell culture systems involve the addition of NPCs as these cells have been shown to play an important role in the manifestation of DILI and survival and maintenance of the hepatic phenotype in culture (Bhandari et al., 2001; Kidambi et al., 2007; Uyama et al., 2002; Zinchenko et al., 2006). These positive effects have been reported to be due to cell-to-cell interactions as well as matrix and diffusible growth factors and cytokines secreted by NPCs (Fausto, 2000). Co-cultures of these two cell types have also been demonstrated and developed through micropatterning approaches, which allows cell-to-cell interactions to be more tightly and accurately regulated (Khetani & Bhatia, 2008). Further development using 3-D models has been made to improve survival and maintenance of a fully differentiated phenotype, as it encompasses additional factors that recapitulate the microenvironment of cells in vivo. The use of spheroids and multi-layer cell aggregates encourages further cell to cell interactions (Hoffman, 1993) and the 3-D architecture allows additional external inputs to add further complexity to the system (Roskelley et al., 1994). Bioreactors have been developed for culturing cells or tissues using a scaffold that allows the formation of tissue-like structures under continuous perfusion (Dash et al., 2009).

With the availability of human-derived cell-based models, complex and informative analytical techniques and the increasing refinement of 3-D platforms, research in drug toxicology and safety pharmacology has never been in a better position. However, the full validation of model systems using hPSC-derived cell types that recapitulate the full cellular function of mature phenotypes for application in drug toxicology and safety pharmacology, remains an elusive but tantalizingly close goal.

Conflict of Interest: The authors have no conflict of interest to declare.

Abbreviations

COX2	cyclooxygenase 2
GSH	gluthatione
ADRs	adverse drug reactions
NHS	National Health Service
hESC	human embryonic stem cells
ESC	embryonic stem cells
PSC	pluripotent stem cells
iPSC	induced pluripotent stem cells
hPSC	human pluripotent stem cells
OECD	Organization for Economic Co-operation and Development
EU	European Union
REACH	Registration, Evaluation, Authorization and Restriction of Chemical substances
EVCAM	European Centre for Validation of Alternative Methods
MM	micromass
WEC	whole-embryo culture
EST	embryonic stem cell test
FBS	fetal bovine serum
PM	prediction model
mESC	mouse embryonic stem cells
EPA	Environmental Protection Agency
CoA	coenzyme A
MAP2	microtubule-associated protein 2
TUBBIII	class III beta tubulin
TNNT2	troponin T type 2
COLIA1	collagen, type I, alpha 1
COL1A2	collagen, type I, alpha 2
DNT	developmental neurotoxicity
RA	retinoic acid

NCE	new chemical entities
TdP	torsade de pointes
CHO	Chinese-hamster ovary
hiPSC	human induced pluripotent stem cells
EBs	embryoid bodies
SIRPA	signal-regulatory protein alpha
FACS	fluorescence-activated cell sorting
hPSC-CM	hPSC-derived cardiomyocytes
NKX2.5	NK2 transcription factor-related
MEF2C	myocyte enhancer factor 2C
MYH7	myosin heavy polypeptide 7
hESC-CM	hESC-derived cardiomyocytes
SR	sarcoplasmic reticulum
MEA	microelectrode array
hERG	human ether-a-go-go-related gene
hiPSC-CM	hiPSC-derived cardiomyocytes
DILI	drug-induced liver injury
PHH	primary human hepatocyte
CYP	cytochrome P450
IR	phosphatidylinositol 3-kinases
NF-κB	nuclear factor kappa-light-chain-enhancer of activated B cells
OCT4	octamer-binding transcription factor 4
SOX2	sex determining region Y-box 2
FOXA2	forkhead box protein 2
FGF	fibroblast growth factor
BMP	bone morphogenetic protein
SOX17	sex determining region Y-box 17
AFP	alpha-fetoprotein
CK19	cytokeratin-19
OSM	oncostatin M
HNF4α	hepatocyte nuclear factor 4 alpha
HNF6	hepatocyte nuclear factor 6
3-D	three-dimensional
2-D	two-dimensional
miRNA	micro ribonucleic acid
miR	micro ribonucleic acid
mRNA	messenger RNA
LETFs	liver-enriched transcription factors
Klf4	Krüppel-like factor 4
TGF-β	transforming growth factor beta
AOF	amine oxidase (flavin containing)
LSD	lysine specific demethylase
KDM	lysine demethylase

DNMT1	DNA (cytosine-5)-methyltransferase 1
DNA	deoxyribonucleic acid
AAT	alpha-1-antitrypsin
ZFN	zinc-finger nucleases
TAT	tyrosine amino-transferase
TO	tryptophan-oxygenase
BF	bufuralol
GSTs	glutathione-S-transferases
GSTM-1	glutathione-S-transferase mu 1
NT2	NTera2
MTT	3-(4,5-dimethylthiazol-2-yl)-2,5-diphenyltetrazolium bromide
HUCB-NSC	human umbilical cord blood neural stem cell
MeHg	methylmercury
NEUROD1	neurogenic differentiation 1
MAP2	microtubule-associated protein 2
rtPCR	reverse transcription polymerase chain reaction
ELISA	enzyme-linked immunosorbent assay
NF68	68kDa neurofilament
BrdU	bromodeoxyuridine
GFAP	glial fibrillary acidic protein
GALC	galactosylceramidase
ATP	adenosine triphosphate
MPP^+	1-methyl-4-phenylpyridinium
PD	Parkinson's disease
LDH	lactate dehydrogenase
NPCs	non-parenchymal cells

References

Adler, S., Lindqvist, J., Uddenberg, K., Hyllner, J., & Strehl, R. (2008a). Testing potential developmental toxicants with a cytotoxicity assay based on human embryonic stem cells. *Alternatives to Laboratory Animals*, *36*(2), 129–140.

Adler, S., Pellizzer, C., Hareng, L., Hartung, T., & Bremer, S. (2008b). First steps in establishing a developmental toxicity test method based on human embryonic stem cells. *Toxicology In Vitro*, *22*(1), 200–211.

Agarwal, S., Holton, K. L., & Lanza, R. (2008). Efficient differentiation of functional hepatocytes from human embryonic stem cells. *Stem Cells*, *26*(5), 1117–1127.

Albini, A., Pennesi, G., Donatelli, F., Cammarota, R., De Flora, S., & Noonan, D. M. (2010). Cardiotoxicity of anticancer drugs: the need for cardio-oncology and cardio-oncological prevention. *Journal of the National Cancer Institute*, *102*(1), 14–25.

Anderson, D., Self, T., Mellor, I. R., Goh, G., Hill, S. J., & Denning, C. (2007). Transgenic enrichment of cardiomyocytes from human embryonic stem cells. *Molecular Theraphy*, *15*(11), 2027–2036.

Andersson, H., Steel, D., Asp, J., Dahlenborg, K., Jonsson, M., Jeppsson, A., et al. (2010). Assaying cardiac biomarkers for toxicity testing using biosensing and cardiomyocytes derived from human embryonic stem cells. *Journal of Biotechnology*, *150*(1), 175–181.

Andrade, R. J., Lucena, M. I., Fernández, M. C., Pelaez, G., Pachkoria, K., García-Ruiz, E., et al. (2005). Drug-induced liver injury: an analysis of 461 incidences submitted to the spanish registry over a 10-year period. *Gastroenterology*, *129*(2), 512–521.

Anokye-Danso, F., Trivedi, C. M., Juhr, D., Gupta, M., Cui, Z., Tian, Y., et al. (2011). Highly efficient miRNA-mediated reprogramming of mouse and human somatic cells to pluripotency. *Cell Stem Cell*, *8*(4), 376–388.

Anson, B. D., Kolaja, K. L., & Kamp, T. J. (2011). Opportunities for use of human iPS cells in predictive toxicology. *Clinical Pharmacology & Therapeutics*, *89*(5), 754–758.

Aoyama, K., Yoshinari, K., Kim, H. J., Nagata, K., & Yamazoe, Y. (2009). Simultaneous expression of plural forms of human cytochrome P450 at desired ratios in HepG2 cells: adenovirus-mediated tool for cytochrome P450 reconstitution. *Drug Metabolism and Pharmacokinetics*, *24*(3), 209–217.

Baek, D. H., Park, S. H., Park, J. H., Choi, Y., Park, K. D., Kang, J. W., et al. (2011). Embryotoxicity of lead (II) acetate and aroclor 1254 using a new end point of the embryonic stem cell test. *International Journal of Toxicology*, *30*(5), 498–509.

Bahadur, G., & Morrison, M. (2010). Patenting human pluripotent cells: balancing commercial, academic and ethical interests. *Human Reproduction*, *25*(1), 14–21.

Baharvand, H., Ashtiani, S. K., Valojerdi, M. R., Shahverdi, A., Taee, A., & Sabour, D. (2004). Establishment and in vitro differentiation of a new embryonic stem cell line from human blastocyst. *Differentiation*, *72*(5), 224–229.

Baharvand, H., Hashemi, S. M., Ashtiani, S. K., & Farrokhi, A. (2006). Differentiation of human embryonic stem cells into hepatocytes in 2D and 3D culture systems in vitro. *International Journal of Developmental Biology*, *50*(7), 645–652.

Baillie, T. A., & Rettie, A. E. (2011). Role of biotransformation in drug-induced toxicity: Influence of intra- and inter-species differences in drug metabolism. *Drug Metabolism and Pharmacokinetics*, *26*(1), 15–29.

Bar-Nur, O., Russ, H. A., Efrat, S., & Benvenisty, N. (2011). Epigenetic memory and preferential lineage-specific differentiation in induced pluripotent stem cells derived from human pancreatic islet beta cells. *Cell Stem Cell*, *9*(1), 17–23.

Barrilleaux, B., & Knoepfler, P. S. (2011). Inducing iPSCs to Escape the dish. *Cell Stem Cell*, *9*(2), 103–111.

Basma, H., Soto-Gutiérrez, A., Yannam, G. R., Liu, L., Ito, R., Yamamoto, T., et al. (2009). Differentiation and transplantation of human embryonic stem cell-derived hepatocytes. *Gastroenterology*, *136*(3), 990–999. e994.

Baxter, M. A., Rowe, C., Alder, J., Harrison, S., Hanley, K. P., Park, B. K., et al. (2010). Generating hepatic cell lineages from pluripotent stem cells for drug toxicity screening. *Stem Cell Research*, *5*(1), 4–22.

Beqqali, A., Kloots, J., Ward-van Oostwaard, D., Mummery, C., & Passier, R. (2006). Genome-wide transcriptional profiling of human embryonic stem cells differentiating to cardiomyocytes. *Stem Cells*, *24*(8), 1956–1967.

Bhandari, R. N., Riccalton, L. A., Lewis, A. L., Fry, J. R., Hammond, A. H., Tendler, S. J., et al. (2001). Liver tissue engineering: a role for co-culture systems in modifying hepatocyte function and viability. *Tissue Engineering*, *7*(3), 345–357.

Biedler, J. L., Helson, L., & Spengler, B. A. (1973). Morphology and growth, tumorigenicity, and cytogenetics of human neuroblastoma cells in continuous culture. *Cancer Research*, *33*(11), 2643–2652.

Bielby, R. C., Boccaccini, A. R., Polak, J. M., & Buttery, L. D. (2004). In vitro differentiation and in vivo mineralization of osteogenic cells derived from human embryonic stem cells. *Tissue Engineering*, *10*(9, 10), 1518–1525.

Bigot, K., de Lange, J., Archer, G., Clothier, R., & Bremer, S. (1999). The relative semi-quantification of mrna expression as a useful toxicological endpoint for the identification of embryotoxic/teratogenic substances. *Toxicology In Vitro*, *13*(4, 5), 619–623.

Birrell, M. A., Hardaker, E., Wong, S., McCluskie, K., Catley, M., De Alba, J., et al. (2005). I{kappa}-B kinase-2 inhibitor blocks inflammation in human airway smooth muscle and a rat model of asthma. *American Journal of Respiratory and Critical Care Medicine*, *172*(8), 962–971.

Bourdi, M., Reilly, T. P., Elkahloun, A. G., George, J. W., & Pohl, L. R. (2002). Macrophage migration inhibitory factor in drug-induced liver injury: a role in susceptibility and stress responsiveness. *Biochemical and Biophysical Research Communications*, *294*(2), 225–230.

Braam, S. R., Tertoolen, L., van de Stolpe, A., Meyer, T., Passier, R., & Mummery, C. L. (2010). Prediction of drug-induced cardiotoxicity using human embryonic stem cell-derived cardiomyocytes. *Stem Cell Research*, *4*(2), 107–116.

Breier, J. M., Radio, N. M., Mundy, W. R., & Shafer, T. J. (2008). Development of a high-throughput screening assay for chemical effects on proliferation and viability of immortalized human neural progenitor cells. *Toxicological Sciences*, *105*(1), 119–133.

Brolén, G., Sivertsson, L., Björquist, P., Eriksson, G., Ek, M., Semb, H., et al. (2010). Hepatocyte-like cells derived from human embryonic stem cells specifically via definitive endoderm and a progenitor stage. *Journal of Biotechnology*, *145*(3), 284–294.

Burridge, P. W., Anderson, D., Priddle, H., Barbadillo Munoz, M. D., Chamberlain, S., Allegrucci, C., et al. (2007). Improved human embryonic stem cell embryoid body homogeneity and cardiomyocyte differentiation from a novel V-96 plate aggregation system highlights interline variability. *Stem Cells*, *25*(4), 929–938.

Burridge, P. W., Thompson, S., Millrod, M. A., Weinberg, S., Yuan, X., Peters, A., et al. (2011). A universal system for highly efficient cardiac differentiation of human induced pluripotent stem cells that eliminates interline variability. *PLoS One*, *6*(4), e18293.

Buzanska, L., Habich, A., Jurga, M., Sypecka, J., & Domanska-Janik, K. (2005). Human cord blood-derived neural stem cell line – possible implementation in studying neurotoxicity. *Toxicology In Vitro*, *19*(7), 991–999.

Buzanska, L., Sypecka, J., Nerini-Molteni, S., Compagnoni, A., Hogberg, H. T., del Torchio, R., et al. (2009). A human stem cell-based model for identifying adverse effects of organic and inorganic chemicals on the developing nervous system. *Stem Cells*, *27*(10), 2591–2601.

Cai, J., Zhao, Y., Liu, Y., Ye, F., Song, Z., Qin, H., et al. (2007). Directed differentiation of human embryonic stem cells into functional hepatic cells. *Hepatology*, *45*(5), 1229–1239.

Caldwell, M. A., He, X., Wilkie, N., Pollack, S., Marshall, G., Wafford, K. A., et al. (2001). Growth factors regulate the survival and fate of cells derived from human neurospheres. *Nature Biotechnology*, *19*(5), 475–479.

Callihan, P., Zitomer, N. C., Stoeling, M. V., Kennedy, P. C., Lynch, K. R., Riley, R. T., et al. (2011). Distinct generation, pharmacology, and distribution of sphingosine 1-phosphate and dihydrosphingosine 1-phosphate in human neural progenitor cells. *Neuropharmacology*.

Carvajal-Vergara, X., Sevilla, A., D'Souza, S. L., Ang, Y. S., Schaniel, C., Lee, D. F., et al. (2010). Patient-specific induced pluripotent stem-cell-derived models of LEOPARD syndrome. *Nature*, *465*(7299), 808–812.

Castell, J. V., Jover, R., Martínez-Jiménez, C. P., & Gómez-Lechón, M. J. (2006). Hepatocyte cell lines: their use, scope and limitations in drug metabolism studies. *Expert Opinion on Drug Metabolism & Toxicology*, *2*(2), 183–212.

Celander, M. C., Goldstone, J. V., Denslow, N. D., Iguchi, T., Kille, P., Meyerhoff, R. D., et al. (2011). Species extrapolation for the 21st century. *Environmental Toxicology and Chemistry*, *30*(1), 52–63.

Chen, R., Chen, J., Cheng, S., Qin, J., Li, W., Zhang, L., et al. (2010). Assessment of embryotoxicity of compounds in cosmetics by the embryonic stem cell test. *Toxicology Mechanisms and Methods*, *20*(3), 112–118.

Chen, Y. -F., Tseng, C. -Y., Wang, H. -W., Kuo, H. -C., Yang, V. W., & Lee, O. K. (2011). Rapid generation of mature hepatocyte-like cells from human induced pluripotent stem cells by an efficient three-step protocol. *Hepatology*.

Chiao, E., Elazar, M., Xing, Y., Xiong, A., Kmet, M., Millan, M. T., et al. (2008). Isolation and transcriptional profiling of purified hepatic cells derived from human embryonic stem cells. *Stem Cells*, *26*(8), 2032–2041.

Chien, K. R. (2006). Herceptin and the heart – a molecular modifier of cardiac failure. *New England Journal of Medicins*, *354*(8), 789–790.

Chung, W. S., Shin, C. H., & Stainier, D. Y. R. (2008). Bmp2 signaling regulates the hepatic versus pancreatic fate decision. *Developmental Cell*, *15*(5), 738–748.

Clarkson, T. W. (1997). The toxicology of mercury. *Critical Reviews in Clinical Laboratory Sciences*, *34*(4), 369–403.

Colleoni, S., Galli, C., Gaspar, J. A., Meganathan, K., Jagtap, S., Hescheler, J., et al. (2011). Development of a neural teratogenicity test based on human embryonic stem cells: response to retinoic acid exposure. *Toxicological Sciences*, *124*(2), 370–377.

Cooke, A., Harrison, D., & Skyring, A. (1963). Use of indocyanine green as a test of liver function. *Digestive Diseases and Sciences*, *8*(3), 244–250.

Coulouarn, C., Factor, V. M., Andersen, J. B., Durkin, M. E., & Thorgeirsson, S. S. (2009). Loss of miR-122 expression in liver cancer correlates with suppression of the hepatic phenotype and gain of metastatic properties. *Oncogene*, *28*(40), 3526–3536.

D'Amour, K. A., Agulnick, A. D., Eliazer, S., Kelly, O. G., Kroon, E., & Baetge, E. E. (2005). Efficient differentiation of human embryonic stem cells to definitive endoderm. *Nature Biotechnology*, *23*(12), 1534–1541.

Dash, A., Inman, W., Hoffmaster, K., Sevidal, S., Kelly, J., Obach, R. S., et al. (2009). Liver tissue engineering in the evaluation of drug safety. *Expert Opinion on Drug Metabolism & Toxicology*, *5*(10), 1159–1174.

de Groot, D. M., Bos-Kuijpers, M. H., Kaufmann, W. S., Lammers, J. H., O'Callaghan, J. P., Pakkenberg, B., et al. (2005). Regulatory developmental neurotoxicity testing: a model study focussing on conventional neuropathology endpoints and other perspectives. *Environmental Toxicology and Pharmacology*, *19*(3), 745–755.

de Jong, E., Barenys, M., Hermsen, S. A., Verhoef, A., Ossendorp, B. C., Bessems, J. G., et al. (2011). Comparison of the mouse embryonic stem cell test, the rat whole embryo culture and the zebrafish embryotoxicity test as alternative methods for developmental toxicity testing of six 1,2,4-triazoles. *Toxicology and Applied Pharmacology*, *253*(2), 103–111.

De Smedt, A., Steemans, M., De Boeck, M., Peters, A. K., van der Leede, B. J., Van Goethem, F., et al. (2008). Optimisation of the cell cultivation methods in the embryonic stem cell test results in an increased differentiation potential of the cells into strong beating myocard cells. *Toxicology In Vitro*, *22*(7), 1789–1796.

Di Guglielmo, C., Lopez, D. R., De Lapuente, J., Mallafre, J. M., & Suarez, M. B. (2010). Embryotoxicity of cobalt ferrite and gold nanoparticles: a first in vitro approach. *Reproductive Toxicology*, *30*(2), 271–276.

Dick, E., Rajamohan, D., Ronksley, J., & Denning, C. (2010). Evaluating the utility of cardiomyocytes from human pluripotent stem cells for drug screening. *Biochemical Society Transactions*, *38*(4), 1037–1045.

Dolci, A., Dominici, R., Cardinale, D., Sandri, M. T., & Panteghini, M. (2008). Biochemical markers for prediction of chemotherapy-induced cardiotoxicity: systematic review of the literature and recommendations for use. *American Journal of Clinical Pathology*, *130*(5), 688–695.

Duan, Y., Catana, A., Meng, Y., Yamamoto, N., He, S., Gupta, S., et al. (2007). Differentiation and enrichment of hepatocyte-like cells from human embryonic stem cells in vitro and in vivo. *Stem Cells*, *25*(12), 3058–3068.

Duan, Y., Ma, X., Zou, W. E.I., Wang, C., Bahbahan, I. S., Ahuja, T. P., et al. (2010). Differentiation and characterization of metabolically functioning hepatocytes from human embryonic stem cells. *Stem Cells*, *28*(4), 674–686.

Duanmu, Z., Locke, D., Smigelski, J., Wu, W., Dahn, M. S., Falany, C. N., et al. (2002). Effects of dexamethasone on aryl (SULT1A1)- and hydroxysteroid (SULT2A1)-sulfotransferase gene expression in primary cultured human hepatocytes. *Drug Metabolism and Disposition*, *30*(9), 997–1004.

Dubois, N. C., Craft, A. M., Sharma, P., Elliott, D. A., Stanley, E. G., Elefanty, A. G., et al. (2011). SIRPA is a specific cell-surface marker for isolating cardiomyocytes derived from human pluripotent stem cells. *Nature Biotechnology*.

Eberhard, D., O'Neill, K., Burke, Z. D., & Tosh, D. (2010). In vitro reprogramming of pancreatic cells to hepatocytes. *Methods in Molecular Biology*, *636*, 285–292.

EC1907/2006.

Eckardt, K., & Stahlmann, R. (2010). Use of two validated in vitro tests to assess the embryotoxic potential of mycophenolic acid. *Archives in Toxicology*, *84*(1), 37–43.

Edwards, I. R., & Aronson, J. K. (2000). Adverse drug reactions: definitions, diagnosis, and management. *Lancet*, *356*(9237), 1255–1259.

Ek, M., Söderdahl, T., Küppers-Munther, B., Edsbagge, J., Andersson, T. B., Björquist, P., et al. (2007). Expression of drug metabolizing enzymes in hepatocyte-like cells derived from human embryonic stem cells. *Biochemical Pharmacology*, *74*(3), 496–503.

Elaut, G., Henkens, T., Papeleu, P., Snykers, S., Vinken, M., Vanhaecke, T., et al. (2006). Molecular mechanisms underlying the dedifferentiation process of isolated hepatocytes and their cultures. *Current Drug Metabolism*, *7*(6), 629–660.

Elsaesser, A., & Howard, C. V. (2011). Toxicology of nanoparticles. *Advanced Drug Delivery Reviews*.

Espandiari, P., Rosenzweig, B., Zhang, J., Zhou, Y., Schnackenberg, L., Vaidya, V. S., et al. (2010). Age-related differences in susceptibility to cisplatin-induced renal toxicity. *Journal of Applied Toxicology*, *30*(2), 172–182.

Eugenin, E. A., King, J. E., Hazleton, J. E., Major, E. O., Bennett, M. V., Zukin, R. S., et al. (2011). Differences in NMDA receptor expression during human development determine the response of neurons to HIV-tat-mediated neurotoxicity. *Neurotoxicological Research*, *19*(1), 138–148.

Fair, J. H., Cairns, B. A., LaPaglia, M., Wang, J., Meyer, A. A., Kim, H., et al. (2003). Induction of hepatic differentiation in embryonic stem cells by co-culture with embryonic cardiac mesoderm. *Surgery*, *134*(2), 189–196.

Fausto, N. (2000). Liver regeneration. *Journal of Hepatology*, *32*(1 Suppl.), 19–31.

Fermini, B., & Fossa, A. A. (2003). The impact of drug-induced QT interval prolongation on drug discovery and development. *Nature Reviews Drug Discovery*, *2*(6), 439–447.

Fleischer, M. (2007). Testing costs and testing capacity according to the REACH requirements – results of a survey of independent and corporate GLP laboratories in the EU and Switzerland. *Journal of Business Chemistry*, *4*(3), 96–114.

Flick, B., & Klug, S. (2006). Whole embryo culture: an important tool in developmental toxicology today. *Current Pharmaceutical Design*, *12*(12), 1467–1488.

Flint, O. P., Orton, T. C., & Ferguson, R. A. (1984). Differentiation of rat embryo cells in culture: response following acute maternal exposure to teratogens and non-teratogens. *J Appl Toxicol*, *4*(2), 109–116.

Fritsche, E., Cline, J. E., Nguyen, N. H., Scanlan, T. S., & Abel, J. (2005). Polychlorinated biphenyls disturb differentiation of normal human neural progenitor cells: clue for involvement of thyroid hormone receptors. *Environmental Health Perspectives*, *113*(7), 871–876.

Gachon, F., & Firsov, D. (2011). The role of circadian timing system on drug metabolism and detoxification. *Expert Opinion on Drug Metabolism & Toxicology*, *7*(2), 147–158.

Genschow, E., Scholz, G., Brown, N., Piersma, A., Brady, M., Clemann, N., et al. (2000). Development of prediction models for three in vitro embryotoxicity tests in an ECVAM validation study. *In Vitro and Molecular Toxicology*, *13*(1), 51–66.

Genschow, E., Spielmann, H., Scholz, G., Seiler, A., Brown, N., Piersma, A., et al. (2002). The ECVAM international validation study on in vitro embryotoxicity tests: results of the definitive phase and evaluation of prediction models. European Centre for the Validation of Alternative Methods. *Alternatives to Laboratory Animals*, *30*(2), 151–176.

Genschow, E., Spielmann, H., Scholz, G., Pohl, I., Seiler, A., Clemann, N., et al. (2004). Validation of the embryonic stem cell test in the international ECVAM validation study on three in vitro embryotoxicity tests. *Alternatives to Laboratory Animals*, *32*(3), 209–244.

Ghodsizadeh, A., Taei, A., Totonchi, M., Seifinejad, A., Gourabi, H., Pournasr, B., et al. (2010). Generation of liver disease-specific induced pluripotent stem cells along with efficient differentiation to functional hepatocyte-like cells. *Stem Cell Reviews and Reports*, *6*(4), 622–632.

Gokhale, M., & Martin, B. C. (2011). Prescription-acquired acetaminophen use and potential overuse patterns: 2001–2008. *Pharmacoepidemiology and Drug Safety*.

Goldring, C. E.P., Kitteringham, N. R., Elsby, R., Randle, L. E., Clement, Y. N., Williams, D. P., et al. (2004). Activation of hepatic Nrf2 in vivo by acetaminophen in CD-1 mice. *Hepatology*, *39*(5), 1267–1276.

Goldring, C. E.P., Kitteringham, N. R., Jenkins, R., Lovatt, C. A., Randle, L. E., Abdullah, A., et al. (2006). Development of a transactivator in hepatoma cells that allows expression of phase I, phase II, and chemical defense genes. *American Journal of Physiology – Cell Physiology*, *290*(1), C104–C115.

González, F., Boué, S., & Belmonte, J. C.I. (2011). Methods for making induced pluripotent stem cells: Reprogramming à la carte. *Nature Reviews Genetics*, *12*(4), 231–242.

Gouon-Evans, V., Boussemart, L., Gadue, P., Nierhoff, D., Koehler, C. I., Kubo, A., et al. (2006). BMP-4 is required for hepatic specification of mouse embryonic stem cell-derived definitive endoderm. *Nature Biotechnology*, *24*(11), 1402–1411.

Graichen, R., Xu, X., Braam, S. R., Balakrishnan, T., Norfiza, S., Sieh, S., et al. (2008). Enhanced cardiomyogenesis of human embryonic stem cells by a small molecular inhibitor of p38 MAPK. *Differentiation*, *76*(4), 357–370.

Greenlee, A. R., Kronenwetter-Koepel, T. A., Kaiser, S. J., & Liu, K. (2005). Comparison of Matrigel and gelatin substrata for feeder-free culture of undifferentiated mouse embryonic stem cells for toxicity testing. *Toxicology In Vitro*, *19*(3), 389–397.

Groebe, K., Hayess, K., Klemm-Manns, M., Schwall, G., Wozny, W., Steemans, M., et al. (2010a). Protein biomarkers for in vitro testing of embryotoxicity. *Journal of Proteome Research*, *9*(11), 5727–5738.

Groebe, K., Hayess, K., Klemm-Manns, M., Schwall, G., Wozny, W., Steemans, M., et al. (2010b). Unexpected common mechanistic pathways for embryotoxicity of warfarin and lovastatin. *Reproductive Toxicology*, *30*(1), 121–130.

Guguen-Guillouzo, C., & Guillouzo, A. (2010). General review on in vitro hepatocyte models and their applications. *Methods in Molecular Biology*, *640*, 1–40.

Guo, L., Abrams, R. M., Babiarz, J. E., Cohen, J. D., Kameoka, S., Sanders, M. J., et al. (2011). Estimating the risk of drug-induced proarrhythmia using human induced pluripotent stem cell-derived cardiomyocytes. *Toxicological Sciences*, *123*(1), 281–289.

Hafner, M., Landthaler, M., Burger, L., Khorshid, M., Hausser, J., Berninger, P., et al. (2010). Transcriptome-wide Identification of RNA-binding protein and MicroRNA target sites by PAR-CLIP. *Cell*, *141*(1), 129–141.

Hamazaki, T., Iiboshi, Y., Oka, M., Papst, P. J., Meacham, A. M., Zon, L. I., et al. (2001). Hepatic maturation in differentiating embryonic stem cells in vitro. *FEBS Letters*, *497*(1), 15–19.

Han, Y., Miller, A., Mangada, J., Liu, Y., Swistowski, A., Zhan, M., et al. (2009). Identification by automated screening of a small molecule that selectively eliminates neural stem cells derived from hESCs but not dopamine neurons. *PLoS One*, *4*(9), e7155.

Hang, H. L., Zhang, L., Shi, X. L., Bian, J. M., & Ding, Y. T. (2011). Isolation, culture and cryopreservation of adult human hepatocytes. *World Chinese Journal of Digestology*, *19*(19), 2016–2021.

Hareng, L., Pellizzer, C., Bremer, S., Schwarz, M., & Hartung, T. (2005). The integrated project ReProTect: a novel approach in reproductive toxicity hazard assessment. *Reproductive Toxicology*, *20*(3), 441–452.

Harrill, J. A., Freudenrich, T. M., Machacek, D. W., Stice, S. L., & Mundy, W. R. (2010). Quantitative assessment of neurite outgrowth in human embryonic stem cell-derived hN2 cells using automated high-content image analysis. *Neurotoxicology*, *31*(3), 277–290.

Hartung, T., & Rovida, C. (2009). Chemical regulators have overreached. *Nature*, *460*(7259), 1080–1081.

Hattori, F., Chen, H., Yamashita, H., Tohyama, S., Satoh, Y. S., Yuasa, S., et al. (2010). Nongenetic method for purifying stem cell-derived cardiomyocytes. *Nature Methods*, *7*(1), 61–66.

Hay, D. C., Fletcher, J., Payne, C., Terrace, J. D., Gallagher, R. C. J., Snoeys, J., et al. (2008). Highly efficient differentiation of hESCs to functional hepatic endoderm requires ActivinA and Wnt3a signaling. *Proceedings of the National Academy of Sciences of the United States of America*, *105*(34), 12,301–12,306.

He, J. Q., Ma, Y., Lee, Y., Thomson, J. A., & Kamp, T. J. (2003). Human embryonic stem cells develop into multiple types of cardiac myocytes: action potential characterization. *Circulation Research*, *93*(1), 32–39.

Hettwer, M., Reis-Fernandes, M. A., Iken, M., Ott, M., Steinberg, P., & Nau, H. (2010). Metabolic activation capacity by primary hepatocytes expands the applicability of the embryonic stem cell test as alternative to experimental animal testing. *Reproductive Toxicology*, *30*(1), 113–120.

Hofer, T., Gerner, I., Gundert-Remy, U., Liebsch, M., Schulte, A., Spielmann, H., et al. (2004). Animal testing and alternative approaches for the human health risk assessment under the proposed new European chemicals regulation. *Archives in Toxicology*, *78*(10), 549–564.

Hoffman, R. M. (1993). To do tissue culture in two or three dimensions? That is the question. *Stem Cells*, *11*(2), 105–111.

Honda, M., Kiyokawa, J., Tabo, M., & Inoue, T. (2011). Electrophysiological characterization of cardiomyocytes derived from human induced pluripotent stem cells. *Journal of Pharmacological Sciences*.

Huangfu, D., Osafune, K., Maehr, R., Guo, W., Eijkelenboom, A., Chen, S., et al. (2008). Induction of pluripotent stem cells from primary human fibroblasts with only Oct4 and Sox2. *Nature Biotechnology*, *26*(11), 1269–1275.

Imai, K., & Nakamura, M. (2006). In vitro embryotoxicity testing of metals for dental use by differentiation of embryonic stem cell test. *Congenital Anomaly (Kyoto)*, *46*(1), 34–38.

Ingelman-Sundberg, M., Sim, S. C., Gomez, A., & Rodriguez-Antona, C. (2007). Influence of cytochrome P450 polymorphisms on drug therapies: Pharmacogenetic, pharmacoepigenetic and clinical aspects. *Pharmacology and Therapeutics*, *116*(3), 496–526.

Ishii, T., Fukumitsu, K., Yasuchika, K., Adachi, K., Kawase, E., Suemori, H., et al. (2008). Effects of extracellular matrixes and growth factors on the hepatic differentiation of human embryonic stem cells. *American Journal of Physiology – Gastrointestinal and Liver Physiology*, *295*(2), G313–G321.

Itoh, K., Igarashi, K., Hayashi, N., Nishizawa, M., & Yamamoto, M. (1995). Cloning and characterization of a novel erythroid cell-derived CNC family transcription factor heterodimerizing with the small Maf family proteins. *Molecular and Cellular Biology*, *15*(8), 4184–4193.

Itoh, K., Chiba, T., Takahashi, S., Ishii, T., Igarashi, K., Katoh, Y., et al. (1997). An Nrf2/small Maf heterodimer mediates the induction of phase II detoxifying enzyme genes through antioxidant response elements. *Biochemical and Biophysical Research Communications*, *236*(2), 313–322.

Itskovitz-Eldor, J., Schuldiner, M., Karsenti, D., Eden, A., Yanuka, O., Amit, M., et al. (2000). Differentiation of human embryonic stem cells into embryoid bodies compromising the three embryonic germ layers. *Molecular Medicine*, *6*(2), 88–95.

Jagtap, S., Meganathan, K., Gaspar, J., Wagh, V., Winkler, J., Hescheler, J., et al. (2011). Cytosine arabinoside induces ectoderm and inhibits mesoderm expression in human embryonic stem cells during multilineage differentiation. *British Journal of Pharmacology*, *162*(8), 1743–1756.

Johnson, G. (1998). Lithium – early development, toxicity, and renal function. *Neuropsychopharmacology*, *19*(3), 200–205.

Jozefczuk, J., Prigione, A., Chavez, L., & Adjaye, J. (2011). Comparative analysis of human embryonic stem cell and induced pluripotent stem cell-derived hepatocyte-like cells reveals current drawbacks and possible strategies for improved differentiation. *Stem Cells and Development*, *20*(7), 1259–1275.

Kamiya, A., Kinoshita, T., & Miyajima, A. (2001). Oncostatin M and hepatocyte growth factor induce hepatic maturation via distinct signaling pathways. *FEBS Letters*, *492*(1, 2), 90–94.

Kang, K. S., Park, J. E., Ryu, D. Y., & Lee, Y. S. (2001). Effects and neuro-toxic mechanisms of 2, 2′, 4, 4′, 5, 5′-hexachlorobiphenyl and endosulfan in neuronal stem cells. *Journal of Veterinary Medical Science*, *63*(11), 1183–1190.

Kang, Y. H., Berthiaume, F., Nath, B. D., & Yarmush, M. L. (2004). Growth factors and nonparenchymal cell conditioned media induce mitogenic responses in stable long-term adult rat hepatocyte cultures. *Experimental Cell Research*, *293*(2), 239–247.

Karginov, F. V., Conaco, C., Xuan, Z., Schmidt, B. H., Parker, J. S., Mandel, G., et al. (2007). A biochemical approach to identifying microRNA targets. *Proceedings of the National Academy of Sciences*, *104*(49), 19,291–19,296.

Kehat, I., Kenyagin-Karsenti, D., Snir, M., Segev, H., Amit, M., Gepstein, A., et al. (2001). Human embryonic stem cells can differentiate into myocytes with structural and functional properties of cardiomyocytes. *Journal of Clinical Investigations*, *108*(3), 407–414.

Kettenhofen, R., & Bohlen, H. (2008). Preclinical assessment of cardiac toxicity. *Drug Discovery Today*, *13*(15, 16), 702–707.

Khetani, S. R., & Bhatia, S. N. (2008). Microscale culture of human liver cells for drug development. *Nature Biotechnology*, *26*(1), 120–126.

Kidambi, S., Sheng, L., Yarmush, M. L., Toner, M., Lee, I., & Chan, C. (2007). Patterned co-culture of primary hepatocytes and fibroblasts using polyelectrolyte multilayer templates. *Macromolecular Bioscience*, *7*(3), 344–353.

Kim, N., Kim, H., Jung, I., Kim, Y., Kim, D., & Han, Y.-M. (2011). Expression profiles of miRNAs in human embryonic stem cells during hepatocyte differentiation. *Hepatology Research*, *41*(2), 170–183.

Kleinstreuer, N. C., Smith, A. M., West, P. R., Conard, K. R., Fontaine, B. R., Weir-Hauptman, A. M., et al. (2011). Identifying developmental toxicity pathways for a subset of ToxCast chemicals using human embryonic stem cells and metabolomics. *Toxicology and Applied Pharmacology*, *257*(1), 111–121.

Kubo, A., Shinozaki, K., Shannon, J. M., Kouskoff, V., Kennedy, M., Woo, S., et al. (2004). Development of definitive endoderm from embryonic stem cells in culture. *Development*, *131*(7), 1651–1662.

Kusuda Furue, M., Tateyama, D., Kinehara, M., Na, J., Okamoto, T., & Sato, J. D. (2010). Advantages and difficulties in culturing human pluripotent stem cells in growth factor-defined serum-free medium. *In Vitro Cellular & Developmental Biology – Animal*, *46*(7), 573–576.

Lagos-Quintana, M., Rauhut, R., Lendeckel, W., & Tuschl, T. (2001). Identification of novel genes coding for small expressed RNAs. *Science*, *294*(5543), 853–858.

Laposa, R. R. (2011). Stem cells for drug screening. *Journal of Cardiovascular Pharmacology*, *58*(3), 240–245.

Lappalainen, R. S., Salomaki, M., Yla-Outinen, L., Heikkila, T. J., Hyttinen, J. A., Pihlajamaki, H., et al. (2010). Similarly derived and cultured hESC lines show variation in their developmental potential towards neuronal cells in long-term culture. *Regenerative Medicine*, *5*(5), 749–762.

Laudadio, I., Manfroid, I., Achouri, Y., Schmidt, D., Wilson, M. D., Cordi, S., et al. (2011). A feedback loop between the liver-enriched transcription factor network and Mir-122 controls hepatocyte differentiation. *Gastroenterology*.

Laurent, L. C., Ulitsky, I., Slavin, I., Tran, H., Schork, A., Morey, R., et al. (2011). Dynamic changes in the copy number of pluripotency and cell proliferation genes in human ESCs and iPSCs during reprogramming and time in culture. *Cell Stem Cell*, *8*(1), 106–118.

Lavon, N., & Benvenisty, N. (2005). Study of hepatocyte differentiation using embryonic stem cells. *Journal of Cellular Biochemistry*, *96*(6), 1193–1202.

Lavon, N., Yanuka, O., & Benvenisty, N. (2004). Differentiation and isolation of hepatic-like cells from human embryonic stem cells. *Differentiation*, *72*(5), 230–238.

Lazarou, J., Pomeranz, B. H., & Corey, P. N. (1998). Incidence of adverse drug reactions in hospitalized patients. *JAMA: The Journal of the American Medical Association*, *279*(15), 1200–1205.

Lee, W. M. (2003). Acute liver failure in the United States. *Seminal Liver Disease*, *23*(03), 217,226.

Lee, E. W., Lai, Y., Zhang, H., & Unadkat, J. D. (2006). Identification of the mitochondrial targeting signal of the human equilibrative nucleoside transporter 1 (hENT1): implications for interspecies differences in mitochondrial toxicity of fialuridine. *Journal of Biological Chemistry*, *281*(24), 16,700–16,706.

Lee, N., Authier, S., Pugsley, M. K., & Curtis, M. J. (2010). The continuing evolution of torsades de pointes liability testing methods: is there an end in sight? *Toxicology and Applied Pharmacology*, *243*(2), 146–153.

Li, S. S.-L., Yu, S. -L., Kao, L. -P., Tsai, Z. Y., Singh, S., Chen, B. Z., et al. (2009). Target identification of microRNAs expressed highly in human embryonic stem cells. *Journal of Cellular Biochemistry*, *106*(6), 1020–1030.

Li, Z. -Y., Xi, Y., Zhu, W. -N., Zeng, C., Zhang, Z. -Q., Guo, Z. -C., et al. (2011). Positive regulation of hepatic miR-122 expression by HNF4α. *Journal of Hepatology*, *55*(3), 602–611.

Liao, B., Bao, X., Liu, L., Feng, S., Zovoilis, A., Liu, W., et al. (2011). MicroRNA cluster 302–367 enhances somatic cell reprogramming by accelerating a mesenchymal-to-epithelial transition. *Journal of Biological Chemistry*, *286*(19), 17,359–17,364.

Lin, S. -L. (2011). Deciphering the mechanism behind iPSC generation. *Stem Cells*.

Lin, S., & Talbot, P. (2011). Methods for culturing mouse and human embryonic stem cells. *Methods in Molecular Biology*, *690*, 31–56.

Lin, S. L., Chang, D. C., Lin, C. H., Ying, S. Y., Leu, D., & Wu, D. T.S. (2011). Regulation of somatic cell reprogramming through inducible mir-302 expression. *Nucleic Acids Research*, *39*(3), 1054–1065.

Lister, R., Pelizzola, M., Kida, Y. S., Hawkins, R. D., Nery, J. R., Hon, G., et al. (2011). Hotspots of aberrant epigenomic reprogramming in human induced pluripotent stem cells. *Nature*, *471*(7336), 68–73.

LoPachin, R. M. (2004). The changing view of acrylamide neurotoxicity. *Neurotoxicology*, *25*(4), 617–630.

Lumelsky, N., Blondel, O., Laeng, P., Velasco, I., Ravin, R., & McKay, R. (2001). Differentiation of embryonic stem cells to insulin-secreting structures similar to pancreatic islets. *Science*, *292*(5520), 1389–1394.

Luyendyk, J. P., Maddox, J. F., Cosma, G. N., Ganey, P. E., Cockerell, G. L., & Roth, R. A. (2003). Ranitidine treatment during a modest inflammatory response precipitates idiosyncrasy-like liver injury in rats. *Journal of Pharmacology and Experimental Therapeutics*, *307*(1), 9–16.

Maddrey, W. C. (2005). Drug-induced hepatotoxicity: 2005. *Journal of Clinical Gastroenterology*, *39*(4 Suppl 2), S83–S89.

Marro, S., Pang, Z. P., Yang, N., Tsai, M. C., Qu, K., Chang, H. Y., et al. (2011). Direct lineage conversion of terminally differentiated hepatocytes to functional neurons. *Cell Stem Cell*, *9*(4), 374–382.

Marx-Stoelting, P., Adriaens, E., Ahr, H. J., Bremer, S., Garthoff, B., Gelbke, H. P., et al. (2009). A review of the implementation of the embryonic stem cell test (EST). The report and recommendations of an ECVAM/ReProTect Workshop. *Alternatives to Laboratory Animals*, *37*(3), 313–328.

Matsa, E., Rajamohan, D., Dick, E., Young, L., Mellor, I., Staniforth, A., et al. (2011). Drug evaluation in cardiomyocytes derived from human induced pluripotent stem cells carrying a long QT syndrome type 2 mutation. *European Heart Journal*, *32*(8), 952–962.

McLean, A. B., D'Amour, K. A., Jones, K. L., Krishnamoorthy, M., Kulik, M. J., Reynolds, D. M., et al. (2007). Activin A efficiently specifies definitive endoderm from human embryonic stem cells only when phosphatidylinositol 3-kinase signaling is suppressed. *Stem Cells*, *25*(1), 29–38.

Meamar, R., Karamali, F., Sadeghi, H. M., Etebari, M., Nasr-Esfahani, M. H., & Baharvand, H. (2010). Toxicity of ecstasy (MDMA) towards embryonic stem cell-derived cardiac and neural cells. *Toxicology In Vitro*, *24*(4), 1133–1138.

Meyer, T., Leisgen, C., Gonser, B., & Gunther, E. (2004). QT-screen: high-throughput cardiac safety pharmacology by extracellular electrophysiology on primary cardiac myocytes. *Assay and Drug Development Technologies*, *2*(5), 507–514.

Misiuta, I. E., Saporta, S., Sanberg, P. R., Zigova, T., & Willing, A. E. (2006). Influence of retinoic acid and lithium on proliferation and dopaminergic potential of human NT2 cells. *Journal of Neuroscience Research*, *83*(4), 668–679.

Mitchell, S. J., Kane, A. E., & Hilmer, S. N. (2011). Age-related changes in the hepatic pharmacology and toxicology of paracetamol. *Current Gerontology and Geriatrics Research*, *2011*, 624,156.

Miyoshi, N., Ishii, H., Nagano, H., Haraguchi, N., Dewi, D. L., Kano, Y., et al. (2011). Reprogramming of mouse and human cells to pluripotency using mature microRNAs. *Cell Stem Cell*, *8*(6), 633–638.

Momose, Y., Matsunaga, T., Murai, K., Takezawa, T., & Ohmori, S. (2009). Differentiation of monkey embryonic stem cells into hepatocytes and mRNA expression of cytochrome P450 enzymes responsible for drug metabolism: Comparison of embryoid body formation conditions and matrices. *Biological and Pharmaceutical Bulletin*, *32*(4), 619–626.

Moore, R. N., & Moghe, P. V. (2009). Expedited growth factor-mediated specification of human embryonic stem cells toward the hepatic lineage. *Stem Cell Research*, *3*(1), 51–62.

Moretti, A., Bellin, M., Jung, C. B., Thies, T. M., Takashima, Y., Bernshausen, A., et al. (2010). Mouse and human induced pluripotent stem cells as a source for multipotent Isl1+ cardiovascular progenitors. *FASEB Journal*, *24*(3), 700–711.

Mummery, C. (2010). Sorting cardiomyocytes: a simple solution after all? *Nature Methods*, *7*(1), 40–42.

Mummery, C., Ward-van Oostwaard, D., Doevendans, P., Spijker, R., van den Brink, S., Hassink, R., et al. (2003). Differentiation of human embryonic stem cells to cardiomyocytes: role of coculture with visceral endoderm-like cells. *Circulation*, *107*(21), 2733–2740.

Mummery, C. L., Ward, D., & Passier, R. (2007). Differentiation of human embryonic stem cells to cardiomyocytes by coculture with endoderm in serum-free medium. *Current Protocols in Stem Cell Biology*. Chapter 1, Unit 1F 2.

Nakanishi, M., Kurisaki, A., Hayashi, Y., Warashina, M., Ishiura, S., Kusuda-Furue, M., et al. (2009). Directed induction of anterior and posterior primitive streak by Wnt from embryonic stem cells cultured in a chemically defined serum-free medium. *FASEB Journal*, *23*(1), 114–122.

Ndountse, L. T., & Chan, H. M. (2008). Methylmercury increases *N*-methyl-D-aspartate receptors on human SH-SY 5Y neuroblastoma cells leading to neurotoxicity. *Toxicology, 249*(2, 3), 251–255.

Nicolson, T. J., Mellor, H. R., & Roberts, R. R. (2010). Gender differences in drug toxicity. *Trends in Pharmacological Sciences, 31*(3), 108–114.

OECD. Guidelines for the testing of chemicals.

Ohi, Y., Qin, H., Hong, C., Blouin, L., Polo, J. M., Guo, T., et al. (2011). Incomplete DNA methylation underlies a transcriptional memory of somatic cells in human iPS cells. *Nature Cell Biology, 13*(5), 541–549.

Olson, H., Betton, G., Robinson, D., Thomas, K., Monro, A., Kolaja, G., et al. (2000). Concordance of the toxicity of pharmaceuticals in humans and in animals. *Regulatory Toxicology and Pharmacology, 32*(1), 56–67.

Osman, A. M., van Dartel, D. A., Zwart, E., Blokland, M., Pennings, J. L., & Piersma, A. H. (2010). Proteome profiling of mouse embryonic stem cells to define markers for cell differentiation and embryotoxicity. *Reproductive Toxicology, 30*(2), 322–332.

Paquette, J. A., Kumpf, S. W., Streck, R. D., Thomson, J. J., Chapin, R. E., & Stedman, D. B. (2008). Assessment of the Embryonic Stem Cell Test and application and use in the pharmaceutical industry. *Birth Defects Research: Part B, Developmental and Reproductive Toxicology, 83*(2), 104–111.

Park, B. K., Kitteringham, N. R., Pirmohamed, M., & Tucker, G. T. (1996). Relevance of induction of human drug-metabolizing enzymes: pharmacological and toxicological implications. *British Journal of Clinical Pharmacology, 41*(6), 477–491.

Park, B. K., Kitteringham, N. R., Maggs, J. L., Pirmohamed, M., & Williams, D. P. (2005). The role of metabolic activation in drug-induced hepatotoxicity. *Annual Review of Pharmacology and Toxicology, 45*, 177–202.

Park, H. R., Kim, M. S., Kim, S. J., Park, M., Kong, K. H., Kim, H. S., et al. (2010). Acrylamide induces cell death in neural progenitor cells and impairs hippocampal neurogenesis. *Toxicological Letters, 193*(1), 86–93.

Pei, H., Yang, Y., Xi, J., Bai, Z., Yue, W., Nan, X., et al. (2009). Lineage restriction and differentiation of human embryonic stem cells into hepatic progenitors and zone 1 hepatocytes. *Tissue Engineering – Part C: Methods, 15*(1), 95–104.

Pellizzer, C., Adler, S., Corvi, R., Hartung, T., & Bremer, S. (2004). Monitoring of teratogenic effects in vitro by analysing a selected gene expression pattern. *Toxicology In Vitro, 18*(3), 325–335.

Peran, M., Sanchez-Ferrero, A., Tosh, D., Marchal, J. A., Lopez, E., Alvarez, P., et al. (2011). Ultrastructural and molecular analyzes of insulin-producing cells induced from human hepatoma cells. *Cytotherapy, 13*(2), 193–200.

Peters, A. K., Wouwer, G. V., Weyn, B., Verheyen, G. R., Vanparys, P., & Gompel, J. V. (2008). Automated analysis of contractility in the embryonic stem cell test, a novel approach to assess embryotoxicity. *Toxicology In Vitro, 22*(8), 1948–1956.

Pfaff, N., Fiedler, J., Holzmann, A., Schambach, A., Moritz, T., Cantz, T., et al. (2011). miRNA screening reveals a new miRNA family stimulating iPS cell generation via regulation of Meox2. *EMBO Reports, 12*(11), 1153–1159.

Phiel, C. J., Zhang, F., Huang, E. Y., Guenther, M. G., Lazar, M. A., & Klein, P. S. (2001). Histone deacetylase is a direct target of valproic acid, a potent anticonvulsant, mood stabilizer, and teratogen. *Journal of Biological Chemistry, 276*(39), 36,734–36,741.

Pick, M., Stelzer, Y., Bar-Nur, O., Mayshar, Y., Eden, A., & Benvenisty, N. (2009). Clone- and gene-specific aberrations of parental imprinting in human induced pluripotent stem cells. *Stem Cells, 27*(11), 2686–2690.

Piersma, A. H. (2006). Alternative methods for developmental toxicity testing. *Basic & Clinical Pharmacology & Toxicology, 98*(5), 427–431.

Piersma, A. H., Genschow, E., Verhoef, A., Spanjersberg, M. Q., Brown, N. A., Brady, M., et al. (2004). Validation of the postimplantation rat whole-embryo culture test in the international ECVAM validation study on three in vitro embryotoxicity tests. *Alternatives to Laboratory Animals*, *32*(3), 275–307.

Pirmohamed, M., James, S., Meakin, S., Green, C., Scott, A. K., Walley, T. J., et al. (2004). Adverse drug reactions as cause of admission to hospital: prospective analysis of 18 820 patients. *BMJ*, *329*(7456), 15–19.

Podolin, P. L., Callahan, J. F., Bolognese, B. J., Li, Y. H., Carlson, K., Davis, T. G., et al. (2005). Attenuation of murine collagen-induced arthritis by a novel, potent, selective small molecule inhibitor of IκB kinase 2, TPCA-1 (2-[(Aminocarbonyl)amino]-5-(4-fluorophenyl)-3-thiophenecarboxamide), occurs via reduction of proinflammatory cytokines and antigen-induced T cell proliferation. *Journal of Pharmacology and Experimental Therapeutics*, *312*(1), 373–381.

Polo, J. M., Liu, S., Figueroa, M. E., Kulalert, W., Eminli, S., Tan, K. Y., et al. (2010). Cell type of origin influences the molecular and functional properties of mouse induced pluripotent stem cells. *Nature Biotechnology*, *28*(8), 848–855.

Ponsoda, X., Pareja, E., Gómez-Lechón, M. J., Fabra, R., Carrasco, E., Trullenque, R., et al. (2001). Drug biotransformation by human hepatocytes. In vitro/in vivo metabolism by cells from the same donor. *Journal of Hepatology*, *34*(1), 19–25.

Pouton, C. W., & Haynes, J. M. (2007). Embryonic stem cells as a source of models for drug discovery. *Nature Reviews Drug Discovery*, *6*(8), 605–616.

Prescott, C. (2011). The business of exploiting induced pluripotent stem cells. *Philosophical Transactions of the Royal Society B: Biological Sciences*, *366*(1575), 2323–2328.

Rashid, S. T., Corbineau, S., Hannan, N., Marciniak, S. J., Miranda, E., Alexander, G., et al. (2010). Modeling inherited metabolic disorders of the liver using human induced pluripotent stem cells. *The Journal of Clinical Investigation*, *120*(9), 3127–3136.

Renaud, H. J., Cui, J. Y., Khan, M., & Klaassen, C. D. (2011). Tissue distribution and gender-divergent expression of 78 cytochrome P450 mRNAs in mice. *Toxicological Sciences*, *124*(2), 261–277.

Romero, A. C., Vilanova, E., & Sogorb, M. A. (2011). Shortening and improving the embryonic stem cell test through the use of gene biomarkers of differentiation. *Journal of Toxicology*, *2011*, 286,034.

Roskelley, C. D., Desprez, P. Y., & Bissell, M. J. (1994). Extracellular matrix-dependent tissue-specific gene expression in mammary epithelial cells requires both physical and biochemical signal transduction. *Proceedings of the National Academy of Sciences of the United States of America*, *91*(26), 12,378–12,382.

Roth, R. A., & Ganey, P. E. (2010). Intrinsic versus idiosyncratic drug-induced hepatotoxicity – two villains or one? *Journal of Pharmacology and Experimental Therapeutics*, *332*(3), 692–697.

Rust, W., Balakrishnan, T., & Zweigerdt, R. (2009). Cardiomyocyte enrichment from human embryonic stem cell cultures by selection of ALCAM surface expression. *Regenerative Medicine*, *4*(2), 225–237.

Saez-Rodriguez, J., Alexopoulos, L. G., Zhang, M., Morris, M. K., Lauffenburger, D. A., & Sorger, P. K. (2011). Comparing signaling networks between normal and transformed hepatocytes using discrete logical models. *Cancer Research*, *71*(16), 5400–5411.

Saldana-Ruiz, S., Soler-Martin, C., & Llorens, J. (2011). Role of CYP2E1-mediated metabolism in the acute and vestibular toxicities of nineteen nitriles in the mouse. *Toxicological Letters*.

Salerno, S., Campana, C., Morelli, S., Drioli, E., & De Bartolo, L. (2011). Human hepatocytes and endothelial cells in organotypic membrane systems. *Biomaterials*, *32*(34), 8848–8859.

Sarafian, T., & Verity, M. A. (1991). Oxidative mechanisms underlying methyl mercury neurotoxicity. *International Journal of Developmental Neuroscience*, *9*(2), 147–153.

Sartiani, L., Bettiol, E., Stillitano, F., Mugelli, A., Cerbai, E., & Jaconi, M. E. (2007). Developmental changes in cardiomyocytes differentiated from human embryonic stem cells: a molecular and electrophysiological approach. *Stem Cells*, *25*(5), 1136–1144.

Satin, J., Kehat, I., Caspi, O., Huber, I., Arbel, G., Itzhaki, I., et al. (2004). Mechanism of spontaneous excitability in human embryonic stem cell derived cardiomyocytes. *Journal of Physiology*, *559*(Pt 2), 479–496.

Satin, J., Itzhaki, I., Rapoport, S., Schroder, E. A., Izu, L., Arbel, G., et al. (2008). Calcium handling in human embryonic stem cell-derived cardiomyocytes. *Stem Cells*, *26*(8), 1961–1972.

Schmidt, M. M., Guan, K., & Wobus, A. M. (2001). Lithium influences differentiation and tissue-specific gene expression of mouse embryonic stem (ES) cells in vitro. *International Journal of Developmental Biology*, *45*(2), 421–429.

Schwartz, C. M., Spivak, C. E., Baker, S. C., McDaniel, T. K., Loring, J. F., Nguyen, C., et al. (2005). NTera2: a model system to study dopaminergic differentiation of human embryonic stem cells. *Stem Cells and Development*, *14*(5), 517–534.

Schwengberg, S., Bohlen, H., Kleinsasser, N., Kehe, K., Seiss, M., Walther, U. I., et al. (2005). In vitro embryotoxicity assessment with dental restorative materials. *Journal of Dentistry*, *33*(1), 49–55.

Seiler, A. E., & Spielmann, H. (2011). The validated embryonic stem cell test to predict embryotoxicity in vitro. *Nature Protocols*, *6*(7), 961–978.

Shen, C. N., & Tosh, D. (2010). Transdifferentiation of pancreatic cells to hepatocytes. *Methods in Molecular Biology*, *640*, 273–280.

Shirahashi, H., Wu, J., Yamamoto, N., Catana, A., Wege, H., Wager, B., et al. (2004). Differentiation of human and mouse embryonic stem cells along a hepatocyte lineage. *Cell Transplantation*, *13*(3), 197–211.

Shiraki, N., Umeda, K., Sakashita, N., Takeya, M., Kume, K., & Kume, S. (2008). Differentiation of mouse and human embryonic stem cells into hepatic lineages. *Genes to Cells*, *13*(7), 731–746.

Si-Tayeb, K., Noto, F. K., Nagaoka, M., Li, J., Battle, M. A., Duris, C., et al. (2010). Highly efficient generation of human hepatocyte-like cells from induced pluripotent stem cells. *Hepatology*, *51*(1), 297–305.

Singh, S., Kumar, V., Singh, P., Banerjee, B. D., Rautela, R. S., Grover, S. S., et al. (2011). Influence of CYP2C9, GSTM1, GSTT1 and NAT2 genetic polymorphisms on DNA damage in workers occupationally exposed to organophosphate pesticides. *Mutation Research*.

Skrzypiec-Spring, M., Grotthus, B., Szelag, A., & Schulz, R. (2007). Isolated heart perfusion according to Langendorff – still viable in the new millennium. *Journal of Pharmacological and Toxicological Methods*, *55*(2), 113–126.

Smith, D. A., & Schmid, E. F. (2006). Drug withdrawals and the lessons within. *Current Opinion in Drug Discovery & Development*, *9*(1), 38–46.

Snir, M., Kehat, I., Gepstein, A., Coleman, R., Itskovitz-Eldor, J., Livne, E., et al. (2003). Assessment of the ultrastructural and proliferative properties of human embryonic stem cell-derived cardiomyocytes. *American Journal of Physiology – Heart and Circulatory Physiology*, *285*(6), H2355–H2363.

Snykers, S., De Kock, J., Rogiers, V., & Vanhaecke, T. (2009). In vitro differentiation of embryonic and adult stem cells into hepatocytes: state of the art. *Stem Cells*, *27*(3), 577–605.

Söderdahl, T., Küppers-Munther, B., Heins, N., Edsbagge, J., Björquist, P., Cotgreave, I., et al. (2007). Glutathione transferases in hepatocyte-like cells derived from human embryonic stem cells. *Toxicology in Vitro*, *21*(5), 929–937.

Song, Z., Cai, J., Liu, Y., Zhao, D., Yong, J., Duo, S., et al. (2009). Efficient generation of hepatocyte-like cells from human induced pluripotent stem cells. *Cell Research*, *19*(11), 1233–1242.

Soto-Gutiérrez, A., Kobayashi, N., Rivas-Carrillo, J. D., Navarro-Álvarez, N., Zhao, D., Okitsu, T., et al. (2006). Reversal of mouse hepatic failure using an implanted liver-assist device containing ES cell-derived hepatocytes. *Nature Biotechnology*, *24*(11), 1412–1419.

Soto-Gutierrez, A., Navarro-Alvarez, N., Zhao, D., Rivas-Carrillo, J. D., Lebkowski, J., Tanaka, N., et al. (2007). Differentiation of mouse embryonic stem cells to hepatocyte-like cells by co-culture with human liver nonparenchymal cell lines. *Nature Protocols*, *2*(2), 347–356.

Spielmann, H. (2005). Predicting the risk of developmental toxicity from in vitro assays. *Toxicology and Applied Pharmacology*, *207*(2 Suppl.), 375–380.

Spielmann, H., & Vogel, R. (2006). REACH testing requirements must not be driven by reproductive toxicity testing. *Alternative to Laboratory Animals*, *34*(4), 365–366.

Spielmann, H., Pohl, I., Doring, B., Liebsch, M., & Moldenhauer, F. (1997). The embryonic stem cells test (EST), an in vitro embryotoxicity test using two permanent mouse cell lines: 3T3 fibroblasts and embyronic stem cells. *In Vitro Toxicology*, *10*, 119–127.

Stadtfeld, M., Apostolou, E., Akutsu, H., Fukuda, A., Follett, P., Natesan, S., et al. (2010). Aberrant silencing of imprinted genes on chromosome 12qF1 in mouse induced pluripotent stem cells. *Nature*, *465*(7295), 175–181.

Stummann, T. C., Hareng, L., & Bremer, S. (2009). Hazard assessment of methylmercury toxicity to neuronal induction in embryogenesis using human embryonic stem cells. *Toxicology*, *257*(3), 117–126.

Subramanyam, D., Lamouille, S., Judson, R. L., Liu, J. Y., Bucay, N., Derynck, R., et al. (2011). Multiple targets of miR-302 and miR-372 promote reprogramming of human fibroblasts to induced pluripotent stem cells. *Nature Biotechnology*, *29*(5), 443–448.

Sudakin, D. L., & Stone, D. L. (2011). Dialkyl phosphates as biomarkers of organophosphates: the current divide between epidemiology and clinical toxicology. *Clinical Toxicology (Philadelphia)*, *49*(9), 771–781.

Sullivan, G. J., Hay, D. C., Park, I. -H., Fletcher, J., Hannoun, Z., Payne, C. M., et al. (2010). Generation of functional human hepatic endoderm from human induced pluripotent stem cells. *Hepatology*, *51*(1), 329–335.

Suzuki, N., Ando, S., Sumida, K., Horie, N., & Saito, K. (2011). Analysis of altered gene expression specific to embryotoxic chemical treatment during embryonic stem cell differentiation into myocardiac and neural cells. *Journal of Toxicological Sciences*, *36*(5), 569–585.

Tada, H., Shiho, O., Kuroshima, K., Koyama, M., & Tsukamoto, K. (1986). An improved colorimetric assay for interleukin 2. *Journal of Immunological Methods*, *93*(2), 157–165.

Takahashi, K., & Yamanaka, S. (2006). Induction of pluripotent stem cells from mouse embryonic and adult fibroblast cultures by defined factors. *Cell*, *126*(4), 663–676.

Tan, S., Guo, J., Huang, Q., Chen, X., Li-Ling, J., Li, Q., et al. (2007). Retained introns increase putative microRNA targets within 3′ UTRs of human mRNA. *FEBS Letters*, *581*(6), 1081–1086.

Tanimizu, N., & Miyajima, A. (2004). Notch signaling controls hepatoblast differentiation by altering the expression of liver-enriched transcription factors. *Journal of Cell Science*, *117*(15), 3165–3174.

Tekin, D., Kayaalti, Z., & Soylemezoglu, T. (2011). The effects of metallothionein 2A polymorphism on lead metabolism: are pregnant women with a heterozygote genotype for metallothionein 2A polymorphism and their newborns at risk of having higher blood lead levels? *International Archives of Occupational and Environmental Health*.

Terrar, D. A., Wilson, C. M., Graham, S. G., Bryant, S. M., & Heath, B. M. (2007). Comparison of guinea-pig ventricular myocytes and dog Purkinje fibres for in vitro assessment of drug-induced delayed repolarization. *Journal of Pharmacological and Toxicological Methods*, *56*(2), 171–185.

The International Conference on Harmonisation. (2011). Safety Guidelines. Available from: http://www.ich.org/products/guidelines/safety/article/safety-guidelines.html (retrieved 26 October 2011).

Thomson, J. A., Itskovitz-Eldor, J., Shapiro, S. S., Waknitz, M. A., Swiergiel, J. J., Marshall, V. S., et al. (1998). Embryonic stem cell lines derived from human blastocysts. *Science*, *282*(5391), 1145–1147.

Tian, X. Y., Xu, M., Deng, B., Leung, K. S., Cheng, K. F., Zhao, Z. Z., et al. (2011). The effects of Boehmeria nivea (L.) Gaud. on embryonic development: in vivo and in vitro studies. *Journal of Ethnopharmacology*, *134*(2), 393–398.

Tohse, N., Seki, S., Kobayashi, T., Tsutsuura, M., Nagashima, M., & Yamada, Y. (2004). Development of excitation-contraction coupling in cardiomyocytes. *The Japanese Journal of Physiology*, *54*(1), 1–6.

Topol, E. J. (2004). Failing the public health–rofecoxib, Merck, and the FDA. *New England Journal of Medicine*, *351*(17), 1707–1709.

Touboul, T., Hannan, N. R.F., Corbineau, S., Martinez, A., Martinet, C., Branchereau, S., et al. (2010). Generation of functional hepatocytes from human embryonic stem cells under chemically defined conditions that recapitulate liver development. *Hepatology*, *51*(5), 1754–1765.

Ungrin, M. D., Joshi, C., Nica, A., Bauwens, C., & Zandstra, P. W. (2008). Reproducible, ultra high-throughput formation of multicellular organization from single cell suspension-derived human embryonic stem cell aggregates. *PLoS One*, *3*(2), e1565.

Uyama, N., Shimahara, Y., Kawada, N., Seki, S., Okuyama, H., Iimuro, Y., et al. (2002). Regulation of cultured rat hepatocyte proliferation by stellate cells. *Journal of Hepatology*, *36*(5), 590–599.

van Dartel, D. A., Zeijen, N. J., de la Fonteyne, L. J., van Schooten, F. J., & Piersma, A. H. (2009). Disentangling cellular proliferation and differentiation in the embryonic stem cell test, and its impact on the experimental protocol. *Reproductive Toxicology*, *28*(2), 254–261.

van Dartel, D. A., Pennings, J. L., de la Fonteyne, L. J., Brauers, K. J., Claessen, S., van Delft, J. H., et al. (2011). Evaluation of developmental toxicant identification using gene expression profiling in embryonic stem cell differentiation cultures. *Toxicological Sciences*, *119*(1), 126–134.

van der Jagt, K., Munn, S., Tørsløv, J., & de Bruijn, J. (2004). *Alternative approaches can reduce the use of test animals under REACH. Addendum to the Report Assessment of Additional Testing Needs Under Reach. Effects of (Q)SARs, Risk-based Testing and Voluntary Industry Initiatives*. Ispra, Italy: European Commission Joint Research Centre. JRC Report EUR 21405 EN, 33 pp.

Van Hoof, D., Dormeyer, W., Braam, S. R., Passier, R., Monshouwer-Kloots, J., Ward-van Oostwaard, D., et al. (2010). Identification of cell surface proteins for antibody-based selection of human embryonic stem cell-derived cardiomyocytes. *J Proteome Res*, *9*(3), 1610–1618.

Vescovi, A. L., Parati, E. A., Gritti, A., Poulin, P., Ferrario, M., Wanke, E., et al. (1999). Isolation and cloning of multipotential stem cells from the embryonic human CNS and establishment of transplantable human neural stem cell lines by epigenetic stimulation. *Experimental Neurology*, *156*(1), 71–83.

Vierbuchen, T., & Wernig, M. (2011). Direct lineage conversions: unnatural but useful? *Nature Biotechnology*, *29*(10), 892–907.

Vierbuchen, T., Ostermeier, A., Pang, Z. P., Kokubu, Y., Sudhof, T. C., & Wernig, M. (2010). Direct conversion of fibroblasts to functional neurons by defined factors. *Nature*, *463*(7284), 1035–1041.

Vittet, D., Prandini, M. H., Berthier, R., Schweitzer, A., Martin-Sisteron, H., Uzan, G., et al. (1996). Embryonic stem cells differentiate in vitro to endothelial cells through successive maturation steps. *Blood*, *88*(9), 3424–3431.

Weinshilboum, R. M. (1978). Human biochemical genetics of plasma dopamine-beta-hydroxylase and erythrocyte catechol-o-methyltransferase. *Human genetics Supplement*, *1*, 101–112.

Wilffert, B., Swen, J., Mulder, H., Touw, D., Maitland-Van der Zee, A. H., & Deneer, V. (2011). From evidence based medicine to mechanism based medicine. Reviewing the role of pharmacogenetics. *International Journal of Clinical Pharmcology*, *33*(1), 3–9.

Wobus, A. M., & Boheler, K. R. (2005). Embryonic stem cells: prospects for developmental biology and cell therapy. *Physiological Reviews*, *85*(2), 635–678.

Wobus, A., & Löser, P. (2011). Present state and future perspectives of using pluripotent stem cells in toxicology research. *Archives of Toxicology*, *85*(2), 79–117.

Wobus, A. M., & Loser, P. (2011). Present state and future perspectives of using pluripotent stem cells in toxicology research. *Archives in Toxicology*, *85*(2), 79–117.

Wobus, A. M., Guan, K., Yang, H. T., & Boheler, K. R. (2002). Embryonic stem cells as a model to study cardiac, skeletal muscle, and vascular smooth muscle cell differentiation. *Methods in Molecular Biology*, *185*, 127–156.

Xu, C., Police, S., Rao, N., & Carpenter, M. K. (2002). Characterization and enrichment of cardiomyocytes derived from human embryonic stem cells. *Circulation Research*, *91*(6), 501–508.

Xu, C., Police, S., Hassanipour, M., & Gold, J. D. (2006). Cardiac bodies: a novel culture method for enrichment of cardiomyocytes derived from human embryonic stem cells. *Stem Cells and Development*, *15*(5), 631–639.

Xu, X. Q., Graichen, R., Soo, S. Y., Balakrishnan, T., Rahmat, S. N., Sieh, S., et al. (2008a). Chemically defined medium supporting cardiomyocyte differentiation of human embryonic stem cells. *Differentiation*, *76*(9), 958–970.

Xu, X. Q., Zweigerdt, R., Soo, S. Y., Ngoh, Z. X., Tham, S. C., Wang, S. T., et al. (2008b). Highly enriched cardiomyocytes from human embryonic stem cells. *Cytotherapy*, *10*(4), 376–389.

Xu, M., Yan, C., Tian, Y., Yuan, X., & Shen, X. (2010). Effects of low level of methylmercury on proliferation of cortical progenitor cells. *Brain Research*, *1359*, 272–280.

Yang, L., Soonpaa, M. H., Adler, E. D., Roepke, T. K., Kattman, S. J., Kennedy, M., et al. (2008). Human cardiovascular progenitor cells develop from a KDR+ embryonic-stem-cell-derived population. *Nature*, *453*(7194), 524–528.

Yarbro, J. W. (1992). Mechanism of action of hydroxyurea. *Seminars in Oncology*, *19* (3 Suppl. 9), 1–10.

Yildirimman, R., Brolen, G., Vilardell, M., Eriksson, G., Synnergren, J., Gmuender, H., et al. (2011). Human embryonic stem cell derived hepatocyte-like cells as a tool for in vitro hazard assessment of chemical carcinogenicity. *Toxicological Sciences*, *124*(2), 278–290.

Yla-Outinen, L., Heikkila, J., Skottman, H., Suuronen, R., Aanismaa, R., & Narkilahti, S. (2010). Human cell-based micro electrode array platform for studying neurotoxicity. *Front Neuroeng, vol. 3*.

Yokoo, N., Baba, S., Kaichi, S., Niwa, A., Mima, T., Doi, H., et al. (2009). The effects of cardioactive drugs on cardiomyocytes derived from human induced pluripotent stem cells. *Biochemical and Biophysical Research Communications*, *387*(3), 482–488.

Yoshida, Y., & Yamanaka, S. (2011). iPS cells: a source of cardiac regeneration. *The Journal of Molecular and Cellular Cardiology*, *50*(2), 327–332.

Yusa, K., Rashid, S. T., Strick-Marchand, H., Varela, I., Liu, P.-Q., Paschon, D. E., et al. (2011). Targeted gene correction of [agr]1-antitrypsin deficiency in induced pluripotent stem cells. *Nature*, *478*(7369), 391–394.

Zeng, X., Chen, J., Deng, X., Liu, Y., Rao, M. S., Cadet, J. L., et al. (2006). An in vitro model of human dopaminergic neurons derived from embryonic stem cells: MPP+ toxicity and GDNF neuroprotection. *Neuropsychopharmacology*, *31*(12), 2708–2715.

Zeng, H., Park, J. W., Guo, M., Lin, G., Crandall, L., Compton, T., et al. (2009). Lack of ABCG2 expression and side population properties in human pluripotent stem cells. *Stem Cells*, *27*(10), 2435–2445.

Zhang, R., & Su, B. (2009). Small but influential: the role of microRNAs on gene regulatory network and 3′UTR evolution. *Journal of Genetics and Genomics*, *36*(1), 1–6.

Zhang, S. C., Wernig, M., Duncan, I. D., Brustle, O., & Thomson, J. A. (2001). In vitro differentiation of transplantable neural precursors from human embryonic stem cells. *Nature Biotechnology*, *19*(12), 1129–1133.

Zhang, J., Wilson, G. F., Soerens, A. G., Koonce, C. H., Yu, J., Palecek, S. P., et al. (2009). Functional cardiomyocytes derived from human induced pluripotent stem cells. *Circulation Research*, *104*(4), e30–41.

Zhao, D., Chen, S., Cai, J., Guo, Y., Song, Z., Che, J., et al. (2009). Derivation and characterization of hepatic progenitor cells from human embryonic stem cells. *PLoS ONE*, *4*(7).

Zhu, M. X., Zhao, J. Y., Chen, G. A., & Guan, L. (2011). Early embryonic sensitivity to cyclophosphamide in cardiac differentiation from human embryonic stem cells. *Cell Biology International*, *35*(9), 927–938.

Zimmer, B., Kuegler, P. B., Baudis, B., Genewsky, A., Tanavde, V., Koh, W., et al. (2011). Coordinated waves of gene expression during neuronal differentiation of embryonic stem cells as basis for novel approaches to developmental neurotoxicity testing. *Cell Death & Differentiation*, *18*(3), 383–395.

Zinchenko, Y. S., Culberson, C. R., & Coger, R. N. (2006). Contribution of non-parenchymal cells to the performance of micropatterned hepatocytes. *Tissue Engineering*, *12*(8), 2241–2251.

Kevin Brady[1] and Rob Webster[2]

[1]Bicycle Therapeutics Ltd., Cambridge, United Kingdom
[2]Pfizer Global Research and Development, Sandwich, Kent, United Kingdom

Disposition of Biologics

Abstract

Drug development is a complex process, requiring scientific and regulatory input at almost all stages from multiple groups of expertise. Small molecule development issues are covered in other parts of this volume. This chapter is devoted to discussing the large molecules, or biologics, and the particular nuances involved in developing these molecules as medicines.

Our definition of biologic, for the purposes of this chapter, differs from that described by the regulatory bodies. Where regulators state that a biologic is a molecule produced by a living organism, be it a mammalian, insect, yeast or bacteria cell, or whole animal, we prefer to include molecules such as oligonucleotides and peptides here, which are usually chemically synthesized. So our definition is that of a molecule whose composition mostly entails naturally occurring amino acids, sugars or nucleotide bases. There are modifications made chemically to oligonucleotides and peptides to improve their drug-like properties, but for this volume, we class them as biologics.

The aim of this chapter is to describe some of the differences, complexities and paradoxically, simplifications in the pharmacokinetics and ADME sciences during drug development of biologics when compared to the more familiar small molecule drug development process. The impact of the particular pharmacokinetics and ADME sciences of biologics on toxicological and pharmacological end points will be discussed.

I. Introduction

During any drug development process, it is critical to demonstrate efficacy and safety of a drug molecule. Underwriting both of these key criteria lie the pharmacokinetics and ADME (absorption, distribution,

Advances in Pharmacology, Volume 63

1054-3589/12 $35.00
http://dx.doi.org/10.1016/B978-0-12-398339-8.00007-0

metabolism and excretion) sciences. These describe what the body, be that animal or human, does to the drug upon administration, with the key goal of eventually producing safe and efficacious medicines in a commercially viable fashion. Pharmacokinetics exists to aid the scientist in choosing the correct dose and dosing frequency to maintain the required concentration of drug in the system, where it can exert its pharmacology in a safe manner. The ADME sciences enable the scientist to choose the appropriate route of administration, understand whether the drug reaches the desired target in the body, and enables safe implementation of the drug into the complex world of clinical management of patients – a world where inter-individual variability, compromised liver and kidney function, polymorphic metabolic enzyme expression and poly-pharmacy all have a potential impact on the ability of the developed drug to act in a safe and efficacious manner.

Over the past 30 years, the portfolio of drugs available to the scientist and physician has changed and expanded. The dominant activities within the pharmaceutical sector over this time period involved traditional medicinal chemistry leading to the development of small molecular weight drugs, or chemically synthesized xenobiotics. A number of these became the blockbuster drugs of the 1980s and 1990s – Tagamet, Zantac, Losec, and Lipitor to name but a few. However, alongside this, the scientific fields of antisense oligonucleotides, therapeutic peptides, recombinant DNA technology and monoclonal antibodies were growing apace with notable clinical successes. These biologic therapeutics (also termed biotherapeutics or biologicals) were beginning to establish themselves within the portfolios of companies. However, where strides were made with these new molecular entities, unforeseen issues arose, such as anaphylaxis with early murine or chimeric antibodies used in clinic or innate immune-system stimulation with oligonucleotide based therapies. Such a balance still remains today, for example whilst due to the advent of fully human monoclonal antibodies, anaphylaxis is now rarely observed in the clinic per se, major toxicities can be observed in humans with super-agonistic antibodies like TGN-1412 (Suntharalingam et al., 2006).

A key point to note for the reader is the definition of a 'biologic'. For the purposes of this chapter, we class biologics as polymeric molecules predominantly consisting of amino acids, nucleic acids or oligosaccharides. This is designated as such to include oligonucleotide and peptides. It should be noted that this differs from the regulatory view, which effectively boils down to how the drug is made. If it is chemically synthesized, as most oligonucleotides and peptides are, the drug is classed as a small molecule, also termed as a New Chemical Entity by the FDA. If the molecule is produced in an organism, for example *Escherichia coli,* or mammalian cell expression, then the drug is classed as a biologic, also known as a New Biological Entity by the FDA.

II. Routes of Administration

One of the most critical parameters for successfully developing drug candidates is absorption from the site of administration. Small molecule drug development is commonly driven by the need for an orally or topically active agent, and the chemical matter explored in pharmaceutical medicinal chemistry is usually focused on physico-chemical properties that lend themselves to this. However, for large molecules, absorption from such routes is challenging, due to their inherent composition, i.e. large size, multiple electrostatic charges, hydrophilicity. Therefore, these molecules are most commonly administered via parenteral routes (subcutaneous, intra-peritoneal, intramuscular and intravenous).

A. Parenteral Routes

Intravenous administration involves direct injection, either as a bolus, or as an infusion. This route is used often in the pre-clinical setting, especially in order to establish key pharmacokinetic parameters, such as clearance and bioavailability (*F*). The route being assessed for bioavailability must be compared to intravenous administration data, in order to calculate *F* using Eq. (1):

$$F = \frac{\text{Dose}_{\text{IV}}}{\text{AUC}_{\text{IV}}} \times \frac{\text{AUC}_{\text{Other}}}{\text{Dose}_{\text{Other}}} \tag{1}$$

With respect to clinical use, intravenous administration is usually only performed in a hospital setting, due to the need for administration to be performed by trained health professionals.

Intra-peritoneal administration is used pre-clinically in smaller animals, i.e. mice, as this is the most facile route of administering an injectable dose. It is used clinically in some instances in oncology, for example, Catumaxomab (Trion Pharma GmbH) is licensed for treatment of gastric cancer and malignant ascites in Europe via the intra-peritoneal route (Removab – EMEA/H/C/000972 – II/0009, EPAR-Product Information).

The intramuscular route is employed most commonly for vaccine therapy. This route is not often considered a mainstream route of administration of therapeutic biologics due to the pain caused to the patient.

The subcutaneous route (S.C.) is the most commonly developed route for biologics, driven mainly by evidence in the diabetic community that it is an acceptable route of drug dosing, where patients can self-administer once informed and instructed by a health professional. The development of pen-like devices has also facilitated the ease with which injectable drugs can be administered. Most injectable programs start with this route in mind for clinical application, and hence this is often employed in the pre-clinical development of a drug.

The subcutaneous space is a region between the skin and the underlying musculature. The region is richly vascularized and has access to lymphatic drainage. Molecules injected into this region either diffuse directly into the microvasculature or enter into the lymphatic drainage system. Which route is taken is primarily driven by molecular weight, although physico-chemical properties can also influence this (Porter et al., 2001; Supersaxo et al., 1990). In cases where the molecular weight of the drug is less than 10kDa, nearly 70% of the dose administered enters the systemic circulation directly, with the remaining 30% entering via the lymphatics. As size increases, restriction of movement into the vasculature becomes more prominent, and the molecule is forced to drain from the subcutaneous depot through the slower lymphatics system into the central blood compartment. As a result, oligonucleotides and peptides administered via the S.C. route are frequently rapidly absorbed, with early T_{max} values. In contrast to this, monoclonal antibodies and Fc-fusion proteins exhibit a slow absorption phase into the blood compartment (Fig. 1).

Some peptides however, can form a depot at the site of injection, and exhibit very slow absorption, e.g. Degarelix. This leads to so-called flip-flop kinetics, where the rate of absorption is the rate-limiting step that drives

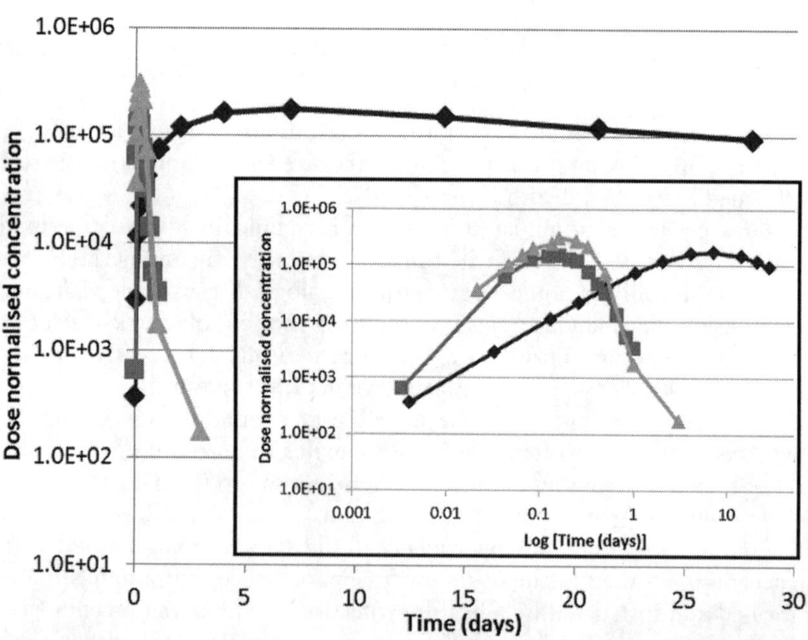

FIGURE 1 Example PK profiles of biotherapeutics delivered via the subcutaneous route. Main graph shows kinetics of a typical monoclonal antibody (diamonds), small protein ~20 kDa (squares) and an oligonucleotide (triangles). Inset graph shows the same data with the x-axis transformed into a logarithmic scale, to allow comparison of each T_{max}.

what seems to be a long half-life in the plasma compartment (Tornøe et al., 2004).

Peptide and protein-based biologics that are not rapidly transiting into the blood will encounter immune surveillance cells in the subcutaneous layer, most notably dendritic cells. These professional antigen presenting cells will engulf, degrade and present fragments of the biologic to T-cells. As some destruction of the dose occurs here, bioavailability is impacted, which at least in part, explains why some proteins do not show appreciable bioavailability when administered subcutaneously. It may also be the case that a biologic can undergo metabolism or receptor mediated clearance in the subcutaneous sites and this may result in bioavailability values by this route of less than 100%. The same can be said for all parenteral routes except intravenous. Precipitation of the biologic can also occur during the time it resides in the subcutaneous depot, which can lead to injection site reactions. Modulating the formulation/concentration can often reduce the risk of this, although in toxicity studies, this may be challenging due to the high concentration frequently required in the dosing solution.

One final point to consider is the fact that if the drug product is pharmacologically active in the subcutaneous space, i.e. target is expressed on cells present in this region, e.g. adipocytes, endothelial cells or dendritic cells, the residence time of the molecule can drive toxicology locally. An example of this is described by Touraine et al. (2009). In a Phase II trial using pegylated growth hormone (peg-GH), injection site lipoatrophy was reported with an incidence of >10%. The authors concluded that the most likely reason for this effect was the local action of peg-GH on adipocytes in the subcutaneous space. Such an effect had previously been reported for growth hormone itself, although the incidence was much lower, arguably because this smaller protein diffuses from the site of injection more rapidly, and hence exerts less pharmacological effect locally.

B. Oral Administration

The gastro-intestinal tract has evolved to break down, and degrade biopolymers in food prior to absorption (see review by Mahato et al., 2003 for a discussion on barriers). As biologics tend to dominantly consist of the same biopolymer components, they are highly susceptible to the degradative environment present in the gut. However, there are a number of examples where biologics, namely peptides, can be successfully administered orally and while oral bioavailability is usually low (<20%), the relative potency of such peptides can ameliorate the barriers to oral delivery, e.g. calcitonin. Chemical strategies can be employed to improve oral bioavailability such as the use of un-natural amino acids to prevent enzymatic degradation and *N*-methylation to the Cα atom in the peptide backbone. Use of this modification can improve enzymatic stability as well as membrane permeability (Biron et al., 2008). Other pharmaceutical solutions are being explored currently in human trials where peptides are formulated in enterically coated dosage forms, along with protease inhibitors and intestinal permeability enhancers. Such strategies may well increase the bioavailability window sufficiently to facilitate oral dosing of biomolecules.

It is also worth noting that to date, only a handful of transporters involved in uptake of peptides have been identified, including PEPT1 and PEPT2 present in the brush border of the gut and kidney endothelia. It is likely that other transporters will be identified in the future, and the impact of drug combinations on the efficacy-toxicology balance of a co-dosed biologic (namely peptides) will need to be considered. Such study may also highlight key mechanisms for uptake, which can then be exploited for delivery.

III. Mechanisms of Biologics Distribution and Clearance, The Importance of Active Processes

Generally passive processes leading to the distribution/clearance of biologics are well conserved. For example, the clearance and distribution of biologics in the kidney by the glomerular filtration is highly conserved and driven by the physico-chemical properties of the molecule (Deen & Satvat, 1981; Strober & Waldmann, 1974).

Perhaps the most important processes, to consider when looking at interpreting toxicological observations and selecting toxicology species, are those that are driven by active processes. As with small molecules, active processes can govern both the distribution and clearance of biologics. However, these processes are perhaps more linked than those seen for small molecule, as discussed below.

Monoclonal antibodies are the most characterized group of biologics with respect to the mechanisms involved in their disposition. Firstly, physicochemical properties such as size, and more specifically Stoke's radius, drive the passive process associated with their distribution and clearance. They are not excreted through the kidney, as they exceed the molecular weight size cut-off deemed to exist in the glomerulus (>50 kDa). Also, due to their size and hydrophilicity, they tend to reside mostly in the blood stream, with some distribution into the tissue extracellular volume. Basement membrane integrity and tight junction formation between endothelial cells in the microvasculature of each location within the body dictates whether or not a biologic will be able to penetrate into that particular tissue. For example, antibodies tend to distribute freely into the liver and spleen, whereas they are excluded extensively from muscle and the brain. As a result, antibody drugs tend to have a low volume of distribution, usually between 0.1 and 0.3 L/kg, which reflects blood volume together with the extracellular volume into which the molecule can distribute.

The active process associated with antibody clearance is driven by the neonatal Fc receptor (FcRn), which is expressed ubiquitously throughout the body. This receptor performs a recycling function, essentially rescuing antibodies from catabolic metabolism within the reticulo-endothelial system. The protein is present in the endosome, where the local pH is lower than that in blood; around pH 6.0 instead of pH 7.4 in blood. This leads to the ionization of histidines within the Fc region of antibodies, that can then bind to negatively charged residues on the surface of the FcRn protein. The complex recycles to the cell surface, where the change in pH leads to deionization of the same histidine residues in the Fc region of the antibody. This causes the complex to disassociate, and returns the rescued antibody to the circulation. FcRn has also been shown to translocate antibodies across cells, and is implicated in the distribution of antibodies in various tissues. Therefore, both distribution and clearance of a given antibody is driven by affinity for this receptor. Understanding this affinity and ensuring comparable potency and distribution of FcRn between species ensures similar distribution/clearance processes will occur in animals. As stated above, because this process is well understood for monoclonal antibodies, species difference in clearance are predictable and can easily be implemented into mathematical predictions of antibody PK/PD performance (Shah & Betts, 2011). However, in order to emphasize the importance of understanding species differences in receptor number and location, the same systems represents an ideal example. There are marked differences in the processes transporting monoclonal antibodies to the fetus in rats and monkeys/human. These differences include differences in location of expressed FcRn (yoke sac versus placenta) and timing of transporter expression/location, leading to differences in the time of fetal transport of IgG in embryo toxicology studies (Roopenian & Akilesh, 2007). These concerns, along with frequently reduced target potency have limited the use of the rodent as an embryo/foetal toxicology species for monoclonal antibodies. Both Fc-fusion proteins and albumin containing fusion proteins use the same recycling process via FcRn and as such similar issues exist for these molecules. The albumin recycling process, however, involves ionization of histidine residues on the FcRn protein in the endosomal environment, and binding occurs at a distal site to the Fc-binding region on FcRn (Andersen et al., 2012). As both antibodies and albumin bind to FcRn in a non-competitive manner, the use of monoclonal antibodies does not interfere with endogenous albumin recycling, in the same way that therapeutic albumin conjugates do not interfere with endogenous IgG recycling (Andersen et al., 2010).

Antisense oligonucleotides must be modified to ensure they are therapeutically useful. The phosphorothioate modification, where one of the phosphate group oxygen atoms is replaced with a sulfur atom, is most commonly used. This modification improves the stability of the molecule with respect to nuclease degradation, and is responsible for protein binding, which retains the molecule within the blood stream instead of being excreted in the urine, as well as facilitating tissue uptake. Studies performed by us have demonstrated single digit micromolar K_D values for phosphorothioate oligonucleotides binding to human albumin, indicating >95% fraction bound. Uptake mechanisms into tissue are not well understood, but it is postulated that oligonucleotides bind with high affinity to various surface tethered proteins on cells, and are internalized via the natural mechanisms involved in cell-surface protein turnover. Oligonucleotides enter into the endosomal pathways, and will eventually escape from here to gain access to the cytoplasm of the cell where they exert their pharmacological effect. However, this is a very inefficient process, with >90% of the drug remaining in the endosomal/lysosomal pathway. Further research is required to understand which proteins and pathways are normally used by oligonucleotides to enter cells, together with enabling more efficient delivery of the drug to the active compartment within the cell.

With peptide therapeutics, strategies are often utilized to increase the systemic exposure through half-life extension. Fatty acid conjugation (Liraglutide), PEGylation (Pegasys) and directed conjugation to antibodies and albumin have all been used. Careful consideration must be given to the impact of these changes on the molecule with respect to the clearance and disposition. For example, the clearance mechanisms of PEGylated growth hormone have been discussed in Webster et al. (2008). The PEGylation of growth hormone with a 40 kDa PEG reduced clearance via glomerular filtration and increased clearance by the growth hormone receptor, present in the liver, relative to that observed for native growth hormone. These changes would clearly lead to markedly different distribution of PEGylated growth hormone relative to growth hormone. This alteration in clearance/distribution indicates that there could be differences in the toxicology of PEGylated growth hormone, relative to growth hormone. However, the key question for a toxicologist is likely to be whether there will be species differences between the toxicity of PEGylated growth hormone. Again this demonstrates the importance of species selection before commencing toxicology species. Therefore, as long as best practice has been followed and there is a robust understanding of the impact of the target receptor and clearance mechanism, it is likely that one can proceed with confidence. This best practice would include understanding the distribution of target receptor and if needs be clearance mechanism in the toxicology species and in human (Webster et al., 2009). This example also demonstrates the principles of target mediated disposition in the clearance and distribution of a biologic, these being important considerations in developing an ADME understanding of a biologic.

From a toxicology standpoint, it is important to consider whether the transporters/processes responsible for the uptake of a molecule are conserved. Failure to consider this could lead to differential distribution/clearance in animals relative to human and could reduce the effective understanding of toxicity in humans.

IV. Distribution Studies with Biologics and Relevance to Toxicology Studies

Many papers have discussed the distribution of biologics, including monoclonal antibodies, peptides, oligos/aptamers, etc. The majority of these studies have been carried out with radiolabels, although studies can be carried out utilizing a range of methodologies, including analysis of compound levels in tissue with immunoassay, mass spectrometry and other end points. Generally for monoclonal antibodies and other protein or amino acid based molecules, distribution tissue concentration differences can be observed at early time points. For example, Vugmeyster et al. (2010), demonstrated apparent tissue-to-serum ratios ranging from <0.01 for brain, fat and muscle at the early time point of 1 h up to approximately 0.1 for heart, kidney, liver and spleen. However, as time post dose increased, the differences between tissues became less apparent with tissue-to-serum ratios approaching 0.1 for most tissues (femur, fat, heart, kidney, large intestine, liver, lung, lymph node, muscle, skin, small intestine, spleen and stomach), except in the brain where concentrations were still low 48 h post dose in mice. These studies have not only been limited to parenteral delivery of proteins. For example, Davis et al., 2011, quantified the oral distribution of proteins (BSA, Casein, CD14) in rats. Finally a limited amount of work has been done in humans where the distribution of indium 111 labeled anti-CD66 IgG (Kletting et al., 2010) has been investigated. This study looked at the distribution of the monoclonal antibody into liver, spleen and bone marrow relative to blood (Fig. 2).

With the amount of available animal data and the presence of limited human data, many authors (Shah & Betts, 2011; Davis et al., 2011; Kletting et al., 2010; Garg & Balthasar, 2007; Heiskanen et al., 2009) have developed mathematical models to describe the distribution of monoclonal antibodies. These physiologically based pharmacokinetic (PBPK) models allow the tissue distribution of a monoclonal antibody to be determined in the absence of binding to its pharmacological target and as such can provide a starting point for understanding the distribution of many monoclonal antibodies and could in fact replace the need for general distribution studies. These efforts also indicate that distribution in animals is similar to that seen

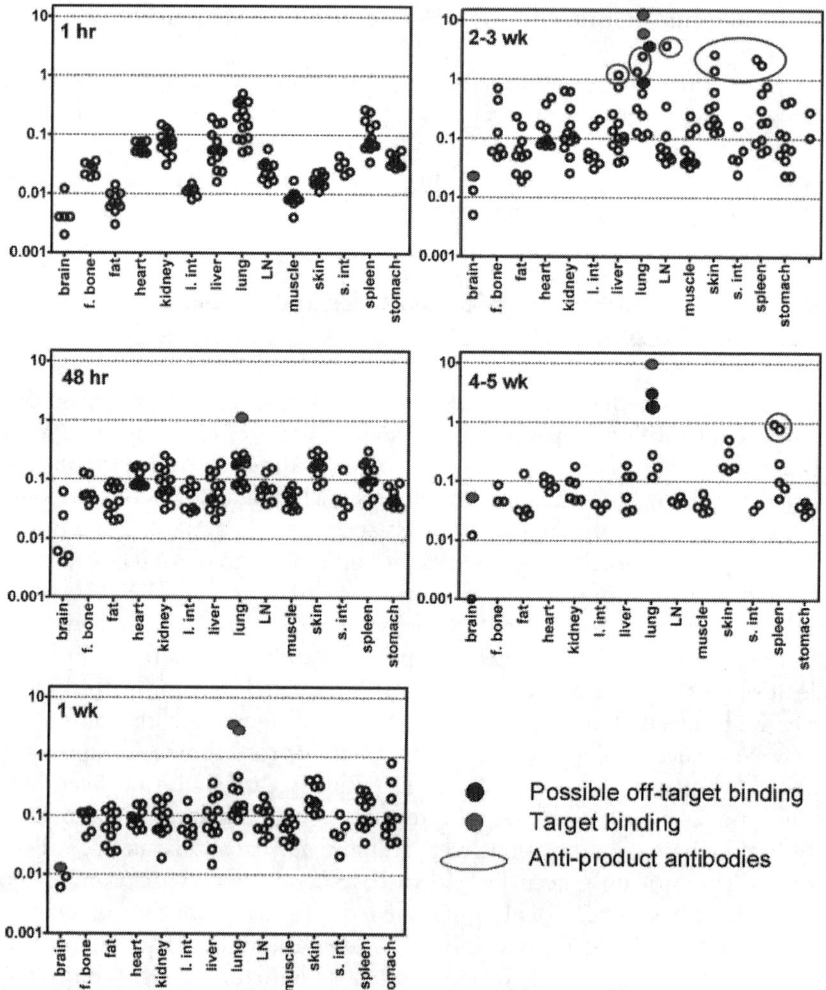

FIGURE 2 Typical tissue-to-serum (T/S) concentration ratios after single IV administration of human or chimeric [^{125}I]-labeled IgG1 antibodies to mice. Various wild-type, knockout or transgenic mouse strains were administered a single IV dose (dose range 1–10 mg/kg) of human or mouse-human chimeric [^{125}I]-labeled IgG1 antibodies (drug candidates at Wyeth, Inc.). T/S ratios were determined as described in the text. High *T/S* ratios that were most likely explained by specific binding to the target are shown in red/light grey circles, while those that were likely related to anti-product antibody formation are encircled. Data points that warranted additional investigation of the off target binding are shown in green/dark grey. LN, lymph node; f. bone, femur bone; l. int, large intestine; and s. int, small intestine. (reproduced with permission from Vugmeyster et al., 2010).

in human (Kletting et al., 2010). In all these distribution studies, one of the key considerations is whether the material present is capable of demonstrating pharmacology. This is particularly an issue for labeled studies (fluorescence or radiolabel). For these studies, products of metabolism may not be active, but will be detected. Several methods have been identified to deal with this question, including precipitation of radiolabel and calculation of the difference between soluble and precipitated radiolabels. The assumption here is that precipitated radiolabel represents intact material and the soluble radiolabel represents small metabolic products. Whilst this approach is valid for many biologic classes, perhaps the most scientifically valid methodology for all biologic classes may be the use of target LC-MS assays to determine the presence of compound or immunoassay designed to detect full length material or key components of the molecule important for efficacy.

The next most studied class of molecules in terms of distribution is oligonucleotides, which includes antisense oligonucleotides, siRNA and aptamers. The abundance of nucleases in plasma prohibits the use of therapeutics oligonucleotides that contain native DNA or RNA. A variety of chemical modifications have been employed to overcome this obstacle, some of which impart other useful properties. For example, the phosphorothioate modification, where a sulfur atom is incorporated in place of one of the oxygen atoms in each phosphate group of the molecule, restricts nuclease degradation, as well as increasing the plasma protein binding potential of the molecule. For example, Yu et al. (2007), demonstrated that a phosphorothioate based oligonucleotide distributed mainly to the liver and kidney in both mice and cynomolgus monkeys, with lower concentrations detected in the spleen, lung, heart and ovaries/testes. No oligonucleotide could be detected in the brain. Similar observations were also made for peptide nucleic acids (PNAs) in the rat and these studies are detailed in Gasser et al. (2010). Finally, Lendvai et al. (2008) demonstrated similar distribution for LNA–DNA mixmers in the rat showing similar distribution for a broad range of oligonucleotide based biologics. To date there has been one published PBPK model for this class. Peng et al. (2001) published a model based on administration of a tritium labeled antisense oligonucleotide to rat. Such a model could form the basis of other pre-clinical PBPK models used during drug development of phosphorothioate oligonucleotides.

It is worth noting at this point that cellular and subcellular distribution assessment is becoming more important, especially for oligonucleotides and cell-penetrating peptides. For example, phosphorothioate antisense oligonucleotides are taken up in the liver initially by endothelial cells, followed by Kupffer cells and hepatocytes (Graham et al., 1998). Such differential uptake must be assessed when targeting other diseased cells, e.g. immune cells. Furthermore, subcellular distribution may aid in the interpretation of toxicity/efficacy issues. When performing pharmacology studies, particular oligonucleotide sequences may demonstrate improved efficacy *in vivo* by being more available for endosomal escape, a pre-requisite for pharmacological activity.

These data indicate that for many classes of biologics, biodistribution has been well studied, particularly for monoclonal antibodies and aptamers/oligos, and in general, distribution seems to be highly conserved. Therefore, a reasonable understanding of the basic distribution of a biologic class can likely be achieved simply using pre-existing literature data or PBPK models. If these data are not available, simple distribution studies using radiolabel, cold compound analysis, etc. can reliably confirm the distribution of a biologic to various tissues.

However, this position does have some exceptions and before pre-existing literature data is used to determine the distribution of a biologic, consideration should be given to the distribution and abundance of the target. The importance of this target distribution/abundance question is discussed in Vugmeyster et al. (2010). They demonstrated differential distribution of a small number of antibodies when compared to a database of a wide range of distribution studies in the mouse. The authors demonstrated that the kidney distribution of this subset of antibodies was 10-fold higher than that seen for a typical antibody and the authors hypothesized that this difference was due to target binding. These observations could be important from a toxicology or efficacy stand point as they demonstrate some off target or target mediated disposition to an organ and as such, potential for pharmacology or exaggerated pharmacology/toxicity in this organ. In a similar vein, this paper also discusses the use of transgenic animals to look at the relationship between the distribution of target and of the biologic. For example, this paper demonstrated the altered distribution of IL21 antibodies using knock out animals.

The paper also highlighted one of the key issues faced by many biologics scientists when conducting biodistribution studies, namely that of relevant target binding and distribution in the species of interest, relative to human. Frequently, the binding of biologics to rodent targets is poor and as such, this species may be completely inappropriate for the study of distribution. In fact this may mean that relevant distribution studies can only be carried out in species with relevant target binding, such as cynomolgus monkey.

This observation does expose the key limitation of distribution studies. Unless they are carried out in a species that has similar target affinity and target distribution, they will limit the understanding of toxicological risk or pharmacological action of a biologic. Alternative approaches to distribution studies may become more insightful over time. The combination of PBPK models combined with a thorough understanding of target distribution could be used to evaluate occupancy in key tissues, informing efficacy/side effect/toxicology profiles. Validation of the estimates of target occupancy against dose in animal experiments using occupancy end points can be translated to a potential human outcome. This methodology may be applicable but a considerable amount of data is required and extrapolations are always complicated in this area. As such, at present it is not clear whether this methodology could be used to make any robust argument on a safety related matter.

In conclusion, distribution studies can be performed for biologics in a range of animals. In order for these studies to be successful in allowing the quantification for risk to human, similar target binding and distribution is required in the study species. The question of target binding and distribution is a key consideration for species selection in the area of biologic toxicology. As the biodistribution properties of the major biologic classes have been well studied and is well conserved, it is unlikely that stand-alone biodistribution studies will add much to the understanding of toxicology within these classes and that well conducted toxicology studies will provide a more than adequate assessment of toxicity. In the cases where new biologic classes develop, performing detailed biodistribution studies may still be warranted.

V. Metabolism of Biologics

As biologics are predominantly natural molecules, the routes of metabolism are frequently those seen for the naturally occurring molecules of any given class. This simplifies the metabolism question for molecules that are made of purely natural constituents, as it is simply sufficient to infer the metabolic fate of the molecule from that of the natural analog. In fact, radiolabel excretion balance studies for these types of molecule may not even be possible, as the biologic molecule is likely to be broken down to simple building blocks, for example amino acids or oligonucleotides, and the fate of these may be either incorporation into new molecules or further degradation to even simpler entities, for example, CO_2, water, etc.

However, this may not be the case for biologics that incorporate non-natural components. It is becoming clear that regulatory authorities can request a more detailed understanding of the fate of the non-natural components of a biologic drug. These requests could include linkers, non-natural amino acids or modified oligonucleotides. In these cases, studies will be required to understand the fate of these molecules. Given the typical properties of biologics, these studies may not be easy and may require long-time courses to develop a solid understanding of the fate of the non-natural portion. It would also be necessary to determine whether the fate of these molecules will be the same in animals as in human. Work in this area is generally at an early stage and whilst the answering of some of these questions will be tractable using traditional approaches such as ^{14}C labeling, etc., it is also likely that more innovative approaches will be necessary such as accelerator mass spectroscopy, NMR, etc. An example of these efforts is detailed in Murphy et al. (2010), where the authors have used a combination of immunoassay and two-dimensional liquid chromatography mass spectrometry to detect and identify biologic metabolites. Whilst these efforts were not targeted at understanding metabolism of the non-natural components per se, they do demonstrate the value of applying non-radiolabel technologies to understanding the metabolism of biologics. Also it is possible that more than one approach will be required to answer these questions potentially incorporating both *in vitro* and *in vivo* sciences. As these questions become more prevalent, it will become clearer which will be the most reliable methods for future use.

An obvious consideration, especially amongst those developing peptides and oligonucleotides, is the role of the more typical metabolic routes involved in small molecule elimination. Due to the intracellular location of cytochrome P450 enzymes (CYPs), along with the host of other phase I and phase II enzymatic processes, the exclusion of biologics from intracellular compartments would normally leave traditional metabolic and drug–drug interaction studies redundant. However, it should be noted that if a biologic is designed to enter a cell, it is critical to establish likely free concentrations of the drug that are present in the same compartment as the metabolic enzymes. For example, oligonucleotides enter into cells in the liver at high concentration, and yet, the overwhelming majority of the drug remains in the endosomal/lysosomal pathways, and never enter the same region of the cell in which CYPs reside. Therefore, direct studies are not usually required.

Drug-biologic interaction studies should be performed in cases where the pharmacology exhibited by the biologic influences the expression of metabolic enzymes e.g. Interferon alpha (IFN-α). Administration of IFN-α downregulates the expression of CYP1A2 when used in anti-viral or anti-tumor chemotherapy. This leads to reduced clearance and subsequent increases in exposure of concomitant medicines such as theophylline which are normally metabolized by this enzyme. It is essential to determine if the desired pharmacology exhibited through the target molecule is linked to the expression profile and activity of metabolic pathways.

VI. Consideration of Immunogenicity – Changes in Disposition and Impact on Toxicology

One major difference between biologics and small molecule drugs is the potential for interaction with multiple components of the host immune system. The immune system has evolved to detect and react to components of invading organisms, namely proteins, peptides, carbohydrates, lipopolysaccharides and nucleic acids. The cellular, humoral and innate immune systems are all involved in sensing the presence of and reaction to the above listed components. The majority of biologics will contain one or more of these, and hence immunogenicity is a key risk during drug development.

TABLE I Description of Potential Impact that Various Biologics may have on the Immune System and Potential Outcomes

Biologic	*Immune System*	*Action*	*Result*
Protein, e.g. MAbs, Fc-Fusions, replacement biologics	Processing of protein to peptides for presentation via MHC class II to CD4+ T-cells (cellular followed by humoral)	Activation of B-cells producing antibodies	(a) Neutralizing antibody production which leads to a reduction of efficacy (b) Accelerated clearance of biologic due to clearance of immune complex (c) Conversely, possible to generate binding antibodies that can increase exposure of a biologic, leading to enhanced pharmacology and toxicity (d) In the case of replacement biologics, potential risk of producing antibodies that cross-react with endogenously expressed protein, leading to accelerated clearance of both endogenous and therapeutic proteins (e) Deposition of immune complexes in microvasculature leading to toxicity – e.g. renal toxicity
Oligonucleotides	Binding to Toll-Like receptors at the cell surface or endosome (innate)	Activation of the anti-viral pathways, usually leading to IFN-α release	Chills, headaches, back pain, aches
MAbs	T-cell specific targeting (e.g. Rituxumab, OXT3) (target related) Direct pharmacological stimulus of cytokine release (e.g. CD28 agonists)	Stimulation of T-cells prior to clearance of the cell Engagement and agonism of CD4+ effector memory cells	Multiple cytokines released causing significant side effects upon dosing
Mabs and Fc-fusions	Fcγ receptor binding (cellular)	(a) At high concentrations, potential to block endogenous antibody–Fcγ interactions. (b) If targeting cellular receptors, use of an ADCC/CDC capable isotype (e.g. IgG1) may be a risk is this pharmacology is not required for normal therapy	(a) Possible immunosuppression by preventing endogenous antibodies from triggering immune reactivity through Fcg receptor binding (e.g. antibody-directed cellular cytotoxicity) (b) Instead of exhibiting desired blockade of a target in an otherwise healthy cell, can lead to destruction of the cell

Another key consideration is whether or not the pharmacological action of the molecule impacts the immune system. Depending on the biologics target molecule *in vivo*, immune system toxicities such as cytokine release syndrome can occur (e.g. CD28 superagonist TGN-1412). Table 1 summarizes the most common potential immunogenicity-related issues arising with biologics.

A. Changes in Disposition

The most obvious alteration in the disposition of biologics upon immune activation is the accelerated clearance of the drug from the circulation. With respect to time-scale, this becomes obvious after 6 days in rats and 10 days in cynomolgus monkeys post administration. This is usually the time taken to raise a robust IgG response to an immunogen. Immunogenicity is also more likely upon repeat dosing (similar to a prime-boost scenario in vaccines). An example of the effect of anti-drug antibodies is shown in Fig. 3.

Such an effect occurs usually when multiple antibodies bind to multiple epitopes on the biologic drug, producing immune complexes that can be rapidly cleared by macrophages (Fig. 4). If the biologic molecule is small, or has a single immunodominant epitope, it is possible to extend the half-life of the therapeutic, i.e. upon complexation with an antibody specific for a single epitope, the therapeutic molecule can exhibit the circulating half-life of the binding antibody itself. This does not necessarily lead to neutralization of the pharmacologically active component of the biologic either. It is possible to dramatically increase the pharmacological effect by increasing the exposure of the drug in this way.

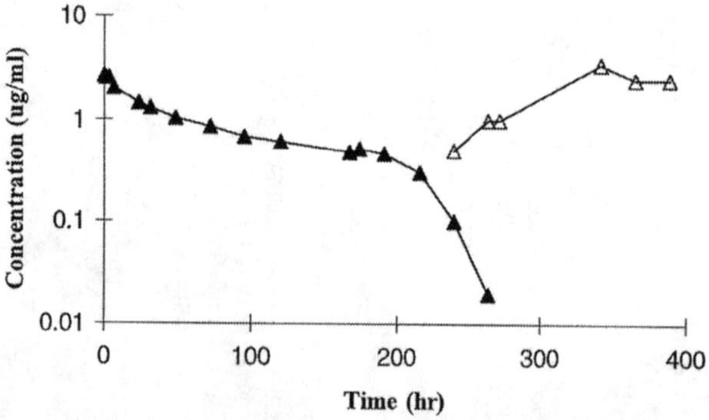

FIGURE 3 Example of the pharmacokinetic impact of anti-drug antibodies on the exposure of the biologic Lenercept in dog (reproduced with permission from Richter et al., 1999). Concentration of lenercept is shown by closed triangles. Anti-drug antibody titer is shown with open triangles. Note that the anti-drug antibody titer appears as the exposure of lenercept rapidly drops, indicating clearance by immune complexation. Also note the time of immune response occurs around 7–10 days.

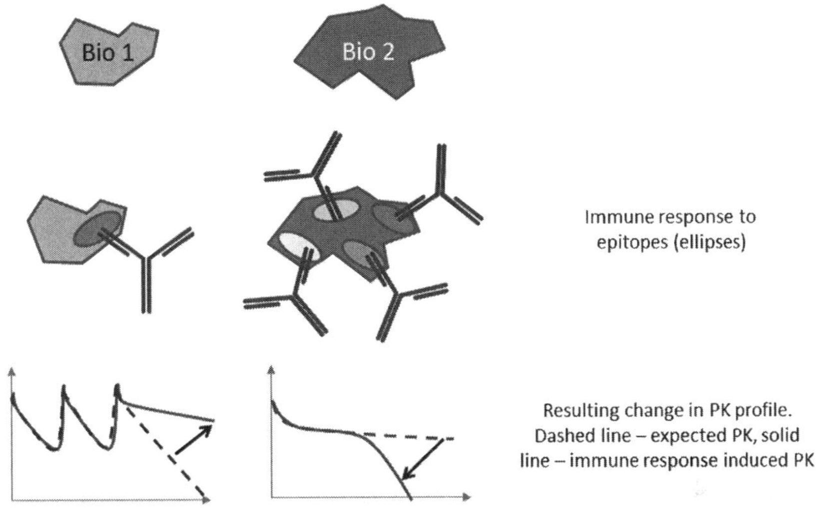

FIGURE 4 Description of potential changes in pharmacokinetics of a biologic, depending on the number of immunoreactive epitopes present on the surface of the protein. Increased exposure driven by binding of a single endogenous antibody to a single epitope on protein Bio 1 – the complex exhibits the same clearance rate as the endogenous antibody, and no longer exhibits the clearance of the biologic. Decreased exposure driven by the presence of multiple epitopes on the surface of Bio 2, leading to a large immune complex. Such complexes are rapidly removed from the circulation by macrophages.

B. Assessment of Immunogenic Risk

First and foremost, if the biologic is being developed to target a key component of the immune system, it is essential to characterize the effector pharmacology in pre-clinical species and in human. In the case of TGN-1412, Eastwood et al., 2010 have recently demonstrated that the target protein for the antibody (CD28) is missing in macaque monkeys on CD4+ effector memory cells that usually reside in tissues. These cells act as fast response cells to immunological attack, releasing pro-inflammatory cytokines rapidly, rather than the slower memory system resident in lymph nodes. They propose this as the key reason why no such toxicity was observed in monkeys during pre-clinical development, and yet led to the severe adverse events observed in the clinical trial. They also propose the continued use of *in vitro* cytokine stimulation assays for biologics, but with the subtle additional interpretation that if a robust IFN-γ response is observed, this may indicate a TGN-1412-like mechanism underlying cytokine release, and should be explored more carefully.

Moving away from immune-system modulation directly, other approaches are used to de-risk molecules with respect to human immunogenicity, namely attempts to characterize and avoid immunogenic epitopes in the protein/peptide. A number of *in silico* and *in vitro* approaches can be used to determine MHC Class I and II binding epitopes that lead to T-cell proliferation. All of these approaches use human sequences, proteins and cells to determine the likely risk. Steps can be taken to modify or 'veneer' regions of high immunogenicity. An example of this is the so-called 'germ-lining' approach used in monoclonal antibody development. Point mutations in the framework regions of the antigen-binding domain of the antibody have occurred during B-cell selection, and these are mutated back to the original human germ-line sequence represented in that particular antibody. This is done to avoid immunological 'hot-spots' within a sequence – somewhat akin to the natural de-selection of B-cell clones *in vivo* that present antibodies with highly immunogenic sequences.

With respect to oligonucleotides, particular motifs in DNA-based molecules are known to activate the innate immune system through toll-like receptor binding. Specifically, the CpG (cytosine-phosphodiester-Guanosine) motif stimulates TLR9, leading to interferon and other pro-inflammatory cytokine production. Modifying the cytosine to 5-methyl cytosine in such a sequence abolishes the recognition by TLR9, and reverts the molecule to an immunologically inert one.

Long double stranded RNA molecules are also recognized by the innate immune system, particularly by TLR3, again leading to interferon-α release. By limiting the length of a therapeutic double stranded RNA molecule to less than 25 bases, this issue can also be avoided.

It should be noted that the currently accepted wisdom (amongst regulators and the industry) is that pre-clinical animal immunogenicity does not predict human immunogenic risk. Pre-clinical immunogenicity does indeed occur in the majority of programs developing human proteins as therapeutics, but this tends to cause problems in interpreting pharmacokinetic or pharmacodynamics endpoints in studies. This can also lead to toxicity through consequences such as immune complex formation and subsequent deposition. While this may describe the potential effect on physiological function as a consequence of immune complex deposition, it is important to gauge the likelihood of risk of this occurring in human.

VII. Conclusion

Drug development of biologics represents some key challenges to the ADME scientist. Whilst in some respects, the ADME issues are simpler than those seen for small molecules, for example metabolism of natural biologics. In many respects, the understanding of the ADME properties can be more complicated and can require the application of new technologies or old technologies in novel ways to provide answers to key questions.

Some of the key biologic questions are related to the clearance/distribution mechanism, which are frequently linked and driven by active receptor mediated processes. In order to fully understand the risks associated with this ADME area, it is critical to have a solid understanding of the processes involved in the clearance and disposition of a biologic. In order to do this, an ADME scientist will not only have to consider the distribution of the target receptor, to understand target mediated disposition and pharmacology in animals and humans, but also an understanding of the clearance mechanism and whether these are conserved between species. Fortunately, building this understanding has been a key criterion for the selection of toxicology species for large molecule toxicology studies and as such it is highly likely that this area can/will be adequately dealt with during the development of the compound.

Another key challenge facing the scientist working with biologics is immunogenicity. At its most simplistic level, the impact on immunogenicity on exposure and toxicology is a frequent, but not overly troubling issue. But this area is indeed complex and in order to successfully pursue a program, key decisions on the immunogenicity assays that will be used to monitor immunogenicity have to be made early in the program and with consideration for the likely risk of an immune response in human. This is one of the many areas where ADME scientists can contribute to the development of a toxicology program.

Finally, metabolism studies, whilst largely unnecessary for natural biologics, are beginning to be required for molecules that contain linkers or non-natural small molecule components. Successfully studying this metabolism will draw on the ingenuity of ADME scientists. Whilst traditional radiolabel excretion balance approaches may provide some data, alternative approaches may be needed for other molecule types, e.g. the use of NMR of PEG. This will require close collaboration between ADME and toxicological scientists in order to frame the key question/s and design the key studies.

Conflict of Interest: Kevin Brady is employed by Bicycle Therapeutics Ltd, a biotechnology company developing peptide-based therapeutics. Rob Wenster is employed by Pfizer Inc., a pharmaceutical company developing small and large molecule therapeutics.

Abbreviations

ADME	Absorption, Distribution, Metabolism and Excretion
CYP	Cytochrome P450 enzyme
DNA	Deoxyribonucleic acid
IgG	Immunoglobulin G
INF	Interferon
K_D	Equilibrium dissociation constant
LNA	Locked nucleic acid
Mab	Monoclonal antibody
MHC	Major histocompatibility complex

PBPK	Physiology based pharmacokinetics
PEG	Polyethylene glycol
PKPD	Pharmacokinetics pharmacodynamics
S.C.	Subcutaneous
T_{max}	Time at which the maximum concentration is observed in a pharmacokinetic profile

References

Andersen, J. T., Daba, M. B., Berntzen, G., Michaelsen, T. E., & Sandlie, I. (2010). Cross-species binding analyses of mouse and human neonatal Fc receptor show dramatic differences in immunoglobulin G and albumin binding. *Journal of Biological Chemistry*, *285*, 4826–4836.

Andersen, J. T., Dalhus, B., Cameron, J., Daba, M. B., Plumridge, A., Evans, L., et al. (2012). Structure-based mutagenesis reveals the albumin-binding site of the neonatal Fc receptor. *Nature Communications*, *3*10.1038/ncomms1607. Article number: 610.

Biron, E., Chatterjee, J., Ovadia, O., Langenegger, D., Brueggen, J., Hoyer, D., et al. (2008). Improving oral bioavailability of peptides by multiple N-methylation: somatostatin analogues. *Angewandte Chemie International Edition*, *47*, 2595–2599.

Davis, L. D., Spencer, W. J., Pham, V. T., Ward, T. L., Blais, D. R., Mack, D. R., et al. (2011). ^{14}C radiolabeling of proteins to monitor biodistribution of ingested proteins. *Analytical Biochemistry*, *410*, 57–61.

Deen, W. M., & Satvat, B. (1981). Determinants of the glomerular filtration of proteins. *American Journal of Physiology*, *241*, F162–F170.

Eastwood, D., Findlay, L., Poole, S., Bird, C., Wadhwa, M., et al. (2010). Monoclonal antibody TGN1412 trial failure explained by species differences in CD28 expression on CD4+ effector memory T-cells. *British Journal of Pharmacology*, *161*, 512–526.

Garg, A., & Balthasar, J. P. (2007). Physiologically-based pharmacokinetic (PBPK) model to predict IgG tissue kinetics in wild-type and FcRn-knockout mice. *Journal of Pharmacokinetics and Pharmacodynamics*, *34*, 687–709.

Gasser, G., Jaeger, K., Zenker, M., Bergmann, R., Steinbach, J., Stephan, H., et al. (2010). Preparation, ^{99m}Tc-labeling and biodistribution studies of a PNA oligomer containing a new ligand derivative of 2,2'-dipicolylamine. *Journal of Inorganic Biochemistry*, *104*, 1133–1140.

Graham, M. J., Crooke, S. T., Monteith, D. K., Cooper, S. R., Lemonidis, K. M., Stecker, K. K., et al. (1998). In vivo distribution and metabolism of a phosphorothioate oligonucleotide within rat liver after intravenous administration. *Journal of Pharmacology and Experimental Therapeutics*, *286*, 447–458.

Heiskanen, T., Heiskanen, T., & Kairemo, K. (2009). Development of a PBPK model for monoclonal antibodies and simulation of human and mice PBPK of a radiolabelled monoclonal antibody. *Current Pharmaceutical Design*, *15*, 988–1007.

Kletting, P., Kull, T., Bunjes, D., Mahren, B., Luster, M., Reske, S. N., et al. (2010). Radioimmunotherapy with anti-CD66 antibody: improving the biodistribution using a physiologically based pharmacokinetic model. *Journal of Nuclear Medicine*, *51*, 484–491.

Lendvai, G., Velikyan, I., Estrada, S., Erikssin, B., Langstrom, B., & Bergstrom, M. (2008). Biodistribution of 68Ga-labelled LNA–DNA mixmer antisense oligonucleotides for rat chromagranin-A. *Oligonucleotides*, *18*, 33–49.

Mahato, R. I., Narang, A. S., Thoma, L., & Miller, D. D. (2003). Emerging trends in oral delivery of peptide and protein drugs. *Critical Reviews in Therapeutic Drug Carrier Systems*, *20*, 153–214.

Murphy, R. E., Kinhikar, A. G., Shields, M. J., Del Rosario, J., Preston, R., Levin, N., et al. (2010). Combined use of immunoassay and two-dimensional liquid chromatography mass spectrometry for the detection and identification of metabolites from biotherapeutic pharmacokinetic samples. *Journal of Pharmaceutical and Biomedical Analysis*, *53*, 221–227.

Peng, B., Andrews, J., Nestorov, I., Brennan, B., Nicklin, P., & Rowland, M. (2001). Tissue distribution and physiologically based pharmacokinetics of antisense phosphorothioate oligonucleotide ISIS 1082 in rat. *Antisense & Nucleic Acid Drug Development*, *11*, 15–27.

Porter, C. J., Edwards, G. A., & Charman, S. A. (2001). Lymphatic transport of proteins after s.c. injection: implications of animal model selection. *Advanced Drug Delivery Reviews*, *50*, 157–171.

Richter, W. F., Gallati, H., & Schiller, C.-D. (1999). Animal pharmacokinetics of the tumor necrosis factor receptor-immunoglobulin fusion protein lenercept and their extrapolation to humans. *Drug Metabolism and Disposition*, *27*, 21–25.

Roopenian, D. C., & Akilesh, S. (2007). FcRn: the neonatal Fc receptor comes of age. *Nature Reviews Immunology*, *7*, 715–725.

Shah, D. K., & Betts, A. M., (2011). Towards a platform PBPK model to characterize the plasma and tissue disposition of monoclonal antibodies in preclinical species and human. *Journal of Pharmacokinetics and Pharmacodynamics*. doi: 10.1007/2 10928-011-9232-2. (Epub ahead of print).

Strober, W., & Waldmann, T. A. (1974). Role of the kidney in the metabolism of plasma proteins. *Nephron*, *13*, 37–68.

Supersaxo, A., Hein, W. R., & Steffen, H. (1990). Effect of molecular weight on the lymphatic absorption of water-soluble compounds following subcutaneous administration. *Pharmaceutical Research*, *7*, 167–169.

Tornoe, C. W., Agerso, H., Nielsen, H. A., Madsen, H., Jonsson, E. N., (2004). Population pharmacokinetic modeling of a subcutaneous depot of GnRH antagonist degarelix. *Pharmaceutical Research*, *21*, 574–584.

Touraine, P., D'Souza, G. A., Kourides, I., Abs, R., Barclay, P., Xie, R., et al. (2009). Lipoatrophy in GH deficient patients treated with a long-acting pegylated GH. *European Journal of Endocrinology*, *161*, 533–540.

Vugmeyster, Y., DeFranco, D., Szklut, P., Wang, Q., & Xu, X. (2010). Biodistribution of [^{125}I]-labeled therapeutic proteins: application in protein drug development beyond oncology. *Journal of Pharmaceutical Sciences*, *99*, 1028–1045.

Webster, R., Xie, R., Didier, E., Finn, R., Finnessy, J., Edgington, A., et al. (2008). PEGylation of somatropin (recombinant human growth hormone): impact on its clearance in humans. *Xenobiotica*, *38*, 1340–1351.

Webster, R., Elliott, V., Park, B. K., Walker, D., Hankin, M., & Taupin, P. (2009). PEG and PEG conjugates toxicity: towards an understanding of the the toxicity of PEG and its relevance to PEGylated biologicals. In F. M. Veronese (Ed.), *PEGylated Protein Drugs: Basic Science and Clinical Application* (pp. 127–146). Birkhäuser Verlag.

Yu, R. Z., Kim, T. W., Hong, A., Watanabe, T. A., Gaus, H. J., & Geary, R. S. (2007). Cross-species pharmacokinetic comparison from mouse to man of a second-generation antisense oligonucleotide, ISIS 301012, targeting human apolipoprotein B-100. *Drug Metabolism and Disposition*, *35*, 460–468.

Index

Note: Page numbers with "t" denote tables; "f" figures.

Recent Volumes in the Serial

Edwards Brothers Malloy
Ann Arbor MI. USA
December 4, 2012